MEDICAL ABBREVIATIONS:

26,000 Conveniences at the Expense of Communication and Safety

12th Edition

Neil M Davis, MS, PharmD, FASHP

Professor Emeritus, Temple University
  School of Pharmacy, Philadelphia, PA,
Editor Emeritus, Hospital Pharmacy
President, Safe Medication Practices
  Consulting, Inc.

published by

Neil M Davis Associates
2049 Stout Drive, B-3
Warminster, PA 18974-3861

Phone (215) 442-7430 or (888) 333-1862
  (9 AM-4 PM EST, Mon-Fri)
FAX (215) 442-7432 or (888) 333-4915
E-mail med@neilmdavis.com
Secure Website www.medabbrev.com

First edition, 1983, titled, "1700 Medical Abbreviations:
   Conveniences at the Expense of Communications and Safety"

Second edition, 1985, titled, "Medical Abbreviations: 2300
   Conveniences ..."
Third edition, 1987, titled, "Medical Abbreviations: 4200 ..."
Fourth edition, 1988, titled, "Medical Abbreviations: 5500 ..."
Fifth edition, 1990, titled, "Medical Abbreviations: 7000 ..."
Sixth edition, 1993, titled, "Medical Abbreviations 8600 ..."
Seventh edition, 1995, titled, "Medical Abbreviations 10,000 ..."
Eighth edition, 1997, titled, "Medical Abbreviations: 12,000 ..."
Ninth edition, 1999, titled, "Medical Abbreviations: 14,000 ..."
Tenth edition, 2001, titled, "Medical Abbreviations: 15,000 ..."
Eleventh edition, 2003, titled, "Medical Abbreviations: 24,000 ..."

Library of Congress Catalog Card Number 2004096392

ISBN 0-931431-12-3

Printed in Canada.

Contents

Dedication

This book is dedicated to Julie, my wife, for her support, patience, assistance, and love.

Acknowledgments

The assistance of Evelyn Canizares, Vicki Bell, Ann Sandt Kishbaugh, Kelly Hogate, Matthew Davis, Robin Miller, and Ben Miller is gratefully acknowledged.

I would like to express my deep appreciation for the many contributions received from readers for their suggested additions and corrections. Please continue to send these to—

Dr. Neil M Davis
2049 Stout Drive, B-3
Warminster, PA 18974
FAX (215) 442-7432 or (888) 333-4915
E-mail   med@neilmdavis.com
Secure Website www.neilmdavis.com

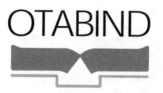

OTABIND

Bound to stay open

The pages in this book open easily and lie flat, a result of the Otabind bookbinding process. Otabind combines advanced adhesive technology and a free-floating cover to achieve books that last longer and are bound to stay open.

Preface
Website-Version Access Information

Along with the purchase of each book, the book owner, at
no extra cost, is entitled to a single-user license for access
to the Internet version of this 12th edition. This license is
valid for 24 months from the date of the initial log-in.
Internet Explorer 4.0, Netscape 4.0, or AOL 5.0 can meet
the minimum browser requirement.

Features of the Web-Version
- Updated monthly (suggestions from users are welcomed
  and will be incorporated).
- Can instantaneously search for the meanings of abbreviations and acronyms.
- Has a reverse-search feature, for example,
  looking for all the abbreviations that contain the word
  "laparoscopic."
- Can search for cross-referenced generic and brand names
  of drugs.
- Can search through the listings of symbols, lists, and normal laboratory values.
- Quick access to a "Do Not Use" list of dangerous abbreviations, an explanation as to why they are dangerous, and
  suggested alternatives to be used. For those facilities that
  obtain multi-user licenses, they may substitute their own
  "Do Not Use" list, which they can control and update.
- Can read the full-text of the introductory chapters of the
  book.

Initial One-time Log-in
- Access the Website at *www.medabbrev.com*
- Click the **Register** button (on the top-left of the screen)
- You will be asked for the 8-letter access code that appears
  on the front inside cover of the book. This will be the
  only time you are asked for this code.
- At this point just follow the directions.
- You must agree to the Single-User License Agreement
  which is presented.
- Note your sign-in name and your self-assigned password.
  This name/password will only permit one access at a
  time, so keep this information confidential to ensure your
  ready access to the site.

Multi-user site licenses are available. A copy of the Multi-User Site License agreement and its price list is available by clicking the "Submit Suggestions" button on *www.medabbrev.com* where you can type a request to receive it or by calling 1 888 333 1862 or 1 215 442 7430.

Searching for the Meaning of an Abbreviation on the Web-version

- Use upper OR lower case letters as the search engine is NOT case sensitive.
- Use normal upper OR lower case letters as the search engine is NOT sensitive to whether the letters are **bold-face** or *italicized.*
- Superscripts and subscripts are to be entered as regular text.
- For other details, just follow the simple instructions shown on the Website. The Web-version of the book is essentially the same as the print version except for the fact that it is searchable and is updated monthly with about 80 new entries.

Chapter 1
Introduction

Listed are current acronyms, symbols, and other abbreviations and 26,000 of their possible meanings. This list has been compiled to assist individuals in reading and transcribing medical records, medically-related communications, and prescriptions. The list, although current and comprehensive, represents a portion of abbreviations in use and their many possible meanings as new ones are being coined every day.

WARNING

Abbreviations are a convenience, a time saver, a space saver, and a way of avoiding the possibility of misspelling words. However, a price can be paid for their use. Abbreviations are sometimes not understood. They can be misread, or are interpreted incorrectly. Their use lengthens the time needed to train individuals in the health fields, wastes the time of healthcare workers in tracking down their meaning, at times delays the patient's care, and occasionally results in patient harm.

The publication of this list of abbreviations is not an endorsement of their legitimacy. It is not a guarantee that the intended meaning has been correctly captured, nor is it an indication that the abbreviation is commonly used. The person who uses an abbreviation must take responsibility for making sure that it is properly interpreted. When an uncommon or ambiguous abbreviation is used and it may not be understood correctly, it should be defined by the writer. Where uncertainty exists, the one who wrote the abbreviation must be contacted for clarification.

There are many variations in how an abbreviation can be expressed. Anterior-posterior has been written as AP, A.P., ap, and A/P. Since there are few standards and those who use abbreviations do not necessarily follow these standards, this book only shows anterior-posterior as AP. This is done to make it easier to find the meaning of an abbreviation as all the meanings of AP are listed together. This elimination of unnecessary duplication also keeps the book at a convenient size, thus enabling it to be sold at a reasonable price.

When an abbreviation is made up of a series of abbreviations, it may not be listed as such. In such instances, the meaning may be determined by looking up each set of abbreviations, as in the example of DTP_a-HIB-PNU-MEN, which means, diphtheria, tetanus toxoids, acellular pertussis; *Haemophilus influenzae* type b conjugate; pneumococcal (*Streptococcus pneumoniae*) conjugate; meningococcal (*Neisseria meningitidis*) conjugate (serogroups unspecified) vaccine.

Lower case letters are used when firm custom dictates as in Ag, Na, mCi, etc. The first letter of brand names are capitalized, whereas nonproprietary names appear in lower case.

The abbreviation AP is listed as meaning doxorubicin and cisplatin. The reason for this apparent disparity is that the official generic names (United States Adopted Names) are shown rather than the brand names Adriamycin® and Platinol AQ®. In the case of LSD, the official name, lysergide, is given, rather than the chemical name, lysergic acid diethylamide. The Latin derivations for older medical and pharmaceutical abbreviations (*t.i.d., ter in die,* three times daily) may be found in *Remington.*[1]

Some abbreviations which have been encountered or that have been suggested for addition to the book have not been added. Some were obscene or completely insensitive.

Abbreviations for medical facility names create problems as they are usually not recognized by the readers in other geographic areas. A clue to the fact that one is dealing with such an abbreviation is when it ends with MC, for Medical Center; HS, for Health System; MH, for Memorial Hospital; CH, for Community Hospital; UH, for University Hospital; and H, for Hospital.

When an abbreviation which ends with "s" can not be found it might be a plural form of a listed abbreviation.

When an abbreviation cannot be found in this book or when the listed meaning(s) do not make sense, there is a possibility that the abbreviation has been misread. As an example, a reader could not find the meaning of HHTS. On closer examination it really was +HTS, not HHTS. Also EWT could not be identified because it was really ENT.

Some common French and Spanish abbreviations are listed in the book. Because of language structure differences, these abbreviations are often reversed, as in the case of HIV, which in Spanish and French is abbreviated as VIH.

Chapter 8 contains a cross-referenced list of 3,400 generic and brand drug names. The list contains names of commonly prescribed and new drugs. Brand names have their first letter capitalized whereas generic names are in lower case. This list will enable readers to obtain the generic name for brand name products or brand names for generic names. It will also serve as a spelling check.

Coded drug names and abbreviations for drug names are found in the chapter on abbreviations (Chapter 5).

Chapter 9 is a table of normal laboratory values. Both the conventional and international values are listed. Each laboratory publishes a list of its normal values. These local lists should be reviewed to see if there are significant differences.

The Council of Biology Editors (CBE), in their 1983 edition of the *CBE Style Manual* listed about 600 abbreviations gathered from 15 internationally recognized authorities and organizations.[2] The majority of these symbols and abbreviations tend to be more scientifically oriented than those which would appear in medical records. In the few situations where the CBE abbreviations differ from what is presented in this book, the CBE abbreviation has been placed in parentheses after the meaning. As is the practice in the United States, mL has been used rather than ml and the spelling of liter, meter, etc. is used rather than litre and metre, even though ml, litre, and metre are listed in the *CBE Style Manual*. A new edition of the *CBE Style Manual* was published in 1995.[3] Again, in this edition, emphasis is placed on scientific abbreviations.

An examination of the abbreviations, acronyms, symbols, and their 26,000 meanings is a testimonial to the problems and dangers associated with most undefined abbreviations.

References

1. Gennaro AR, ed. Remington's Pharmaceutical Sciences, 20th ed. Phila., PA: Lippincott Williams and Wilkins, 2000.

2. CBE Style Manual, 5th ed. Bethesda, MD: Council of Biology Editors; 1983.

3. Scientific Style and Format: The CBE Manual for Authors, Editors, and Publishers, 6th Ed. Council of Biological Editors-Cambridge University Press. Cambridge UK, New York, Victoria Australia: 1995.

Additions, Corrections, and Suggestions are Welcomed

Please send them via any means shown below:

Neil M Davis
2049 Stout Drive, B-3
Warminster PA 18974-3861

FAX 1 888 333 4915 or 1 215 442 7432
Email med@neilmdavis.com
Web site www.medabbrev.com

Thank you for your help in the past.

Have You Used the Web-Version of This Book?

- It is instantaneously searchable for the meanings of abbreviations
- It is reverse searchable (search for all the abbreviations containing a particular word)
- Each month, about 80 new entries are added

See the preface (page vii) for access instructions. A two-year, single-user access is included in the purchase price of the book.

PDA Versions are Available

See pricing and ordering information in the pricing section on page 461.

Multi-User Site Licenses are Available

Medical facilities can substitute their own "Do Not Use" list of dangerous abbreviations for the one present. This list would be controlled by the facility. Demonstrations and pricing information are available by calling 1 888 333 1862 or 1 215 442 7430 or via an e-mail request to ev@neilmdavis.com

Chapter 2

Dangerous, Contradictory, and/or Ambiguous Abbreviations

Healthcare organizations are directed by the Joint Commission on Accreditation of Healthcare Organizations to formulate a "Do Not Use" list of dangerous abbreviations which should NOT be used. An example of such a list, which has been adopted from the Institute of Safe Medication Practice Inc. (ISMP) list, is shown as Table 1.

Many inherent problems associated with abbreviations contribute to or cause errors. Reports of such errors have been published routinely.[1–5]

Abbreviations and symbols can easily be misread or interpreted in an unintended manner. For example:

(1) "HCT250 mg" was intended to mean hydrocortisone 250 mg but was interpreted as hydrochlorothiazide 50 mg (HCTZ50 mg).

(2) Flucytosine was improperly abbreviated as 5 FU, causing it to be read as fluorouracil. Flucytosine is abbreviated 5 FC and fluorouracil is 5 FU.

(3) Floxuridine was improperly abbreviated as 5 FU, causing it to be read as fluorouracil. Floxuridine is abbreviated FUDR and fluorouracil is 5 FU.

(4) MTX was thought to be mechlorethamine. MTX is methotrexate and mechlorethamine is abbreviated HN2.

(5) **The abbreviation "U" for unit is the most dangerous one in the book, having caused numerous tenfold insulin and heparin overdoses. The word unit should never be abbreviated.** The handwritten U for unit has been mistaken for a zero, causing tenfold errors. The handwritten U has also been read as the number four, six, and as "cc."

Table 1. Dangerous abbreviations and dosage designations

Problem term	Reason	Suggested term
O.D. for once daily	Interpreted as right eye	Write "once daily"
q.o.d. for every other day	Interpreted as meaning "every once a day" or read as q.i.d.	Write "every other day"
q.d. for once daily	Read or interpreted as q.i.d.	Write "once daily"
q.n. for every night	Read as every hour	Write "every night," "HS" or nightly
q hs for once daily at bedtime, each day	Read as every hour	Use "HS" or "at bedtime"
TIW for three times a week	Interpeted as T/W (Tuesday & Wednesday); as twice a week; as TID (three times daily)	Write "three times a week"
U for Unit	Read as 0, 4, 6, or cc	Write "unit"
O.J. for orange juice	Read as OD or OS	Write "orange juice"
µg (microgram)	When handwritten, misread as mg	Write "mcg"
sq or sub q for subcutaneous	The q is read as every	Use "subcut"
IU for international unit	Misread as IV (intravenous) also the I is read as a one (6 IU is read as 61 units)	Use "units" or spell out "international units," using a lowercase i.
AU for each ear	Read as OU (each eye)	Spell out "each ear"
ss for sliding scale or half in the Apothecary system	Read as the number 55	Spell out "sliding scale" or "1/2"
Chemical symbols	Not understood or misunderstood	Write full name
cc	Read as u (unit)	Write "mL"

Table 1. Dangerous abbreviations and dosage designations (continued)

Problem term	Reason	Suggested term
Lettered abbreviations for drug names such as MS and MS04 for morphine sulfate or DPH, ASA, APAP, AZT, CPZ, and others and for protocols	Not understood or misunderstood	Use generic or brand name(s). For protocols, follow the facility's procedures.
Apothecary symbols or terms	Not understood or misunderstood	Use metric system
per os for by mouth	OS read as left eye	Use "by mouth," "orally," or "PO"
D/C for discharge	Interpreted as discontinue (orders for discharge medications result in premature discontinuance of current medication)	Write "discharge"
T/d for one per day	Read as t.i.d.	Use "once daily"
/ (a slash mark) for with, and, or per	Read as a one	Use, "and," "with," or "per"
Roman numerals	Not understood or misinterpreted (iv read as intravenous rather than 4; iii, X, L, and M, are not understood)	Use Arabic numerals (4, 3, 10, 50, 100, etc.)
> and <	Not understood or the meaning is reversed	Use "greater than" or "less than"
Drug name and dosage not separated by space	Inderal40 mg misread as Inderal 140 mg	Always leave a space between a drug name, dose, and unit of measure
Trailing zeros; 1.0 mg	Decimal point not seen causing tenfold overdose	Omit zero; 1 mg
Naked decimal point; .5 mL	Decimal point not seen causing tenfold overdose	Add zero; 0.5 mL

(6) OD, meant to signify once daily, has caused Lugol's solution to be given in the right eye.

(7) OJ meant to signify orange juice, looked like OS and caused saturated solution of potassium iodide to be given in the left eye.

(8) IVP, meant to signify intravenous push (Lasix 20 mg IVP), caused a patient to be given an intravenous pyelogram which is the usual meaning of this abbreviation.

(9) Na Warfarin (sodium warfarin) was read as "No Warfarin."

(10) The abbreviation "s" for "without" has been thought to mean "with" (c).

(11) The order for PT, intended to signify a laboratory test order for prothrombin time, resulted in the ordering of a physical therapy consultation.

(12) The abbreviation "TAB," meant to signify Triple Antibiotic (a coined name for a hospital sterile topical antibiotic mixture), caused patients to have their wounds irrigated with a diet soda. At another facility, with the same set of circumstances, they did not have TAB®, so they used Diet Shasta.®

(13) A slash mark (/) has been mistaken for a one, causing a patient to receive a 100 unit overdose of NPH insulin when the slash was used to separate an order for two insulin doses:

6 units regular insulin/20 units NPH insulin

(14) Vidarabine, an antiviral agent, was ordered as ara-A; however, ara-C, which is cytarabine, an antineoplastic agent, was given.

(15) On several occasions, pediatric strength diphtheria-tetanus toxoids (DT) have been confused with adult strength tetanus-diphtheria toxoids (Td).

(16) DTP is commonly understood to refer to diphtheria-tetanus-pertussis vaccine, but in some hospitals it is also used as shorthand for a sedative cocktail of Demerol, Thorazine, and Phenergan. Several cases have occurred where a child was vaccinated rather than given the sedative mixture.

(17) What does the abbreviation MR mean? Some will guess measles-rubella vaccine (M-R-Vax II, Merck), while others will assume mumps-rubella vaccine (Biavax II, Merck).

(18) The abbreviation TIW (three times a week) was thought to mean Tuesday and Wednesday when the I was read as a slash mark. Due to confirmation bias (you see what you know), this uncommon abbreviation is seen as the more commonly used TID (three times a day).

(19) PCA, meant to be procainamide, was interpreted as patient-controlled analgesia.

(20) PGE$_1$ (alprostadil, Caverject) was read as P6 E1 (Alcon's ophthalmic 6% pilocarpine and 1% epinephrine solution).

(21) A nurse transcribed an oral order for the antibiotic aztreonam as AZT, which was subsequently thought to be the antiviral drug zidovudine.

(22) An order for TAC 0.1%, intended to mean triamcinolone cream, was interpreted as tetracaine, Adrenalin, and cocaine solution.

(23) An order for SPA (salt poor albumin) was overlooked because it was not recognized as a drug order.

(24) Therapy was delayed and considerable professional time was wasted when an order for "Bactrim SS q 12 h on S/S" had to be clarified (Bactrim Single Strength every 12 hours on Saturday and Sunday).

(25) A physician wrote an order stating "may take own supply of EPO". The physician meant evening primrose oil, not Epogen (epoetin alfa).

(26) 4-MP was recommended to treat ethylene glycol poisoning. The medical resident mistakenly interpreted this as 6-MP (6-mercaptopurine). 4-MP is fomepizole (4 methylpyrazole) and 6-MP is mercaptopurine (6-mercaptopurine).

(27) An order for lomustine stated it was to be given at "hs". This was misinterpreted as to mean every night. After continuous administration, toxicity resulted in the patient's death. The drug is normally given once every 6 weeks. State complete orders such as "HS $\times$ 1 dose today," "HS nightly," or "HS nightly PRN for sleep."

(28) The directions for an order for Cortisporin Otic Solution indicated "Three drops in ® ear TID." The patient was given the drops in the rear rather than the right ear.

(29) There have been mix-ups between IL-2 and IL-11 when IL-2 is expressed as IL-II (Roman numeral 2). The II has been read as "IL eleven," and vice versa.

IL-2 (interleukin 2) is aldesleukin (Proleukin) and IL-11 is oprelvekin (Neumega).

(30) A drug was ordered "Q 10 h." It was read as QID (four times daily). Drugs should not be ordered at unusual hourly intervals such as every 10, 18, or 36 hours, as this has resulted in a host of errors. Standard times are every 2, 3, 4, 6, 8, or 12 hours; once, twice, three, or four times daily; every other day, or Monday, Wednesday, and Friday and once weekly.

(31) 6 IU was read 61 units instead of the intended 6 international units.

(32) A dose of phenytoin was modified and expressed as mg/Kg/d. The d was read as "dose" rather than the intended "day" resulting in 3 extra doses being given.

(33) An order appeared as "If no BM in PM, give MOM in AM p.r.n."

(34) Sometimes ambiguous abbreviations cause financial loses to health providers. For example, all insurance provider may pay less for an office visit for mental retardation than it does for mitral regurgitation. This can happen if the coder is faced with the abbreviation MR.

The author would appreciate receiving other examples of abbreviations that have been misinterpreted causing error or delays so that this section can be expanded.

A prescription could be written with directions as follows: "OD OD OD," to mean one drop in the right eye once daily!

Abbreviations should not be used for drug names as they are particularly dangerous. As previously illustrated, there is the possibility that the writer may, through mental error, confuse two abbreviations and use the wrong one. Similarly, the reader may attribute the wrong meaning to an abbreviation. To further confound the problem, some drug name abbreviations have multiple meanings (see ATR, CPM, CPZ, FLU, GEM, NITRO, and PBZ in Table 2). The abbreviation AC has been used for three different cancer chemotherapy combinations to mean Adriamycin and either cyclophosphamide, carmustine, or cisplatin.

Beside causing medication errors and incorrect interpretation of medical records, abbreviations can create problems because treatment is delayed while a health professional seeks clarification for the meaning of the abbreviation used. Abbreviations should not be used to designate drugs or combinations of drugs.

Table 2. Examples of abbreviations that have contradictory or ambiguous meanings

ABP	=	ambulatory blood pressure
		arterial blood pressure
ACU	=	acute receiving unit
		ambulatory care unit
AMI	=	amifostine
		amitriptyline
APC	=	advanced pancreatic cancer
		advanced prostate cancer
ATR	=	atropine
		atracurium
AZT	=	zidovudine
		azathioprine
BO	=	bowel open
		bowel obstruction
CAS	=	carotid artery stenosis
		cerebral arteriosclerosis
		coronary artery stenosis
CIA	=	chemotherapy-induced amenorrhea
		chemotherapy-induced anemia
CLD	=	chronic liver disease
		chronic lung disease
CPM	=	cyclophosphamide
		chlorpheniramine maleate
CPZ	=	chlorpromazine
		Compazine
CRU	=	cardiac rehabilitation unit
		catheterization recovery unit
		clinical research unit
DW	=	dextrose in water
		distilled water
		deionized water

DXM	= dexamethasone dextromethorphan
ESLD	= end-stage liver disease end-stage lung disease
FEC	= fluorouracil, epirubicin, and cyclophosphamide fluorouracil, etoposide, and cisplatin
FGAs	= first generation antihistamines first generation antipsychotics
FLU	= fluconazole (Diflucan) fludarabine (Fludara) flunisolide (Aero Bid) fluoxetine (Prozac) fluticasone propionate (Flonase) influenza
GD	= Graves disease Gaucher disease
GEM	= gemfibrozil gemicitabine
HD	= Hansen disease Hodgkin disease Huntington disease
HRF	= hypertensive renal failure hypoxic respiratory failure
ICA	= internal carotid artery intracranial abscess intracranial aneurysm
IAI	= intra-abdominal infection intra-abdominal injury intra-amniotic infection
I & D	= incision and drainage irrigation and debridement
IT	= intrathecal intratracheal intratumoral

Table 2. Examples of abbreviations that have contradictory or ambiguous meanings (*continued*)

KET	= ketamine ketoconazole
LFD	= lactose-free diet low fat diet low fiber diet
MP	= melphalan; prednisone mitoxantrone; prednisone
MPM	= malignant peritoneal mesothelioma malignant pleural mesothelioma
MS	= morphine sulfate multiple sclerosis mitral stenosis musculoskeletal medical student minimal support muscle strength
MS	= mental status milk shake mitral sound morning stiffness
MTD	= maximum tolerated dose minimum toxic dose
MTZ	= mirtazapine mitoxantrone
MV	= mechanical ventilation manual ventilation
NBM	= no bowel movement normal bowel movement nothing by mouth
NE	= no effect no enlargement not evaluated
NITRO	= nitroglycerin sodium nitroprusside

OLB	= open-liver biopsy open-lung biopsy
PBL	= primary breast lymphoma primary brain lymphoma
PBZ	= phenylbutazone pyribenzamine phenoxybenzamine
PD	= Paget disease panic disorder Parkinson disease personality disorder
PORT	= postoperative radiotherapy postoperative respiratory therapy
PVO	= peripheral vascular occlusion portal vein occlusion pulmonary venous occlusion
RS	= Reiter syndrome Rett syndrome Reye syndrome Raynaud disease (syndrome) rumination syndrome
S & S	= swish and spit swish and swallow
SA	= suicide alert suicide attempt
SAD	= schizoaffective disorder social anxiety disorder seasonal affective disorder
SDBP	= seated, standing, or supine diastolic blood pressure
SGAs	= second generation antihistamines second generation antipsychotics
SJS	= Schwartz-Jampel syndrome Stevens-Johnson syndrome Swyer-James syndrome

Table 2. Examples of abbreviations that have contradictory or ambiguous meanings (*continued*)

SSE	= saline solution enema soapsuds enema
STF	= special tube feeding standard tube feeding
TICU	= thoracic intensive care unit transplant intensive care unit trauma intensive care unit
TMZ	= temazepam temozolomide
TS	= Tay-Sachs (disease) Tourette syndrome Turner syndrome
VAD	= vincristine, doxorubicin, (Adriamycin) and dexamethasone vincristine, doxorubicin (Adriamycin) and dactinomycin
VAP	= vincristine, Adriamycin, and prednisone vincristine, Adriamycin, and procarbazine vincristine, actinomycin D, and Platinol AQ vincristine, asparaginase, and prednisone

Certain meanings of abbreviations in the book are followed by a warning, "this is a dangerous abbreviation." This warning could be placed after many abbreviations, but was reserved for situations where errors have been published because these abbreviations were used or where the meaning is critical and not likely to be known. If no alternative abbreviation is suggested, then the term should be spelled out rather than abbreviated. Such warning statements should also appear after every abbreviation for a drug or drug combination.

References

1. Davis NM, Cohen MR. Medication errors: causes and prevention. Huntingdon Valley, PA: Neil M Davis Associates; 1983.

2. Cohen MR. Medication error reports. Hosp Pharm (appears monthly from 1975 to the present).

3. Cohen MR. Medication errors. Nursing 2005 (appears monthly, starting in Nursing 77, to the present).

4. Davis NM. Med Errors. Am J Nursing (appears monthly from 1994 to 1995).

5. Cohen MR. Medication Errors. American Pharmaceutical Assoc. Wash. DC, 1999.

Additions, Corrections, and Suggestions are Welcomed

Please send them via any means shown below:

Neil M Davis
2049 Stout Drive, B-3
Warminster PA 18974-3861

FAX 1 888 333 4915 or 1 215 442 7432
Email med@neilmdavis.com
Web site www.medabbrev.com

Thank you for your help in the past.

Have You Used the Web-Version of This Book?

- It is instantaneously searchable for the meanings of abbreviations
- It is reverse searchable (search for all the abbreviations containing a particular word)
- Each month, about 80 new entries are added

See the preface (page vii) for access instructions. A two-year, single-user access is included in the purchase price of the book.

Chapter 3

A Healthcare Controlled Vocabulary

Presently there are no standards for abbreviations used in prescribers' orders, consultations, written prescriptions, standing orders, computer order sets, nurse's medication administration records, pharmacy profiles, hospital formularies, etc. Because in the healthcare field everyone does their own thing, there are many variations. These variations in the way abbreviations are expressed are not always understood and at times are misinterpreted. They cause delays in initiating therapy, cause accidents, waste time for everyone in clarifying these documents, lengthen the time it takes to train those working in the healthcare field, lengthen hospital stays, and waste money.

A controlled vocabulary similar to what is used in the aviation industry is needed. Everyone in the aviation industry "follows the book," and uses a controlled vocabulary. All pilots and air traffic controllers say, "alfa", "bravo", "charlie." See Table 1, the phonetic alphabet. They do not go off on their own and say "adam", "beef", "candy!" They say "one three," not thirteen, because thirteen sounds like thirty. Radio transmission in the aviation industry is not easy to decipher, yet because precision is critical everything possible is done to eliminate error. To prevent errors all radio transmissions are given only in English, every transmission is given in the same order and must be immediately repeated by the receiver to make sure it was heard correctly. Written and oral communication in the medical professions are just as critical and are also not easy to decipher, so establishing a controlled vocabulary is also necessary in this industry.

Listed below are six organizations that have ongoing projects related to standardizing medical terminology:

Computer-Based Patient Record Institute, Inc.
1000 East Woodfield Rd. Suite 102
Schuamburg, IL 60173

The United States Pharmacopeial Convention, Inc.
12601 Twinbrook Parkway
Rockville, MD, 20852

National Library of Medicine
Unified Medical Language Systems
8600 Rockville Pike
Bethesda, MD, 20894

Council of Biological Editors, through their Scientific Style and Format: The CBE Manual for Authors, Editors, and Publishers, 6th Ed. Council of Biological Editors; Cambridge University Press, Cambridge UK, New York, Victoria Australia: 1995

American Medical Association, through their American Medical Assoc. Manual of Style, 9th Edition. AMA, Chicago, 1998

American Association of Medical Transcriptionists through their AAMT Book of Style for Medical Transcriptions, 2nd Edition. American Assoc. for Medical Transcriptions, Modesta CA, 2002

Listed below (Table 2) is the start of a Healthcare Controlled Vocabulary. The basis for this controlled vocabulary is established standard terminology and the result of 37 years of studying medical errors by this author.

It is anticipated that a Healthcare Controlled Vocabulary, with professional organizations' input and backing, will grow and someday evolve into an "official standard." Your suggestions and comments are vital to this growth and eventual recognition. It is always safest to avoid the use of abbreviations unless they are well known in your work environment.

Table 1. Phonetic Alphabet

The International Civil Aviation Organization phonetic alphabet is used by the aviation industry when communications conditions are such that the information cannot be readily received without their use. Health professionals also should use it when it is necessary to orally spell critical information.

Character	Telephony	Phonic
A	Alfa	(AL-FAH)
B	Bravo	(BRAH-VOH)
C	Charlie	(CHAR-LEE)
		or (SHAR-LEE)
D	Delta	(DELL-TA)
E	Echo	(ECK-OH)
F	Foxtrot	(FOKS-TROT)
G	Golf	(GOLF)
H	Hotel	(HOH-TEL)
I	India	(IN-DEE-AH)
J	Juliett	(JEW-LEE-ETT)
K	Kilo	(KEY-LOH)
L	Lima	(LEE-MAH)
M	Mike	(MIKE)
N	November	(NO-VEM-BER)
O	Oscar	(OSS-CAH)
P	Papa	(PAH-PAH)
Q	Quebec	(KEH-BECK)
R	Romeo	(ROW-ME-OH)
S	Sierra	(SEE-AIR-RAH)
T	Tango	(TANG-GO)
U	Uniform	(YOU-NEE-FORM)
		or (OO-NEE-FORM)
V	Victor	(VIK-TAH)
W	Whiskey	(WIS-KEY)
X	X-ray	(ECKS-RAY)
Y	Yankee	(YANG-KEY)
Z	Zulu	(ZOO-LOO)
1	One	(WUN)
2	Two	(TOO)
3	Three	(TREE)
4	Four	(FOW-ER)
5	Five	(FIFE)
6	Six	(SIX)
7	Seven	(SEV-EN)
8	Eight	(AIT)
9	Nine	(NIN-ER)
0	Zero	(ZEE-RO)

Table 2. Examples of a Controlled Vocabulary

Standard	What **not** to use or do	Comments
100 mg (100 space mg)	100mg (100 no space mg)	The USP* standard way of expressing a strength is to leave a space between the number and its units. Leaving this space makes it easier to read the number as can be seen below. 1mg 1 mg 10mg 10 mg 100mg 100 mg
1 mg	1.0 mg	This is a USP standard. When a trailing zero is used, the decimal point is sometimes not seen thus causing a tenfold overdose. These overdoses have caused injury and death.
0.1 mL	.1 mL	When the decimal point is not seen, this is read as 1 mL, causing a ten fold overdose.
once daily (Do not abbreviate.)	The abbreviation OD	The classic meaning for OD is right eye. Liquids intended to be given once daily are mistakenly given in the right eye.
	The abbreviation QD	When the Q in QD is dotted too aggressively it looks like Q.I.D. and the medication is given four times daily. When a lower case q is used, the tail of the q has come up between the q and the d to make it look like qid. In the United Kingdom, Q.D. means four times daily
unit (Do not abbreviate. Write "unit" using a lower-case u)	The abbreviation U	The handwritten U is mistaken for a zero when poorly written causing a 10 fold overdose (i.e. 6 U regular insulin is read as 60). The poorly written U has also been read as a 4, 6, and cc. Write "unit," leaving a space between the number and the word unit.

Table 2. (cont.)

Standard	What **not** to use or do	Comments
mg (lower case mg with no period)	mg., Mg., Mg, MG, mgm, mgs	The USP standard expression is the mg
mL (lower case m with a capital L, no period)	mL., ml, ml., mls, mLs, cc	The USP standard expression is the mL
Use generic names or brand names	Do not abbreviate drug names or combinations of drugs, such as CPZ, PBZ, NTG, MS, MSO₄, 5FC, MTX, 6MP, MOPP, ASA, HCTZ, etc. Do not use shortened names or chemical names in patient-related documents	Abbreviated drug names and acronyms are not always known to the reader; at times they have more than one possible meaning, or are thought to be another drug. When the chemical name "6 mercaptopurine" has been used, six doses of mercaptopurine have been mistakenly administered. The generic name, mercaptopurine, should be used. MgSO₄ has been read as morphine sulfate. When an unofficial shortened version of the name norfloxacin, norflox was used, Norflex was mistakenly given. An order for Aredia was read as Adriamycin, as some professionals abbreviated the name Adriamycin as "Adria" which looks like Aredia.
The metric system	The apothecary system (grains, drams, minims, ounces, etc.)	The Apothecary system is so rarely used it is not recognized or understood. The symbol for minim (m̥) is read as mL; the symbol for one dram (Ʒ T) is read as 3 tablespoons, and gr (grain) is read as gram.
Use properly placed commas for numbers above 999, as in 10,000, or 5,000,000	5000000	Some healthcare workers have difficulty in reading large numbers such as 5000000. The use of commas helps the reader to read these numbers correctly.

(continued)

Table 2. (cont.)

Standard	What **not** to use or do	Comments
600 mg When possible, do not use decimal expressions. 25 mcg	0.6 g 0.025 mg	A USP standard. The elimination of decimals lessens the chance for error. Mistakes are made when reading numbers less than 1 with decimals.
Use specific concentrations and the time in which intravenous potassium chloride should be administered.	Do not use the term "bolus" in conjunction with the administration of potassium chloride injection.	Some physicians will erroneously indicate that potassium chloride injection should be "bolused" or be given "IV push," vaguely meaning that it should not be dripped in slowly. Many deaths have been reported when prescribers have been taken literally and the potassium chloride was given by bolus or IV push for fluid-restricted patients. Orders should be specific such as, "20 mEq of potassium chloride in 50 mL of 5% dextrose to run over 30 minutes."
use "and"	Do not use a slash (/) mark or the symbol "&"	A slash mark looks like a one. An order written "6 units regular insulin/20 units NPH insulin", was read as 120 units of NPH insulin. The symbol "&" has been read as a 4.
Orally transmitted medical orders should be read back as heard for verification.	Do not assume that one has spoken or heard correctly.	During oral communications, speakers misspeak and/or transcribers mishear. To minimize these errors, the transmitter must speak clearly and slowly, the transcriber must repeat what was transcribed, and the transmitter must listen attentively when this is being done. Errors are less likely to occur when the prescription is complete. When spelling out words, use the phonetic alphabet shown in Table 1. Oral orders should be avoided whenever possible.

Table 2. (cont.)

Standard	What **not** to use or do	Comments
When prescriptions are written or orally transmitted they must be complete. • dosage form must be specified • strength must be specified • directions must be specified • included in the directions must be the purpose or indication.	Incomplete orders	Prescribers on occasion think of one drug and mistakenly order another. Nurses and pharmacists on occasion misread prescriptions because of error, poor handwriting or poor oral communications, or look-alike or sound-alike drugs.[1] When the prescription is complete and the purpose or indication is included, these errors are less likely to occur. Listing the purpose or indication on the prescription label will assist in increasing patient adherence.
Written communications must be legible.	Illegible handwriting	Those who cannot or will not write legibly must print (if this would be legible), type, use a computer, or have an employee write for them and then immediately verify and sign the document.
Prescribe specific doses.	Do not prescribe 2 ampuls or 2 vials	There is often more than one size or concentration of drug available. Failing to be specific will lead to unintended doses being administered.
As required by the Joint Commission on Accreditation of Healthcare Organizations, establish a list of dangerous abbreviations which should not be used	Use dangerous abbreviations.	See Chapter 2 of this book "Dangerous, Contradictory, and/or Ambiguous Abbreviations."
Use h or hr for hour	°	An order written as q 4° has been read as q 40 or the symbol ° has not been understood.
Specify amount of drug to be given in a single dose.[2]	Specify total amount of drug to be administered over a period of time.	Orders such as . . . 1,600 mg over 4 days have caused death when mistakenly given as a single dose. Order should state . . . 400 mg once daily for four days (2-1-04 to 2-4-04)

*USP = United States Pharmacopeia
1. Davis NM. Look-alike and sound alike drug names. Hosp Pharm 2004, 37, No. 2, Supplement Wall-chart (Call 1-800-223-0554)
2. Kohler D. Standardizing the expression & nomenclature of cancer treatment regimens. Am J Health-System Pharm. 1998;55;137–44

PDA Versions are Available

See pricing and ordering information in the pricing section on page 461.

Multi-User Site Licenses are Available

Medical facilities can substitute their own "Do Not Use" list of dangerous abbreviations for the one present. This list would be controlled by the facility. Demonstrations and pricing information are available by calling 1 888 333 1862 or 1 215 442 7430 or via an e-mail request to ev@neilmdavis.com

Additions, Corrections, and Suggestions are Welcomed

Please send them via any means shown below:

Neil M Davis
2049 Stout Drive, B-3
Warminster PA 18974-3861

FAX 1 888 333 4915 or 1 215 442 7432
Email med@neilmdavis.com
Web site www.medabbrev.com

Thank you for your help in the past.

Have You Used the Web-Version of This Book?

- It is instantaneously searchable for the meanings of abbreviations
- It is reverse searchable (search for all the abbreviations containing a particular word)
- Each month, about 80 new entries are added

See the preface (page vii) for access instructions. A two-year, single-user access is included in the purchase price of the book.

Chapter 4

Medical Abbreviation Primer

When first entering a medically related field, one must learn the language in order to function. Part of learning this language is to learn the meaning of the abbreviations, acronyms, and symbols in use. This chapter is intended to introduce newcomers to this commonly used medically related shorthand.

The determination of which abbreviations (refers also to acronyms and symbols) are most commonly used is based on the selection by the author with the consultation of experts in various health-related fields. The categorizing of the abbreviations is arbitrary, but is intended to represent the most common use, as the abbreviations could have been placed in many different categories.

This list could have been expanded to include many hundreds-more commonly used abbreviations, but then the list would have been too long to serve as a primer. The absence of an abbreviation from this listing does not mean it is not in common use. Each area of practice and specialty could have added their own commonly used abbreviations.

A few of the abbreviations below have more than one meaning listed. This was done when several meanings are in common use. Many abbreviations have more than one meaning and they must be viewed in their clinical context to arrive at their intended meaning. See Chapter 5 of this book for additional meanings for the abbreviations listed below.

In practice, there are inconsistencies as to how abbreviations are written. They may appear in all capital letters, lower case, or in capital letters and lower case. They may or may not have periods after each letter.

The readers are urged to read Chapter 2, Dangerous, Contradictory, and/or Ambiguous Abbreviations.

Two Hundred and Seventy-Five Commonly Used Medical Abbreviations Arranged by Category—a Primer

Physical Examination, History Portion of the Medical Record, and Discharge Summary

C/O	complains of	RUQ	right upper quadrant (also there is RLQ, LUQ, and LLQ)
CC	chief complaint(s)		
CTA	clear to auscultation		
Dx	diagnosis	TM	tympanic membrane
F/U	follow-up	AAO X 3	awake and oriented to time, place, and person
FH	family history		
H/O	history of		
HPI	history of present illness	BM	bowel movement
		BP	blood pressure
Hx	history	CVAT	costovertebral angle tenderness
PE	physical examination; pelvic examination; pulmonary embolism		
		DTR	deep tendon reflex
		EOMI	extraocular muscles intact
PH/SH	personal and social history		
		HJR	hepatojugular reflux
PI	present illness	JVD	jugular venous distention
PMH	past medical history		
ROS	review of systems	IBW	ideal body weight
SH	social history	LBW	lean body weight
Tx	treatment	BSA	body surface area
CV	cardiovascular	LMP	last menstrual period
GI	gastrointestinal	NAD	no apparent distress; no apparent disease
GU	genitourinary		
EENT	ears, eyes, nose, and throat	NC/AT	normocephalic, atraumatic
HEENT	head, ears, eyes, nose, and throat	NKA	no known allergies
		NKDA	no known drug allergies
Ob/Gyn	obstetrics and gynecology	OD	right eye
		OS	left eye
Peds	pediatrics	OU	both eyes
UCD	usual childhood diseases	PERRLA	pupils equal, round, reactive to light and accommodation
A & P	auscultation and percussion		
		IOP	intraocular pressure
ADL	activities of daily living	ROM	range of motion
CN III	third cranial nerve (there are CN I to XII)	VS	vital signs
		P	pulse
		T	temperature
RCM	right costal margin (there is also a LCM)	RR	respiratory rate; recovery room

HR	heart rate	YO	year old
RRR	regular rate and rhythm (heart)	DOB	date of birth
		+	positive; present; plus
WDWNWM	well developed, well nourished, white male (also there are abbreviations for females and other races [WF= white female; AAF= African-American female]	−	negative; absent; minus
		c̄	with
		s̄	negative; without
		W/O	without

Diseases and Symptoms

AD	Alzheimer disease	URI	upper respiratory infection
AIDS	acquired immunodeficiency syndrome	TB	tuberculosis
		CVA	cerebrovascular accident; costovertebral angle
HIV	human immuno-deficiency virus		
AMI	acute myocardial infarction	DVT	deep vein thrombosis
		NV	nausea and vomiting
MI	myocardial infarction	NVD	nausea, vomiting, and diarrhea; neck vein distention
CHF	congestive heart failure		
ACS	acute coronary syndrome		
		PONV	postoperative nausea and vomiting
HT	hypertension (also HTN); height	PUD	peptic ulcer disease
DM	diabetes mellitus	GERD	gastroesophageal reflux disease
AODM	adult onset diabetes mellitus		
		RA	rheumatoid arthritis
IDDM	insulin dependent diabetes mellitus	OA	osteoarthritis
		SLE	systemic lupus erythematosus
NIDDM	noninsulin-dependent diabetes mellitus		
		TIA	transient ischemic attack
PD	Parkinson disease		
AOM	acute otitis media	HA	headache
Ca	cancer	BPH	benign prostatic hypertrophy (hyperplasia)
COAD	chronic obstructive airway disease		
COPD	chronic obstructive pulmonary disease	UTI	urinary tract infection
		STD	sexually transmitted disease
DOE	dyspnea on exertion		
SOB	shortness of breath	MVA	motor vehicle accident

Clinical Laboratory

ANA	antinuclear antibody	aPTT	activated partial thromboplastin time
Alb	albumin		
ALT	alanine aminotransferase	AST	aspartate aminotransferase
LFT	liver function test		

BG	blood glucose; blood gases	TP	total protein
BS	blood sugar; bowel sounds; breath sounds	Ca	Calcium (also Ca^{++})
		Cl	Chloride (also Cl^-)
		K	Potassium (also K^+)
BUN	blood urea nitrogen	Mg	Magnesium (also Mg^{++})
CK-MB	creatine kinase, MB fraction	Na	Sodium (also Na^+)
CO_2	carbon dioxide	OGTT	oral glucose tolerance test
CPK	creatinine phosphokinase	PSA	prostate-specific antigen
CrCl	creatinine clearance	UA	urinalysis
SCr	serum creatinine	VDRL	Venereal Disease Research Laboratory (test for syphilis)
C & S	culture and sensitivity		
ESR	erythrocyte sedimentation rate	CBC	complete blood count
Gluc	glucose	Diff	differential (blood count)
FBS	fasting blood sugar	Eos	eosinophil
HbA_{1c}	glycosylated hemoglobin	Fe	iron
CHOL	cholesterol	Hct	hematocrit
HDL	high-density lipoprotein	Hgb	hemoglobin
LDL	low-density lipoprotein	Plt	platelets
LDH	lactic dehydrogenase	MCV	mean corpuscular volume
Trig	trigylcerides	RBC	red blood cell (count)
INR	international normalized ratio	Segs	segmented neutrophils
		WBC	white blood cell (count)
DB	direct bilirubin	ABG	arterial blood gases
TB	total bilirubin	WNL	within normal limits

Other Diagnostic Tests, Procedures, and Treatments

ECG	electrocardiogram	CT	computer tomography
EEG	electroencephalogram	IVP	intravenous pyelogram
FEV_1	forced expiratory volume in one second	MRI	magnetic resonance imaging
IPPB	intermittent positive-pressure breathing	PET	positron emission tomography
		US	ultrasound
PFT	pulmonary function tests	CABG	coronary artery bypass graft
PEEP	positive end-expiratory pressure	PCTA	percutaneous transluminal coronary angioplasty
MUGA	multigated (radionuclide) angiogram	PT	physical therapy
		D & C	dilatation and curettage

Physicians' Orders and Prescriptions

ASAP	as soon as possible	CPR	cardiopulmonary resuscitation
OOB	out of bed		
BRP	bathroom privileges	DNR	do not resuscitate

DAW	dispense as written	h	hour(s)
DC or D/C	discharge; discontinue	*b.i.d.*	*twice daily*
I/O	intake and output	*t.i.d.*	*three times daily*
LD	loading dose	*q.i.d.*	*four times daily*
NAS	no salt added	*QAM*	every morning
NPO	nothing by mouth	QPM	every evening
PO	by mouth; postoperative	*AC*	*before meals*
IM	intramuscular	*PC*	*after meals*
IV	intravenous	*HS*	*bedtime*
SC	subcutaneous	NR	no refills (prescriptions)
SQ	subcutaneous (SC preferred)	*PRN*	*as required; whenever necessary*
PICC	percutaneous indwelling central catheter	MRx1	may repeat one time
		Rx	*prescription; pharmacy*
IVPB	intravenous piggyback	OTC	over-the-counter (no prescription required)
NGT	nasogastric tube		
cap	capsule		
tab	tablet	*Stat*	*immediately*
inj	injection	TKO	to keep (vein) open
i	one	TO	telephone order
ii	two	VO	verbal order
q	*every (as in q 6 hours)*		

Drug Names (It is dangerous to abbreviate drug names)

APAP	acetaminophen	KCl	potassium chloride
ASA	aspirin	$MgSO_4$	magnesium sulfate
5D/W	dextrose 5% injection (in water)	MOM	milk of magnesia
		NaCl	sodium chloride
Dig	digoxin	NS	normal saline (0.9% sodium chloride; same as NSS)
ETOH	alcohol (ethyl alcohol)		
$FeSO_4$	ferrous sulfate		
H_2O	water	NSS	normal saline solution (0.9% sodium chloride)
H_2O_2	hydrogen peroxide		
HCl	hydrochloride (when following a drug name, as in thiamine HCl [thiamine hydrochloride]) hydrochloric acid (when it appears separately [not as part of a drug name])	O_2	oxygen
		PCN	penicillin
		tPA	tissue plasminogen activator
		IVF	intravenous fluids
		TPN	total parenteral nutrition
		lytes	electrolytes (sodium, potassium, chloride, etc.)

Drug Classes

ABX	antibiotic(s)	OC	oral contraceptive
COX-2 I	cyclooxygenase-2 inhibitor	PPI	proton pump inhibitor
		SSRI	selective serotonin reuptake inhibitor
MOAI	monoamine oxidase inhibitor		
		TCA	tricyclic antidepressant
NSAID	nonsteroidal anti-inflammatory drug		

Units of Measure

cm	centimeter (2.54 cm = 1 inch)	mcg	microgram (1,000 mcg = 1 milligram [mg])
g	gram (28.35 g = 1 ounce)	mEq	milliequivalent
Kg	kilogram (1 Kg = 2.2 pounds)	mg	milligram (1,000 mg = 1 gram [g])
L	liter (l L = 1,000 mL = 1 quart plus about 2 ounces)	mL	milliliter (1,000 mL = 1 liter [L])
		mmHg	millimeters of mercury
		°C	degrees Centigrade
lb	pound (1 lb = 0.454 Kg)	°F	degrees Fahrenheit

Hospital Locations

CCU	caridac care unit	NICU	neonatal intensive care unit
DR	delivery room		
ED	emergency department	OB	obstetrics
ER	emergency room (same as ED)	OR	operating room
		PACU	postanesthesia care unit
ICU	intensive care unit	PICU	pediatric intensive care unit; pulmonary intensive care unit
L & D	labor and delivery		
LDR	labor, delivery, and recovery		
		RD	radiology department
MICU	medical intensive care unit	SICU	surgical intensive care unit

Miscellaneous

ARNP	Advanced Registered Nurse Practitioner	MD	Doctor of Medicine
		OD	Doctor of Osteopathy
LPN	Licensed Practical Nurse	PA	Physician Assistant
		RPh	Registered Pharmacist
MA	Medical Assistant	RN	Registered Nurse
MAR	medication administration record		

Chapter 5

Lettered Abbreviations and Acronyms

Where an abbreviation contains numbers, symbols, punctuation, spaces, etc., they are *not* considered during alphabetizing (6 MP is listed under MP). Entries beginning with a *Greek letter* are alphabetized where the name of the letter would be found alphabetically.

The letter-by-letter (dictionary) system of alphabetizing is used ("*ad lib*" is listed under ADL).

Brand names (proprietary names) have their first letter capitalized, whereas nonproprietary (generic) names are in lower-case letters.

Drug names should not be abbreviated as the meaning may not be known to the reader or interpreted as intended.

The listing of symbols, numbers, and Greek letters can be found in Chapter 6.

See WARNING in chapter 1.

A

A	accommodation
	Acinetobacter
	adenine
	age
	alive
	ambulatory
	angioplasty
	anterior
	anxiety
	apical
	arterial
	artery
	Asian
	assessment
	auscultation

A+	blood type A positive (A positive is preferred)
A−	blood type A negative (A negative is preferred)
A′	ankle
@	at
(a)	axillary temperature
$\overline{a}$	before
A_1	aortic first heart sound
A_2	aortic second sound
A250	5% albumin 250 mL
A1000	5% albumin 1000 mL
A II	angiotensin II
AA	acetic acid
	achievement age
	active assistive
	acute asthma
	affected area
	affirmative action
	African American

A

	Alcoholics Anonymous		antimicrobial
	alcohol abuse		agent-associated colitis
	alopecia areata		augmentative and
	alveolar-arterial gradient		alternative
	amino acid		communication
	anaplastic astrocytoma	AACD	aging-associated cognitive
	androgenetic alopecia		decline
	anesthesiologist assistant	AACG	acute-angle closure
	anti-aerobic		glaucoma
	antiarrhythmic agent	AACLR	arthroscopic anterior
	aortic aneurysm		cruciate ligament
	aplastic anemia		reconstruction
	arachidonic acid	AAD	acid-ash diet
	arm ankle (pulse ratio)		antibiotic-associated
	ascending aorta		diarrhea
	audiologic assessment	A_1AD	alpha$_1$-antitrypsin
	Australia antigen		deficiency
	authorized absence	AADA	Abbreviated Antibiotic
	automobile accident		Drug Application
	cytarabine (ara-C)	[A-a]Do$_2$	alveolar-arterial oxygen
	and doxorubicin		tension gradient
	(Adriamycin)	AAE	active assistance exercise
aa	of each		acute allergic encephalitis
A&A	aid and attendance	AAECS	amino acid enriched
	arthroscopy and arthrotomy		cardioplegic solution
	awake and aware	A/AEX	active assistive exercise
A-a	alveolar arterial (gradient)	AAF	African-American
a/A	arterial-alveolar (gradient)		female
AIIA	Angiotensin II antagonist	AAFB	alcohol acid-fast bacilli
AAA	abdominal aortic	AAFO	active ankle-foot orthoses
	aneurysmectomy	AAG	alpha-1-acid glycoprotein
	(aneurysm)	AAH	acute alcoholic hepatitis
	acute anxiety attack		atypical adenomatous
	Area Agencies on Aging		hyperplasia
	aromatic amino acids	AAI	acute alcohol intoxication
A&AA	active and active assistive		arm-ankle index
AAAASF	American Association for		atlantoaxial instability
	Accreditation of		atrial demand-inhibited
	Ambulatory Surgery		(pacemaker)
	Facilities	AAK	atlantoaxial kyphosis
AAAE	amino acid activating	AAL	anterior axillary line
	enzyme	AAM	African-American male
AAAHC	Accreditation Association		amino acid mixture
	of Ambulatory Health	AAMI	age-associated memory
	Care		impairment
AABB	American Association of	AAMS	acute aseptic meningitis
	Blood Banks		syndrome
AABR	automated auditory	AAN	AIDS-associated
	brainstem response		neutropenia
AAC	Adrenalin, atropine, and		analgesic abuse
	cocaine		nephropathy
	advanced adrenocortical		analgesic-associated
	cancer		nephropathy

	attending's admission notes	AASV	antibody-associated systemic vasculitis
AANA	American Association of Nurse Anesthetists	AAT	activity as tolerated alpha-antitrypsin
AAO	alert, awake, & oriented		androgen ablation therapy
AAO × 3	awake and oriented to time, place, and person		at all times atrial demand-triggered (pacemaker)
AAOC	antacid of choice		atypical antibody titer
AAP	acute anterior poliomyelitis American Academy of Pediatrics (guidelines)		automatic atrial tachycardia
	assessment adjustment pass	A_1AT	alpha$_1$-antitrypsin
AAPC	antibiotic-associated pseudomembranous	A_1AT-P_i	alpha$_1$-antitrypsin (phenotyping)
	colitis	AAU	acute anterior uveitis
AAPMC	antibiotic-associated	AAV	adeno-associated vector adeno-associated virus
	pseudomembranous colitis	AAVV	accumulated alveolar ventilatory volume
a/ApO$_2$	arterial-alveolar oxygen tension ratio	AAWD	antiandrogen withdrawal
AAPSA	age-adjusted prostate-specific antigen	AB	abortion Ace® bandage
AAR	antigen-antiglobulin reaction		antibiotic antibody
	automated anesthesia record		Aphasia Battery apical beat
AARF	atlantoaxial rotatory fixation (subluxation; dislocation)		armboard attentional blink products meeting bioequivalence requirements for
AAROM	active-assistive range of motion		generic pharmaceuticals
AAS	acute abdominal series	Aβ	beta-amyloid peptide
	allergic Aspergillus sinusitis	A/B	acid-base ratio apnea/bradycardia
	androgenic-anabolic steroid	A > B	air greater than bone (conduction)
	Ann Arbor stage (Hodgkin disease staging system)	A & B	apnea and bradycardia assault and battery
	aortic arch syndrome	AB+	AB positive blood type (AB positive preferred)
	atlantoaxis subluxation atypical absence seizure	AB−	AB negative blood type (AB negative preferred)
AASCRN	amino acid screen	ABA	applied behavioral
AASH	adrenal androgen-stimulating hormone		analysis
AAST	American Association for the Surgery of Trauma (trauma grading)	ABBI	Advanced Breast Biopsy Instrumentation
AAST-OIS	American Association for the Surgery of Trauma—Organ Injury Scale	ABC	abacavir (Ziagen) abbreviated blood count absolute band counts absolute basophil count advanced breast cancer

airway, breathing, and circulation

all but code (resuscitation order)

aneurysmal bone cyst

antigen-binding capacity

apnea, bradycardia, and cyanosis

applesauce, bananas, and cereal (diet)

argon-beam coagulator

aspiration, biopsy and cytology

artificial beta cells

automated blood count (no differential)

avidin-biotin complex

ABCD amphotericin B cholesteryl sulfate complex (Amphotec; amphotericin B colloid dispersion)

asymmetry, **b**order irregularity, **c**olor variation, and **d**iameter more than 6 mm (melanoma warning signs in a mole)

automated blood count (differential done manually)

ABCDE botulism toxoid pentavalent

ABCS automated blood count, STKR (differential done by machine)

ABD after bronchodilator

automated border detection detection

type of plain gauze dressing

Abd abdomen

abdominal

abductor

ABDCT atrial bolus dynamic computer tomography

ABD GR abdominal girth

ABD PB abductor pollicis brevis

ABD PL abductor pollicis longus

ABE acute bacteria endocarditis

adult basic education

average bioequivalence

botulism equine trivalent antitoxin

ABECB acute bacterial exacerbations of chronic bronchitis

ABEP auditory brain stem-evoked potentials

aortic blood flow

ABF aortobifemoral (bypass)

ABG air/bone gap

aortoiliac bypass graft

arterial blood gases

axiobuccogingival

ABH Ativan, Benadryl, and Haldol

ABI ankle brachial index (ankle-to-arm systolic blood pressure ratio)

atherothrombotic brain infarction

auditory brainstem implant

ABID antibody identification

A Big atrial bigeminy

ABK aphakic bullous keratopathy

ABL abetalipoproteinemia

allograft bound lymphocytes

axiobuccolingual

ABLB alternate binaural loudness balance

ABLC amphotericin B lipid complex (Abelcet)

ABLV Australian bat lyssavirus

A/B Mods apnea/bradycardia moderate stimulation

ABMS autologous bone marrow support

A/B MS apnea/bradycardia mild stimulation

ABMT autologous bone marrow transplantation

ABN abnormality(ies)

advance beneficiary notice

abnl bld abnormal bleeding

ABNM American Board of Nuclear Medicine

abnor. abnormal

ABO absent bed occupant

blood group system (A, AB, B, and O)

ABP	ambulatory blood pressure		antecubital
	androgen-binding protein		anticoagulant
	arterial blood pressure		anticonvulsant
ABPA	allergic bronchopulmo- nary aspergillosis		arm circumference assist control
ABPB	axillary brachial plexus block		autologous cell before meals
ABPM	axillary brachial plexus block		(*a.c.* preferred) doxorubicin (Adriamycin)
ABPM	allergic bronchopulmo- nary mycosis	*a.c.*	and cyclophosphamide before meals
	ambulatory blood pressure monitoring	A-C	Astler-Coller (stages of colorectal cancer
ABQAURP	American Board of Quality Assurance and	A/C	anterior chamber of the eye assist/control
	Utilization Review	A & C	alert and cooperative
	Physicians	A_{1C}	glycosylated hemoglobin
ABR	absolute bed rest		A_{1C}
	auditory brain-stem	5-AC	azacitidine (Vidaza)
	response	9AC	rubitecan (9-aminocamp-
ABRS	acute bacterial		tothecin; Orathecin)
	rhinosinusitis	ACA	acrodermatitis chronica
ABS	absent		atrophicans
	absorbed		acyclovir
	absorption		adenocarcinoma
	Accuchek® blood sugar		against clinical advice
	acute brain syndrome		aminocaproic acid
	admitting blood sugar		(Amicar)
	Alterman-Bishop stent		anterior cerebral artery
	antibody screen		anterior communicating
	at bedside		artery
ABSS	Anderson Behavioral		anticanalicular antibodies
	State Scale	AC/A	accommodation
A/B SS	apnea/bradycardia self- stimulation		convergence– accommodation (ratio)
ABT	aminopyrine breath test	ACABS	acute community-acquired
	antibiotic therapy		bacterial sinusitis
	autologous blood therapy	ACAD	anterior circulation arterial
ABVD	doxorubicin		dissection
	(Adriamycin)®,	ACAS	acute community-acquired
	bleomycin, vinblastine,		sinusitis
	and dacarbazine (DTIC)		asymptomatic carotid
ABW	actual body weight		artery study
ABx	antibiotics	ACAT	acyl coenzyme A:
AC	abdominal circumference		cholesterol
	acetate		acyltransferase
	acromioclavicular	ACB	alveolar-capillary block
	activated charcoal		antibody-coated bacteria
	acute		aortocoronary bypass
	African Caribbean		before breakfast
	air conditioned	AcB	assist with bath
	air conduction	AC & BC	air and bone conduction
	anchored catheter	ACBE	air contrast barium enema

ACBG	aortocoronary bypass graft	ACDFs	adult children from dysfunctional families
ACBT	active cycle of breathing techniques	ACDK	acquired cystic disease of the kidney
ACC	acalculous cholecystitis	ACDs	anticonvulsant drugs
	accident	ACE	adrenocortical extract
	accommodation		adverse clinical event
	adenoid cystic carcinomas		aerosol-cloud enhancer
	administrative control center		angiotensin-converting enzyme
	advanced colorectal cancer		antegrade colonic enema
	ambulatory care center		antegrade continence enema
	American College of Cardiology (guidelines)		doxorubicin (Adriamycin), cyclophosphamide, and etoposide
	amylase creatinine clearance	ACEI	angiotensin-converting enzyme inhibitor
	anterior cingulate cortex	ACF	aberrant crypt focus
	automated cell count		accessory clinical findings
ACCE	Academic Clinical Coordinator Educator		acute care facility
AcCoA	acetyl-coenzyme A		anterior cervical fusion
ACCP	American College of Chest Physicians	ACG	accelerography
			angiocardiography
ACCR	amylase creatinine clearance ratio	ACGME	Accreditation Council for Graduate Medical Education
ACCU	acute coronary care unit		
ACCU✔	Accucheck® (blood glucose monitoring)	ACH	adrenal cortical hormone
			aftercoming head
ACD	absolute cardiac dullness		arm girth, chest depth, and hip width
	absorbent cover dressing	ACh	acetylcholine
	acid-citrate-dextrose	ACHA	air-conduction hearing aid
	allergic contact dermatitis	AChE	acetylcholinesterase
	anemia of chronic disease	AChEIs	acetylcholinesterase inhibitors
	anterior cervical diskectomy	ACHES	abdominal pain, chest pain, headache, eye problems, and severe leg pains (early danger signs of oral contra-ceptive adverse effects)
	anterior chamber depth		
	anterior chamber diameter		
	anterior chest diameter		
	before dinner		
	dactinomycin (actinomycin D; Cosmegen)		
ACDC	antibody complement-dependent cytolysis	AC & HS	before meals and at bedtime
AC-DC	bisexual (homo- and heterosexual)	ACI	acceleration index
			adrenal cortical insufficiency
ACDDS	Alcoholism/Chemical Dependency Detoxification Service		aftercare instructions
			anabolic-catabolic index
ACDF	anterior cervical diskectomy and fusion		anemia of chronic illness
			autologous chondrocyte implantation

ACIOL	anterior chamber intraocular lens	A COMM A	anterior communicating artery
ACIP	Advisory Committee on Immunization Practices (of the Centers for Disease Control and Prevention)	ACOS-OG	American College of Surgeons Oncology Group
		ACP	accessory conduction pathway
ACIS	automated cellular imaging system		acid phosphatase adamantinomatous craniopharyngioma
ACJ	acromioclavicular joint		adenocarcinoma of the prostate
A/CK	Accuchek®		
ACL	accessory collateral ligament (hand)		ambulatory care program anesthesia-care provider
	American cutaneous leishmaniasis		anterior cervical plate antrochoanal polyp
	anterior cruciate ligament (knee)	ACPA	anticytoplasmic antibodies
aCL	anticardiolipin (antibody)	AC-PC line	anterior commissure-posterior commissure line
ACLA	aclarubicin		
ACLF	adult congregate living facility	AC-PH	acid phosphatase
		ACPO	acute colonic pseudo-obstruction
ACLR	anterior cruciate ligament repair	ACPP	adrenocorticopolypeptide
ACLS	advanced cardiac (cardio-pulmonary) life support	ACPPD	average cost per patient day
		ACPP PF	acid phosphatase prostatic fluid
	Allen Cognitive Level Screen	ACPS	anterior cervical plate stabilization
ACM	alternative/complementary medicine	ACQ	acquired Areas of Change Questionnaire
	Arnold-Chiari malformation		
ACME	aphakic cystoid macular edema	ACR	adenomatosis of the colon and rectum
	Automated Classification of Medical Entities		albumin to creatinine ratio American College of Rheumatology
ACMT	advanced combined modality therapy		
ACMV	assist-controlled mechanical ventilation		anterior chamber reformation
ACN	acute conditioned neurosis		anticonstipation regimen
		ACR20	American College of Rheumatology rating scale (20% or more improvement)
ACNP	Acute Care Nurse Practitioner		
ACNU	nimustine HCl (Nidran; Acnu)		
		ACRC	advanced colorectal cancer
ACO	anterior capsular opacification	ACRES	amplification created restriction enzyme site
ACOA	Adult Children of Alcoholics	ACS	anterior compartment syndrome
ACOG	American College of Obstetricians and Gynecologists		acute confusional state acute coronary syndromes

American Cancer Society
anodal-closing sound
automated corneal shaper
before supper

ACSF anterior cervical spine fixation
artificial cerebrospinal fluid

ACSL automatic computerized solvent litholysis

ACSVBG aortocoronary saphenous vein bypass graft

ACSW Academy of Certified Social Workers

ACT activated clotting time
aggressive comfort treatment
allergen challenge test
anticoagulant therapy
artemisinin-based combination therapy
assertive community treatment (program)
doxorubicin (adriamycin), cyclophosphamide, and paclitaxel (Taxol)

ACT-D dactinomycin (Cosmegen)

Act Ex active exercise

ACTG AIDS Clinical Trial Group

ACTH corticotropin (adrenocorticotropic hormone)

ACT-Post activated clotting time post-filter

ACT-Pre activated clotting time pre-filter

ACTSEB anterior chamber tube shunt encircling band

ACU ambulatory care unit

ACUP adenocarcinoma of unknown primary (origin)

ACUV air-contrast ultrasound venography

ACV acyclovir (Zovirax)
amifostine, cisplatin, and vinblastine
assist control ventilation
atrial/carotid/ventricular

A-C-V A wave, C wave, and V wave

ACVD acute cardiovascular disease

ACVP doxorubicin (Adriamycin), cyclophosphamide, vincristine, and prednisone

ACW anterior chest wall
apply to chest wall

acyl-CoA acyl coenzyme A

AD accident dispensary
admitting diagnosis
advance directive (living will)
air dyne
alternating days (this is a dangerous abbreviation)
Alzheimer disease
androgen deprivation
antidepressant
assistive device
atopic dermatitis
axillary dissection
axis deviation
right ear

A&D admission and discharge
alcohol and drug
ascending and descending
vitamins A and D

ADA adenosine deaminase
American Dental Association
American Diabetes Association
Americans with Disabilities Act
anterior descending artery
awareness during anesthesia

ADAM adjustment disorder with anxious mood

ADAS Alzheimer Disease Assessment Scale

ADAS-COG Alzheimer Disease Assessment Scale-Cognitive Subscale

ADAT advance diet as tolerated

ADAU adolescent drug abuse unit

ADB amorous disinhibited behavior

ADC Aid to Dependent Children
AIDS (acquired immune deficiency syndrome) dementia complex
anxiety disorder clinic

	apparent diffusion coefficient (radiology)	ADI	acute diaphragmatic injury
			allowable (acceptable) daily intake
	average daily census		axiodistoincisal
	average daily consumption	A-DIC	doxorubicin (Adriamycin) and dacarbazine
ADCA	autosomal dominant cerebellar ataxia		
ADCC	antibody-dependent cellular cytotoxicity	Adj Dis	adjustment disorder
		Adj D/O	adjustment disorder
A.D.C. VAAN DIML	mnemonic for formatting physician orders: Admit, Diagnosis, Condition, Vitals, Activity, Allergies, Nursing procedures, Diet, Ins and outs, Medication, Labs	ADL	activities of daily living
		ADLG	average duration of life gained
		ad lib	as desired
			at liberty
		ADM	abductor digiti minimi (muscle)
			acceptance of disability modified
ADD	adduction		administered (dose)
	annual disability density		admission
	arrest in dilation/descent		adrenomedullin
	attention-deficit disorder		doxorubicin (Adriamycin)
	average daily dose	ADMA	asymmetrical dimethyl arginine
ADDH	attention-deficit disorder with hyperactivity		
ADDL	additional	ADME	absorption, distribution, metabolism, and excretion
ADDM	adjustment disorder with depressed mood		
		ADO	axiodisto-occlusal
ADDP	adductor pollicis	Ad-OAP	doxorubicin (Adriamycin), vincristine, (Oncovin) cytarabine, (Ara C) and prednisone
ADDs	AIDS (acquired immune deficiency syndrome)-defining diseases		
ADDU	alcohol and drug dependence unit	ADOL	adolescent
		ADON	Assistant Director of Nursing
ADE	acute disseminated encephalitis		
		ADP	arterial demand pacing
	adverse drug event		adenosine diphosphate
ADEM	acute disseminating encephalomyelitis	ADPKD	autosomal dominant polycystic kidney disease
ADE-NOCA	adenocarcinoma		
		ADPV	anomaly of drainage of pulmonary vein
ADEPT	antibody-directed enzyme prodrug therapy		
		ADQ	abductor digiti quinti
ADFT	atrial defibrillation threshold		adequate
		ADR	acute dystonic reaction
ADFU	agar diffusion for fungus		adverse drug reaction
ADG	atrial diastolic gallop		alternative dispute resolution
	axiodistogingival		doxorubicin (Adriamycin)
ADH	antidiuretic hormone	ADRB2	beta-2 adrenergic receptor
	atypical ductal hyperplasia	ADRD	Alzheimer disease and related disorders
ADHD	attention-deficit hyperactivity disorder		
		ADRIA	doxorubicin (Adriamycin)
ADHF	acute decompensated heart failure	ADRV	adult diarrhea rotavirus

ADS	admission day surgery	AEB	as evidenced by
	anatomical dead space		atrial ectopic beat
	anonymous donor's sperm	AEC	absolute (blood)
	antibody deficiency		eosinophil count
	syndrome		at earliest convenience
ADs	advance directives (living	AECB	acute exacerbations of
	wills)		chronic bronchitis
ADSU	ambulatory diagnostic	AECG	ambulatory
	surgery unit		electrocardiogram
ADT	admission, discharge, and	AECOPD	acute exacerbation of
	transfer		chronic obstructive
	alternate-day therapy		pulmonary disease
	androgen deprivation	AED	antiepileptic drug
	treatment (therapy)		automated (automatic)
	anticipate discharge		external defibrillator
	tomorrow	AEDD	anterior extradural defects
	any damn thing (a placebo)	AEDF	absent end-diastolic flow
	Auditory Discrimination		(umbilical-artery
	Test		Doppler
ADTP	Adolescent Day Treatment		ultrasonography)
	Program	AEDP	assisted end-diastolic
	Alcohol-Dependence		pressure
	Treatment Program		automated external
ADTR	Academy of Dance		defibrillator pacemaker
	Therapists, Registered	AEE	asthma-exacerbation
ADU	automated dispensing unit		episodes
ADV	adenovirus vaccine, not	AEEU	admission entrance and
	otherwise specified		evaluation unit
adv	adventitious sounds	AEG	air encephalogram
	(wheezes and rhonchi)		Alcohol Education
ADV$_4$	adenovirus vaccine, type		Group
	4, live, oral	AEIOU	mnemonic for the
ADV$_7$	adenovirus vaccine, type	TIPS	diagnosis of coma:
	7, live, oral		**A**lcohol,
A5D5W	alcohol 5%, dextrose 5%		**E**ncephalopathy,
	in water for injection		**I**nsulin, **O**piates,
ADX	audiological diagnostic		**U**remia, **T**rauma,
AE	above elbow (amputation)		**I**nfection, **P**sychiatric,
	accident and emergency		and **S**yncope
	(department)	AELBM	after each loose bowel
	acute exacerbation		movement
	adaptive equipment	AEM	active electrode monitor
	adverse event		ambulatory electrogram
	air entry		monitor
	anoxic encephalopathy		antiepileptic medication
	antiembolitic	AEP	auditory evoked potential
	arm ergometer	AEq	age equivalent
	aryepiglottic (fold)	AER	acoustic evoked response
A&E	accident and emergency		albumin excretion rate
	(department)		auditory evoked response
AEA	above-elbow amputation	AERD	aspirin-exacerbated
	anti-endomysium		respiratory disease
	antibody	Aer. M.	aerosol mask

AERS	adverse event reporting system	A Flu	atrial flutter
AERs	adverse event reports	AFM	acute *Plasmodium falciparum* malaria
Aer. T.	aerosol tent		aerosol face mask
AES	adult emergency service		atomic force microscopy
	anti-embolic stockings		doxorubicin (Adriamycin),
AEs	adverse events		fluorouracil, and
AET	alternating esotropia		methotrexate
	atrial ectopic tachycardia	AFM×2	double-aerosol face mask
AF	acid-fast	AFO	ankle-fixation orthotic
	afebrile		ankle-foot orthosis
	amniotic fluid	AFOF	anterior fontanelõopen
	anterior fontanel		and flat
	antifibrinogen	AFP	acute flaccid paralysis
	aortofemoral		alpha-fetoprotein
	ascitic fluid		anterior faucial pillar
	atrial fibrillation		ascending frontal parietal
AFB	acid-fast bacilli	AFQT	Armed Forces
	aorto-femoral bypass		Qualification Test
	aspirated foreign body	AFRD	acute febrile respiratory
AFB₁	aflatoxin B₁		disease
AFBG	aortofemoral bypass graft	AFRIMS	Armed Forces Research
AFBY	aortofemoral bypass (graft)		Institute of Medical Sciences
AFC	adult foster care	AFRRI	Armed Forces
	air filled cushions		Radiological Research
	alveolar fluid clearance		Institute
AFDC	Aid to Families with Dependent Children	AFRS	allergic fungal rhinosinusitis
AFE	amniotic fluid embolization	AFS	allergic fungal sinusitis
			atomic fluorescence
AFEB	afebrile		spectrometry
AFEU	ante partum fetal evaluation unit	Aft/Dis	aftercare/discharge
		AFV	amniotic fluid volume
AF/FL	atrial fibrillation/atrial flutter	AFVSS	afebrile, vital signs stable
		AFX	air-fluid exchange
aFGF	acidic fibroblast growth factor	AG	abdominal girth
			adrenogenital
AFH	angiomatoid fibrous histiocytoma		aminoglycoside
			Amsler grid
	anterior facial height		anion gap
AFI	acute febrile illness		antigen
	amniotic fluid index		antigravity
A fib	atrial fibrillation		atrial gallop
AFIP	Armed Forces Institute of Pathology	Ag	silver
		A/G	albumin to globulin ratio
AFKO	ankle-foot-knee orthosis	AGA	accelerated growth area
AFL	air/fluid level		acute gonococcal arthritis
	atrial flutter		androgenetic alopecia
AFLP	acute fatty liver of pregnancy		antigliadin antibody
			appropriate for gestational age
	amplified fragment length polymorphism		average gestational age

AGAS	accelerated graft atherosclerosis	AH	abdominal hysterectomy
			amenorrhea and hirsutism
AG/BL	aminoglycoside/beta-lactam		amenorrhea-hyperprolac-tinemia
AGC	absolute granulocyte count		antihyaluronidase
	advanced gastric cancer		auditory hallucinations
	atypical glandular cells	A&H	accident and health (insurance)
AGCUS	atypical glandular cells of undetermined significance	AHA	acetohydroxamic acid (Lithostat®)
AGD	agar gel diffusion		acquired hemolytic anemia
AGE	acute gastroenteritis		American Health Association (guidelines)
	advanced glycation end product(s)		autoimmune hemolytic anemia
	angle of greatest extension		
	anterior gastroenterostomy	AHAs	alpha hydroxy acids
	arterial gas embolism	AHase	antihyaluronidase
AGECAT	automatic geriatric exami-nation for computer-assisted taxonomy	AHB_c	hepatitis B core antibody
		AHC	acute hemorrhagic conjunctivitis
AGF	angle of greatest flexion		acute hemorrhagic cystitis
AGG	agammaglobulinemia		Adolescent Health Center
aggl.	agglutination		alternating hemiplegia of childhood
AGI	alpha-glucosidase inhibitor		
AGL	acute granulocytic leukemia		avoidable hospitalization conditions
A GLAC-TO-LK	alpha galactoside leukocytes	AHCA	Agency for Healthcare Administration
AGN	acute glomerulonephritis		American Healthcare Association
AGNB	aerobic gram-negative bacilli	AHCPR	Agency for Health Care Policy and Research
$AgNO_3$	silver nitrate		
AgNORs	argyrophilic nucleolar organizer regions (staining)	AHCs	academic health centers
		AHD	alien-hand syndrome
			antecedent hematological disorder
α_1-AGP	alpha$_1$-acid glycoprotein		arteriosclerotic heart disease
AGPT	agar-gel precipitation test		
AGS	adrenogenital syndrome		autoimmune hemolytic disease
	Alagille syndrome		
AG SYND	adrenogenital syndrome	AHE	acute hemorrhagic encephalomyelitis
AGT	alanine-glyoxylate aminotransferase		amygdalo-hippocampectomy
	angiotensinogen		
AGTT	abnormal glucose tolerance test	AHEC	Area Health Education Center
AGU	aspartylglycosaminuria	AHF	antihemophilic factor
AGUS	atypical glandular cells of uncertain significance		Argentine hemorrhagic fever (Junin virus) vaccine
AGV	Ahmed glaucoma valve		
AGVHD	acute graft-versus-host disease	AHF-M	antihemophilic factor (human), method M, (monoclonal purified)
AGVI	Ahmed glaucoma valve implantation		

AHFS	American Hospital Formulary Service
AHG	antihemophilic globulin
AHGS	acute herpetic gingival stomatitis
AHHD	arteriosclerotic hypertensive heart disease
AHI	apnea-hypopnea index
AHJ	artificial hip joint
AHL	apparent half-life
AHM	ambulatory Holter monitoring
AHMO	anterior horizontal mandibular osteotomy
AHN	adenomatous hyperplastic nodule
	Assistant Head Nurse
AHO	Albright hereditary osteodystrophy
AHP	acute hemorrhagic pancreatitis
	acute hepatic panel (see page 392)
	American Herbal Pharmacopeia and Therapeutic Compendium
AhpF	alkyl hydroperoxide reductase, F isomer
AHR	airway hyperresponsiveness
AHRE	atrial high-rate event
AHRF	acute hypoxemic respiratory failure
AHS	adaptive hand skills
	allopurinol hypersensitivity syndrome
	Alpers-Huttenlocher syndrome
	antiepileptic hypersensitivity syndrome
AHSA	Assistant Health Services Administrator
AHSCT	autologous hemopoietic stem-cell transplantation
AHSG	fetuin-A (alpha2-Heremans Schmid glycoprotein
AHST	autologous hematopoietic stem cell transplantation

AHT	alternating hypertropia
	autoantibodies to human thyroglobulin
AHTG	antihuman thymocyte globulin
AI	accidentally incurred
	accommodative insufficiency
	allelic imbalance
	American Indian
	allergy index
	aortic insufficiency
	apical impulse
	artificial insemination
	artificial intelligence
A & I	Allergy and Immunology (department)
	auscultation and inspection
AIA	Accommodation Independence Assessment
	allergen-induced asthma
	allyl isopropyl acetamide
	anti-insulin antibody
	aspirin-induced asthma
AI-Ab	anti-insulin antibody
AIBF	anterior interbody fusion
AICA	anterior inferior cerebellar artery
	anterior inferior communicating artery
AICBG	anterior interbody cervical bone graft
AICD	activation-induced cell death
	automatic implantable cardioverter/defibrillator
AICM	anti-inflammatory controller medication
AICS	acute ischemic coronary syndromes
AID	absolute iron deficiency
	acute infectious disease
	aortoiliac disease
	artificial insemination donor
	automatic implantable defibrillator
AIDH	artificial insemination donor husband
AIDKS	acquired immune deficiency syndrome with Kaposi sarcoma

AIDP	acute inflammatory demyelinating polyradiculoneuropathy		acute intermittent porphyria
AIDS	acquired immuno-deficiency syndrome		acute interstitial pneumonia
AIE	acute inclusion body encephalitis		asymptomatic inflammatory prostatitis
AIED	autoimmune inner-ear Disease		autoimmune pancreatitis
AIEOP	Italian Association of Pediatric Hematology and Oncology (cancer study group)	AIPC	androgen-independent prostate cancer
		AIR	accelerated idioventricular rhythm
AIF	aortic-iliac-femoral		acetylcholine-induced relaxation
AIGHL	anterior band of the inferior glenohumeral ligament	AIRE	autoimmune regulator (gene)
		AIRR	acute infusion-related reaction
AIH	artificial insemination with husband's sperm	AIS	Abbreviated Injury Score
			acute ischemic stroke
	autoimmune hepatitis		adolescent idiopathic scoliosis
AIHA	autoimmune hemolytic anemia		anti-insulin serum
AIHD	acquired immune hemolytic disease	AISA	acquired idiopathic sideroblastic anemia
AIIS	anterior inferior iliac spine	AIS/ISS	Abbreviated Injury Scale/Injury Severity Score
AILD	angioimmunoblastic lymphadenopathy with dysproteinemia		
		AIT	adoptive immunotherapy
AILT	angioimmunoblastic T-cell lymphoma		Advanced Individual Training (Army)
AIM	anti-inflammatory medication		auditory integration therapy
AIMS	Abnormal Involuntary Movement Scale	AITD	autoimmune thyroiditis
		AITN	acute interstitial tubular nephritis
	Arthritis Impact Measurement Scales	AITP	autoimmune thrombocytopenia purpura
AIN	acute interstitial nephritis		
	anal intraepithelial neoplasia	AIU	absolute iodine uptake
			adolescent inpatient unit
	anterior interosseous nerve	AIVC	absence of the inferior vena cava
AINS	anti-inflammatory non-steroidal		
AIO	all-in-one (lipid emulsion, protein, carbohydrate, and electrolytes	AIVR	accelerated idioventricular rhythm
		AJ	ankle jerk
	combined total parenteral nutrition)	AJCC	American Joint Committee on Cancer
AIOD	aortoiliac occlusive disease	AJO	apple juice only
		AJR	abnormal jugular reflex
AION	anterior ischemic optic neuropathy	AK	above-knee (amputation)
			actinic keratosis
AIP	acute infectious polyneuritis		artificial kidney
		AKA	above-knee amputation

	alcoholic ketoacidosis		alternate level of care
	all known allergies		Alternate Lifestyle
	also known as (a.k.a.		Checklist
	preferred)		axiolinguocervical
a.k.a.	also known as	ALCA	anomalous left coronary
AKP	anterior knee pain		artery
AKS	alcoholic Korsakoff	ALCL	anaplastic large-cell
	syndrome		lymphoma
	arthroscopic knee	ALC R	alcohol rub
	surgery	ALD	adrenoleukodystrophy
AKU	artificial kidney unit		alcoholic liver disease
AL	acute leukemia		aldolase
	argon laser	ALDH	aldehyde dehydrogenase
	arterial line	ALDO	aldosterone
	assisted living	ALDOST	aldosterone
	axial length	ALF	acute liver failure
	left ear		arterial line filter
Al	aluminum		assisted living facility
ALA	adrenalin (epinephrine),	ALFT	abnormal liver function
	lidocaine, and		tests
	amethocaine	ALG	antilymphoblast globulin
	(tetracaine)		antilymphocyte globulin
	alpha-linolenic acid (α-	ALGB	adjustable laparoscopic
	linolenic acid)		gastric banding
	alpha-lipoic acid	ALH	atypical lobular
	amebic liver abscess		hyperplasia
	aminolevulinic acid	ALI	Abbott Laboratories,
	(Levulan)		Inc.
	antileukotriene agent		acute lung injury
	antilymphocyte antibody		argon laser iridotomy
	as long as	ALIF	anterior lumbar interbody
ALAC	antibiotic-loaded acrylic		fusion
	cement	A-line	arterial catheter
ALAD	abnormal left axis	ALJ	administrative law judge
	deviation	ALK	alkaline
ALA-GLN	alanyl-glutamine		automated lamellar
ALARA	as low as reasonably		keratoplasty
	achievable	ALK Ø	alkaline phosphatase
ALAT	alanine aminotransferase	ALK ISO	alkaline phosphatase
	(also ALT; SGPT)		isoenzymes
ALAX	apical long axis	ALK-P	alkaline phosphatase
ALB	albumin	ALK PHOS	alkaline phosphatase
	albuterol	ISO	isoenzyme
	anterior lenticular	ALL	acute lymphoblastic
	bevel		leukemia
ALBUMS	aldehyde linker-based		acute lymphocytic
	ultrasensitive mismatch		leukemia
	scanning		allergy
ALC	acute lethal catatonia	ALLD	arthroscopic lumbar laser
	alcohol		diskectomy
	alcoholic liver cirrhosis	ALLO	allogeneic
	allogeneic lymphocyte	Allo-BMT	allogeneic bone marrow
	cytotoxicity		transplantation

Allo-HCT	allogenic hematopoietic cell transplant	2 *alt*	every other day (this is a dangerous abbreviation)
ALM	acral lentiginous melanoma	ALTB	acute laryngotracheobronchitis
	alveolar lining material autoclave-killed *Leishmania major*	ALTE	acute (aberrant, apparent) life threatening event
ALMI	anterolateral myocardial infarction	*alt hor*	every other hour (this is a dangerous abbreviation)
ALN	anterior lower neck	ALTP	argon laser trabeculoplasty
	anterior lymph node	ALUP	Alupent
	axillary lymph nodes	ALv	attachment level (dental)
ALND	axillary lymph node dissection	ALVAD	abdominal left ventricular assist device
ALNM	axillary lymph node metastasis	ALWMI	anterolateral wall myocardial infarct
ALO	apraxia of eyelid opening	ALZ	Alzheimer disease
	axiolinguo-occlusal	AM	adult male
ALOC	altered level of consciousness		aerosol mask
			amalgam
Al(OH)₃	aluminum hydroxide		anovulatory menstruation
ALOS	average length of stay		anterior midpapillary
ALP	alkaline phosphatase		morning (a.m.)
	argon laser photocoagulation		myopic astigmatism
		AMA	advanced maternal age
	Alupent		against medical advice
ALPS	autoimmune lymphoproliferative syndrome		American Medical Association
			antimitochondrial antibody
ALPSA	anterior labroligamentous periosteal sleeve avulsion	AMAC	adults molested as children
ALPZ	alprazolam (Xanax)	AMAD	activity median aerodynamic diameter
ALR	adductor leg raise		
ALRI	acute lower-respiratory-tract infection	AMBI	acute multiple brain infarcts
	anterolateral rotary instability	AM Care	brushing teeth, washing face and hands
ALS	acid-labile subunit	AMAD	morning admission
	acute lateral sclerosis	AM/ADM	morning admission
	advanced life support	AMAG	adrenal medullary autograft
	amyotrophic lateral sclerosis	AMAL	amalgam
	antilymphocyte serum	AMAN	acute motor axonal neuropathy
ALSG	Australian Leukemia Study Group	AMAP	American Medical Accreditation Program
ALT	alanine aminotransferase (SGPT)		as much as possible
	antibiotic lock technique (catheter infection prevention)	Amask	aerosol mask
		AMAT	anti-malignant antibody test
	argon laser trabeculoplasty		Arm Motor Ability Test
	autolymphocyte therapy	A-MAT	amorphous material

AMB	ambulate
	ambulatory
	amphotericin B (Fungizone)
	as manifested by
AMBER	advanced multiple beam equalization radiography
AMC	arm muscle circumference
	arthrogryposis multiplex congenita
AM/CR	amylase to creatinine ratio
AMD	age-related macular degeneration
	arthroscopic microdiskectomy
	axiomesiodistal
	dactinomycin (actinomycin D; Cosmegen)
	methyldopa (alpha methyldopa)
AME	agreed medical examination
	anthrax meningoencephalitis
	apparent mineralocorticoid excess (syndrome)
	Aviation Medical Examiner
AMegL	acute megakaryoblastic leukemia
AMES-LAN	American sign language
AMF	aerobic metabolism facilitator
	amifostine (Ethyol)
	autocrine motility factor
AMG	acoustic myography
	aminoglycoside
	axiomesiogingival
	Federal Republic of Germany's equivalent to United States Food, Drug, and Cosmetic Act
AMGA	American Medical Group Association
AMI	acute myocardial infarction
	amifostine (Ethyol)
	amitriptyline
	axiomesioincisal
AMKL	acute megakaryocytic leukemia

AML	acute myelogenous leukemia
	angiomyolipoma
	anterior mitral leaflet
AMLOS	arithmetic mean length of stay
AMLR	auditory midlatency response
	Marketing Authorization Application (French)
AMM	agnogenic myeloid metaplasia
AMML	acute myelomonocytic leukemia
AMMOL	acute myelomonoblastic leukemia
AMN	adrenomyeloneuropathy
amnio	amniocentesis
AMN SC	amniotic fluid scan
AMOL	acute monoblastic leukemia
AMOVA	analysis of molecular variance
AMP	adenosine monophosphate
	ampere
	ampicillin
	ampul
	amputation
	antipressure mattress
AMPLE	allergies, medications, past medical history, last meal, events leading to admission (used for history and physical examination)
AMPPE	acute multifocal placoid pigment epitheliopathy
A-M pr	Austin-Moore prosthesis
AMPS	Assessment of Motor and Process Skills
AMPT	metyrosine (alphamethylpara tyrosine)
AMR	acoustic muscle reflex
	alternating motion rates
	amrubicin
AMRI	anterior medial rotary instability
AMS	accelerator mass spectrometry
	acute maxillary sinusitis
	acute mountain sickness
	aggravated in military service

A

47

	altered mental status
	amylase
	aseptic meningitis syndrome
	atypical mole syndrome
	auditory memory span
m-AMSA	amsacrine (acridinyl anisidide)
AMSAN	acute motor sensory axonal neuropathy
AMSIT	portion of the mental status examination: A—appearance, M—mood, S—sensorium, I—intelligence, T—thought process
AMT	abbreviated mental test
	Adolph's Meat Tenderizer
	allogeneic (bone) marrow transplant
	alpha-methyltryptamine
	aminopterin
	amniotic membrane transplantation
	amount
AMTS	Abbreviated Mental Test Score
AMU	accessory-muscle use
AMV	alveolar minute ventilation
	assisted mechanical ventilation
AMY	amylase
AMY/CR	amylase/creatinine ratio
AN	acoustic neuromas
	Alaska Native
	amyl nitrate
	anorexia nervosa
	anticipatory nausea
	Associate Nurse
	avascular necrosis
ANA	American Nurses Association
	antinuclear antibody
ANAD	anorexia nervosa and associated disorders
ANADA	Abbreviated New Animal Drug Application
ANAG	acute narrow angle glaucoma
ANA SWAB	anaerobic swab

ANC	absolute neutrophil count
ANCA	antineutrophil cytoplasmic antibody
anch	anchored
ANCN	absolute neutrophil count nadir
ANCOVA	analysis of covariance
AND	anterior nasal discharge
	axillary node dissection
ANDA	Abbreviated New Drug Application
anes	anesthesia
ANF	antinuclear factor
	atrial natriuretic factor
ANG	angiogram
ANG II	angiotensin II
ANGIO	angiogram
ANH	acute normovolemic hemodilution
	artificial nutrition and hydration
ANISO	anisocytosis
ANK	ankle
	appointment not kept
ANLL	acute nonlymphoblastic leukemia
ANM	Assistant Nurse Manager
ANN	artificial neural network(s)
	axillary node-negative
ANNA	artificial neural network analysis
ANOVA	analysis of variance
ANP	Adult Nurse Practitioner
	atrial natriuretic peptide (anaritide acetate)
	axillary node–positive
ANPR	advanced notice of proposed rule making
ANS	answer
	autonomic nervous system
ANSER	Aggregate Neurobehavioral Student Health and Education Review
ANSI	American National Standards Institute
ANT	anterior
	anthrax vaccine, not otherwise specified
	enpheptin (2-amino-5-nitrothiazol)
ANT_a	anthrax vaccine, absorbed

ante	before	AOBS	acute organic brain syndrome
ANTI A:AGT	anti–blood group A antiglobulin test		
Anti bx	antibiotic	AOC	abridged ocular chart
anti-D	anti-D immune globulin		advanced ovarian cancer
anti-GAD	antibodies to glutamic acid decarboxylase		amoxicillin, omeprazole, and clarithromycin
anti-HBc	antibody to hepatitis B core antigen (HBcAg)		anode opening contraction antacid of choice
anti-HBe	antibody to hepatitis B e antigen (HBeAg)	AOCD	area of concern anemia of chronic disease
anti-HBs	antibody to hepatitis B surface antigen (HBsAg)	AOCL AOD	anodal opening clonus adult-onset diabetes
ant sag D	anterior sagittal diameter		alcohol and (and/or) other drugs
ANTU	alpha naphthylthiourea		alleged onset date
ANUG	acute necrotizing ulcerative gingivitis		anaplastic oligodendroglioma
ANV	acute nausea and vomiting		arterial occlusive disease
ANX	anxiety		Assistant-Officer-of-the- Day
	anxious	AODA	alcohol and other drug abuse
ANZDATA	Australia and New Zealand Dialysis and Transplant Registry	AODM	adult-onset diabetes mellitus
AO	abdominal obesity	A of 1	assistance of one
	acridine orange (stain)	A of 2	assistance of two
	Agent Orange	AOI	area of induration
	anaplastic oligoden- drogliomas	ao-il AOIVM	aorta-iliac angiographically occult intracranial vascular malformation
	anterior oblique		
	aorta		
	aortic opening	AOL	augmentation of labor
	aortography	AOLC	acridine-orange leukocyte cytospin
	axio-occlusal		
	plate, screw (orthopedics)	AOLD	automated open lumbar diskectomy
	right ear		
A-O	atlanto-occipital (joint)	AOM	acute otitis media
A/O	alert and oriented		alternatives of management
A & O	alert and oriented		
A&O × 3	awake and oriented to person, place, and time	AONAD	alert, oriented, and no acute distress
A&O × 4	awake and oriented to person, place, time, and object	AOO	anodal opening odor continuous arterial asynchronous pacing
AOA	anaplastic oligoastrocytoma	AOP	anemia of prematurity anodal opening picture
AOAA	aminooxoacetic acid		aortic pressure
AOAP	as often as possible		apnea of prematurity
AOAs	adult offspring of alcoholics	AOR	adjusted odds ratio Alvarado Orthopedic
AOB	alcohol on breath		Research
AOBC	aortic occlusion balloon catheter		at own risk auditory oculogyric reflex

AORT REGURG	aortic regurgitation
AORT STEN	aortic stenosis
AOS	ambulatory outpatient surgery
	anode opening sound
	antibiotic order sheet
	aortic ostial stenoses
	arrived on scene
AOSC	acute obstructive suppurative cholangiotomy
AOSD	adult-onset Still disease
AOTB	alcohol on the breath
AOTe	anodal opening tetanus
AP	abdominal pain
	abdominoperineal
	acute pancreatitis
	aerosol pentamidine
	alkaline phosphatase
	angina pectoris
	antepartum
	anterior-posterior (x-ray)
	apical pulse
	appendectomy
	appendicitis
	arterial pressure
	arthritis panel (see page 392)
	atrial pacing
	attending physician
	doxorubicin (Adriamycin); cisplatin (Platinol AQ)
A&P	active and present
	anterior and posterior
	assessment and plans
	auscultation and percussion
A/P	ascites/plasma ratio
$A_2 > P_2$	second aortic sound greater than second pulmonic sound
APA	aldosterone-producing adenoma
	American Psychiatric Association
	anticipatory postural adjustment
	antiphospholipid antibody
APAA	anterior parietal artery aneurysm
APACHE	Acute Physiology and Chronic Health Evaluation

APAD	anterior-posterior abdominal diameter
APAG	antipseudomonal aminoglycosidic
APAP	acetaminophen (N acetyl-para-aminophenol; Tylenol; paracetamol)
APB	abductor pollicis brevis
	atrial premature beat
APBSCT	autologous peripheral blood stem cell transplantation
APC	absolute phagocyte count
	activated protein C
	acute pharyngoconjunctiivitis (fever)
	adenoidal-pharyngeal-conjunctival
	adenomatous polyposis of the colon and rectum
	advanced pancreatic cancer
	advanced prostate cancer
	Ambulatory Payment Classification
	antigen-presenting cell
	argon plasma coagulator
	aspirin, phenacetin, and caffeine (no longer marketed in the US)
	asymptomatic prostate cancer
	atrial premature contraction
	autologous packed cells
APCD	adult polycystic disease
APCE	affinity probe capillary electrophoresis
APCIs	atrial peptide clearance inhibitors
APCKD	adult polycystic kidney disease
AP-CT	abdominal and pelvic computer tomography
APD	acid peptic disease
	action potential duration
	afferent pupillary defect
	anterior-posterior diameter
	atrial premature depolarization
	automated peritoneal dialysis

pamidronate disodium (aminohydroxypropylidene diphosphate)

anterior pituitary-like (hormone)

chorionic gonadotropin

APDC	Anxiety and Panic Disorder Clinic	AP & L	anteroposterior and lateral
APDT	acellular pertussis vaccine with diphtheria and tetanus toxoids	APLA	antiphospholipid antibody
		APLD	automated percutaneous lumbar diskectomy
APE	absolute prediction error	APLS	antiphospholipid syndrome
	acute psychotic episode	APME	acute postinfectious measles encephalitis
	acute pulmonary edema		
	anterior pituitary extract	APMPPE	acute posterior multifocal placoid pigment epitheliopathy
	doxorubicin (Adriamycin), cisplatin (Platinol-AQ), and etoposide		
APECED	autoimmune polyendo-crinopathy-candidiasis ectodermal dystrophy	APMS	acute pain management service
		APN	acquired pendular nystagmus
			acute panautonomic neuropathy
APER	abdominoperineal excision of the rectum		acute pyelonephritis
			Advanced Practice Nurse
APG	ambulatory patient group	APO	adverse patient occurrence
	Apgar (score)		apolipoprotein A-1
Apgar	appearance (color), pulse (heart rate), grimace (reflex irritability), activity (muscle tone), and respiration (score reflecting condition of newborn)		doxorubicin (Adriamycin), prednisone, and vincristine (Oncovin)
		APO(a)	apolipoprotein (A)
		APOE	apolipoprotein E
		APOE-4	apolipoprotein-E (gene)
APH	adult psychiatric hospital	APOLT	auxiliary partial orthotopic liver transplantation
	alcohol-positive history		
	antepartum hemorrhage	APOPPS	adjustable postoperative protective prosthetic socket
APhA	American Pharmacists Association		
APHIS	Animal and Plant Health Inspection Service	APP	alternating pressure pad
			amyloid precursor protein
API	active pharmaceutical ingredients		appetite
		APPG	aqueous procaine penicillin G (dangerous terminology; since it is for intramuscular use only; write as penicillin G procaine)
	Asian-Pacific Islander		
APIS	Acute Pain Intensity Scale		
APIVR	artificial pacemaker-induced ventricular rhythm		
		appr.	approximate
		appt.	appointment
APKD	adult polycystic kidney disease	APPY	appendectomy
		APR	abdominoperineal resection
	adult-onset polycystic kidney disease		acute radiation proctitis
APL	abductor pollicis longus	AP & R	apical and radial (pulses)
	accelerated painless labor	APRN	Advanced Practice Registered Nurse
	acute promyelocytic leukemia		

APRT	abdominopelvic radiotherapy		aortic regurgitation
APRV	airway pressure release ventilation		apoptotic rate
APS	acute pain service		Argyll Robertson (pupil)
	Acute Physiology Scoring (system)		assisted respiration
	adult protective services		at risk
	Adult Psychiatric Service	Ar	aural rehabilitation
	antiphospholipid syndrome	A&R	adenoidectomy with radium
APSAC	anistreplase (anisoylated plasminogen streptokinase activator complex)	A-R	advised and released
			apical-radial (pulses)
		ARA	Action Research Arm (test)
APSD	Alzheimer presenile dementia		adenosine regulating agent
APSP	assisted peak systolic pressure	ara-A	vidarabine (Vira-A)
		ara-AC	fazarabine
APSS	Associated Professional Sleep Societies	ara-C	cytarabine (Cytosar-U)
		ARAD	abnormal right axis deviation
aPTT	activated partial thromboplastin time	ARAS	ascending reticular activating system
APU	ambulatory procedure unit		atherosclerotic renal-artery stenosis
	antepartum unit	ARB	angiotensin II receptor blocker
APUD	amine precursor uptake and decarboxylation		antibiotic-resistant bacteria
APV	amprenavir (Agenerase)		any reliable brand
APVC	partial anomalous pulmonary venous connection	ARBOR	arthropod-borne virus
		ARBOW	artificial rupture of bag of water
APVR	aortic pulmonary valve replacement	ARC	abnormal retinal correspondence
APW	aortopulmonary window		AIDS-related complex
AQ	amodiaquine		Alcohol Rehabilitation Center
aq	water		anomalous retinal correspondence
AQ	accomplishment quotient		American Red Cross
aq dest	distilled water		autologous red cells
AQLQ-J	Asthma Quality of Life Questionnaire—Juniper	ARCBS	American Red Cross Blood Services
AQLQ-M	Asthma Quality of Life Questionnaire—Marks	ARD	acute respiratory disease
AQOL	acne quality of life		adult respiratory distress
A quad	atrial quadrageminy		antibiotic removal device
AR	Achilles reflex		antibiotic retrieval device
	acoustic reflex		aphakic retinal detachment
	active resistance	ARDMS	American Registry of Diagnostic Medical Sonographers
	airway resistance		
	alcohol related		
	allergic rhinitis		
	androgen receptor		
	ankle reflex		

ARDS	adult respiratory distress syndrome		alcohol rehabilitation program
ARE	active-resistive exercises	ARPE	amylase-rich pleural effusion
ARF	acute renal failure		
	acute respiratory failure	ARPF	anterior release posterior fusion
	acute rheumatic fever		
	amylase-rich food (flour)	ARPKS	autosomal recessive poly-cystic kidney disease
ARG	alkaline reflux gastritis	ARPT	acid reflux provocation test
	arginine		
ARGNB	antibiotic-resistant gram-negative bacilli	ARR	absolute risk reduction
			anterior rectal resection
ARH	autosomal recessive hypercholesterolemia		arrive
		ARROM	active resistive range of motion
ARHL	age-related hearing loss		
ARHNC	advanced resected head and neck cancer	ARRT	American Registry of Radiologic Technologists
ARI	acute renal insufficiency		
	acute respiratory infection	ARS	antirabies serum
	aldose reductase inhibitor	ART	Accredited Record Technician (for newer title, see RHIT)
	arousal index		
ARIF	arthroscopic reduction and internal fixation		Achilles (tendon) reflex test
ARIMA	autoregressive integrated moving average (model)		acoustic reflex threshold(s)
			antiretroviral therapy
ARL	acquired immunodeficiency syndrome(AIDS)-related lymphoma		arterial
			assessment, review, and treatment
	average remaining lifetime		assisted reproductive technology
ARLD	alcohol-related liver disease		automated reagin test (for syphilis)
ARM	anxiety reaction, mild		
	artificial rupture of membranes	ARTIC	articulation
ARMD	age-related macular degeneration	Art T	art therapy
		ARU	acute receiving unit
ARMS	alveolar rhabdomyosarcoma		alcohol rehabilitation unit
		ARV	AIDS-related virus
	amplification refractory mutation system		antiretroviral
ARN	acute retinal necrosis	ARVC	arrhythmogenic right ventricular cardiomyopathy
ARND	alcohol-related neurodevelopmental disorder		
		ARVD	arrhythmogenic right ventricular dysplasia
ARNP	Advanced Registered Nurse Practitioner		atherosclerotic renovascular disease
AROM	active range of motion	ARVMB	anomalous right ventricular muscle bundles
	artifical rupture of membranes		
ARP	absolute refractory period	ARVs	antiretroviral drugs
		ARW	Accredited Rehabilitation Worker
	acute radiation proctitis		

ARWY	airway	5-ASA	mesalamine (5-aminosalicylic acid; Asacol; Rowasa) (this is a dangerous abbreviation as it is mistaken for five aspirin tablets)
AS	activated sleep		
	alpha-synuclein		
	anabolic steroid		
	anal sphincter		
	androgen suppression		
	Angelman syndromes		
	ankylosing spondylitis	ASAA	acquired severe aplastic anemia
	anterior synechia		
	anxiety sensitivity	ASACL	American Society of Anesthesiologists Classification (see ASA I)
	aortic stenosis		
	Asperger syndrome		
	atherosclerosis		
	atropine sulfate AutoSuture®	ASAD	arthroscopic subacromial decompression
	doctor called through answering service	AS/AI	aortic stenosis/aortic insufficiency
	left ear	A's & B's	apnea and bradycardia
ASA	American Society of Anesthesiologists	ASAP	Alcohol and Substance Abuse Program
	American Statistical Association		as soon as possible
	argininosuccinate	ASAT	aspartate aminotransferase (also AST; SGOT)
	aspirin (acetylsalicylic acid)	ASB	anesthesia standby
	as soon as		asymptomatic bacteriuria
	atrial septal aneurysm	ASBO	adhesive small-bowel obstruction
ASA I	**American Society of anesthesiologists' classification**	ASBS	American Society of Bariatric Surgery
	Healthy patient with localized pathological process	ASBs	artificially sweetened beverages
		ASC	altered state of consciousness
ASA II	A patient with mild to moderate systemic disease		ambulatory surgery center
			anterior subcapsular cataract
ASA III	A patient with severe systemic disease limiting activity but not incapacitating		antimony sulfur colloid
			apocrine skin carcinoma
			ascorbic acid (vitamin C)
		ASCAD	atherosclerotic coronary artery disease
ASA IV	A patient with incapacitating systemic disease	ASCCC	advanced squamous cell cervical carcinoma
ASA V	Moribund patient not expected to live. (These are American Society of Anesthesiologists' patient classifications. Emergency operations are designated by "E" after the classification.)	ASCCHN	advanced squamous cell carcinoma of the head and neck
		ASCI	acute spinal cord injury
		ASCO	American Society of Clinical Oncology
		ASCR	autologous stem cell rescue
		ASCS	autologous stem cell support

ASCT	allogeneic stem cell transplantation		B-Incomplete—Preserved sensation
	autologous stem cell transplantation		C-Incomplete—Preserved motor (nonfunctional)
ASCUS	atypical squamous cell of undetermined significance		D-Incomplete—Preserved motor (functional)
			E-Complete Recovery
ASCVD	arteriosclerotic cardiovascular disease	ASIH	absent, sick in hospital
		ASIMC	absent, sick in medical center
ASCVR	arteriosclerotic cardiovas-cular renal disease	ASIS	anterior superior iliac spine
ASD	air-space disease	ASK	antistreptokinase
	aldosterone secretion defect	ASKase	antistreptokinase
	androstenedione	ASL	American Sign Language
	annual summary dose (ionizing radiation)		antistreptolysin (titer)
	atrial septal defect	ASLO	antistreptolysin-O
	autism spectrum disorder(s)	ASLV	avian sarcoma and leukosis virus (Rous virus)
ASD I	atrial septal defect, primum		
ASD II	atrial septal defect, secundum	AsM	myopic astigmatism
		ASMA	antismooth-muscle antibody
ASDA	American Sleep Disorders Association (criteria)	ASMI	anteroseptal myocardial infarction
ASDH	acute subdural hematoma		
ASE	abstinence symptom evaluation	ASO	accessory sinus ostia
	acute stress erosion		AIDS (acquired immunodeficiency syndrome) service organization(s)
ASEX	Arizona Sexual Experiences (sexual dysfunction scale)		aldicarb sulfoxide
ASF	anterior spinal fusion		allele-specific oligodeoxy-nucleotide (probes)
	asymmetric screen film (radiology)		Amplatzer Septal Occluder
ASFR	age-specific fertility rate		antisense oligonucleotides
ASG	atrial septal graft		antistreptolysin-O titer
ASH	asymmetric septal hypertrophy		arterial switch operation
			arteriosclerosis obliterans
AsH	hypermetropic astigmatism		automatic stop order
ASHD	arteriosclerotic heart disease	As₂O₃	arsenic trioxide (Trisenox)
		ASOT	antistreptolysin-O titer
ASI	active specific immunotherapy	ASOTP	Affiliate Sex Offender Treatment Provider
	Anxiety Status Inventory	ASP	acute suppurative parotitis
aSi	amorphous silicon		acute symmetric polyarthritis
ASIA	**American Spinal Injury Association (Score)**		antisocial personality
	A-Complete—No preservation of any motor and/or sensory function below the zone of injury		application service provider
			asparaginase
			aspartic acid

ASPDV	anterior superior pancreaticoduodenal vein
ASPVD	arteriosclerotic peripheral vascular disease
ASR	aldosterone secretion rate
	automatic speech recognition
ASRA	Alcohol Severity Rating Scale
ASS	anterior superior supine
	aspirin (some European countries)
	assessment
ASST	autologous serum skin test
asst	assistant
AST	allergy skin test
	Aphasia Screening Test
	aspartate aminotransferase (SGOT)
	astemizole (Hismanal)
	astigmatism
AstdVe	assisted ventilation
ASTH	asthenopia
ASTI	acute soft tissue injury
AS TOL	as tolerated
ASTIG	astigmatism
ASTRO	astrocytoma
ASTM	American Society for Testing and Materials
ASTZ	antistreptozyme test
ASU	acute stroke unit
	ambulatory surgical unit
ASV	antisnake venom
ASVD	arteriosclerotic vessel disease
ASYM	asymmetric(al)
ASX	asymptomatic
AT	abdominothoracic
	activity therapy (therapist)
	Addiction Therapist
	anaerobic threshold
	antithrombin
	applanation tonometry
	ataxia-telangiectasia
	atraumatic
	atrial tachycardia
AT1	angiotensin II type 1
AT 10	dihydrotachysterol (Hytakerol; DHT®)
ATA	atmosphere absolute
	authority to administer

ATB	antibiotic
	aquatic therapy bar
	atypical tuberculosis
ATBF	African tick-bite fever
ATC	acute toxic class
	aerosol treatment chamber
	alcoholism therapy classes
	all-terrain cycle
	antituberculous chemoprophylaxis
	around-the-clock
	Arthritis Treatment Center
	Athletic Trainer, Certified
ATCC	American Type Culture Collection
ATD	antithyroid drug(s)
	anticipated time of discharge
	aqueous tear deficiency
	asphyxiating thoracic dystrophy
	autoimmune thyroid disease
ATE	adipose tissue extraction
AT-EI	assistive technology and environmental interventions
ATEM	analytical transmission electron microscopy
ATF	Alcohol, Tobacco, and Firearms (Bureau)
At Fib	atrial fibrillation
ATFL	anterior talofibular ligament
AT III FUN	antithrombin III functional
ATG	antithymocyte globulin
ATHR	angina threshold heart rate
ATI	Abdominal Trauma Index
	acute traumatic ischemia
ATL	Achilles tendon lengthening
	adult T-cell leukemia
	anterior temporal lobectomy
	anterior tricuspid leaflet
	antitension line
	atypical lymphocytes
ATLL	adult T-cell leukemia lymphoma
ATLP	anterior thoracolumbar locking (implant) plate
ATLS	acute tumor lysis syndrome

	advanced trauma life support
ATM	acute transverse myelitis
	ataxia telangiectasia mutated (gene)
	atmosphere
At ma	atrial milliamp
ATN	acute tubular necrosis
ATNC	atraumatic normocephalic
aTNM	autopsy staging of cancer
ATNR	asymmetrical tonic neck reflex
ATO	arsenic trioxide (Trisenox)
ATOD-C	Alcohol, Tobacco and Other Drugs, Certified addiction treatment program
ATP	adenosine triphosphate
	anterior tonsillar pillar
	autoimmune thrombocytopenia purpura
ATP III	Adult Treatment Panel III
ATPase	adenosine triphosphatase
ATPS	ambient temperature & pressure, saturated with water vapor
ATR	Achilles tendon reflex
	atracurium (Tracrium)
	atrial
	atropine
ATRA	all-*trans* retinoic acid (tretinoin-Vesanoid®)
atr fib	atrial fibrillation
ATRO	atropine
ATRX	acute transfusion reaction
ATU	alcohol treatment unit
ATV	all-terrain vehicle
ATS	American Thoracic Society (guidelines)
	antimony trisulfide
	antitetanus serum (tetanus antitoxin)
	anxiety tension state
ATSO	admit to (the) service of
ATSO4	atropine sulfate
ATSP	asked to see patient
ATT	alternating triple therapy
	antitetanus toxoid
	arginine tolerance test
ATTN	attention
ATTR	amyloid transtyretin

at. wt	atomic weight
ATX	atelectasis
ATZ	anal transitional zone
AU	allergenic (allergy) units
	arbitrary units
	both ears (this is a dangerous abbreviation, as it may be seen as OU [both eyes])
Au	gold
A/U	at umbilicus
198Au	radioactive gold
AUA score	American Urological Association—pertains to benign prostatic hypertrophy symptoms
AUB	abnormal uterine bleeding
AuBMT	autologous bone marrow transplant
AUC	area under the curve
AUC$_t$	area under the curve to last time point
AUD	amplifiable units of DNA (deoxyribonucleic acid)
	arthritis of unknown diagnosis
	auditory
AUD COMP	auditory comprehension
AUDIT	Alcohol Use Disorders Identification Test
AUG	acute ulcerative gingivitis
AUGIB	acute upper gastrointestinal bleeding
AUIC	area under the inhibitory curve
AUL	acute undifferentiated leukemia
AUR	acute urinary retention
AUS	acute urethral syndrome
	artificial urinary sphincter
	auscultation
AutD	autistic disorder
AUTO	autologous
AUTO SP	automatic speech
AV	anteverted
	anticipatory vomiting
	arteriovenous
	atrioventricular
	auditory visual
	auriculoventricular
A:V	arterial-venous (ratio in fundi)

AVA	anthrax vaccine, adsorbed	AVNB	atrioventricular nodal block
	aortic valve atresia		
	arteriovenous anastomosis	AVNR	atrioventricular nodal re-entry
AVB	atrioventricular block		
	Aventis Behring	AVNRT	atrioventricular node recovery time
AVC	acrylic veneer crown		
	aortic valve classification		atrioventricular nodal re-entry tachycardia
	atrioventricular conduction		
AVD	aortic valve disease	A-VO$_2$	arteriovenous oxygen difference
	apparent volume of distribution		
		AVOC	avocation
	arteriosclerotic vascular disease	AVP	arginine vasopressin
			Aventis Pasteur
	atrioventricular delay	AVPU	alert, (responds to) verbal (stimuli), (responds to) painful (stimuli), unresponsive (mnemonic used by EMTs to judge patients' level of consciousness)
	cerebrovascular accident (French, Spanish)		
AVDP	asparaginase, vincristine, daunorubicin, and prednisone		
	avoirdupois		
AVDO$_2$	arteriovenous oxygen difference	AVR	aortic valve replacement
			augmented unipolar right (right arm)
AVE	aortic valve echocardiogram		
		AVRP	atrioventricular refractory period
	atrioventricular extrasystole		
AVED	ataxia with isolated vitamin E deficiency	AVRT	atrioventricular reciprocating tachycardia
AVF	arteriovenous fistula		
	augmented unipolar foot (left leg)	AVS	aortic valve sclerosis
			atriovenous shunt
avg	average	AVSD	atrioventricular septal defect
AVGS	autologous vein graft stent		
		AVSS	afebrile, vital signs stable
AVGs	ambulatory visit groups		
AVH	acute viral hepatitis	AVT	atrioventricular tachycardia
AVHB	atrioventricular heart block		
			atypical ventricular tachycardia
AVJA	atrioventricular junction ablation		
		AvWS	acquired von Willebrand syndrome
AVJR	atrioventricular junctional rhythm		
		AW	abdominal wall
AVL	American visceral leishmaniasis		abnormal wave
			airway
	augmented unipolar left (left arm)	A/W	able to work
		A&W	alive and well
AVLT	auditory verbal learning test	AWA	alcohol withdrawal assessment
AVM	arteriovenous malformation		as well as
		A waves	atrial contraction wave
AVN	arteriovenous nicking	AWB	autologous whole blood
	atrioventricular node	AWD	alcohol withdrawal delirium
	avascular necrosis		

AWDW	assault with a deadly weapon
AWE	acetowhite epithelium
AWI	anterior wall infarct
AWMI	anterior wall myocardial infarction
AWO	airway obstruction
AWOL	absent without leave
AWP	airway pressure
	average wholesale price
AWRU	active wrist rotation unit
AWS	alcohol withdrawal seizures (syndrome)
AWSA	Alcohol Withdrawal Severity Assessment (scale)
AWU	alcohol withdrawal unit
ax	axillary
AXB	axillary block
AXC	aortic cross clamp
ax-fem.fem.	axilla-femoral-femoral (graft)
AXND	axillary node dissection
AXR	abdomen x-ray
AxSYM®	immunodiagnostic testing equipment
AXT	alternating exotropia
AY	acrocyanotic (infant color)
AZA	azathioprine (Imuran)
AZA-CR	azacitidine (Vidaza)
5-AZC	azacitidine (Vidaza)
AzdU	azidouridine
AZE	azelastine hydrochloride (Astelin)
AZM	acquisition zoom magnification
	azithromycin (Zithromaz; Z-Pak)
AZQ	diaziquone
AZT	zidovudine (azidothymidine; Retrovir)
A-Z test	Aschheim-Zondek test (diagnostic test for pregnancy)

B

B	bacillus
	bands
	bilateral
	black
	bloody
	bolus
	both
	botulism (Vaccine B is botulism toxoid)
	brother
	buccal
	See "Plan B"
Ⓑ	both
B+	blood type B positive (B positive is preferred)
B−	blood type B negative (B negative is preferred)
B_1	thiamine HCl
B I	Billroth I (gastric surgery)
B II	Billroth II (gastric surgery)
B_2	riboflavin
B_3	nicotinic acid
b/4	before
B_5	pantothenic acid
B_6	pyridoxine HCl
B_7	biotin
B_8	adenosine phosphate
B_9	benign
B_{12}	cyanocobalamin
B19	parvovirus B19
BA	backache
	Baker Act (Florida mental health act enabling involuntary commitment)
	Baptist
	benzyl alcohol
	bile acid
	biliary atresia
	bioavailability
	blood agar
	blood alcohol
	bone age
	Bourns assist
	branchial artery
	broken appointment
	bronchial asthma

	buccoaxial	BAEDP	balloon aortic end diastolic pressure
	butyric acid		
Ba	barium	BAEP	brain stem auditory evoked potential
B > A	bone greater than air		
B < A	bone less than air	BAERs	brain stem auditory evoked responses
B & A	brisk and active		
BAA	beta-adrenergic agonist	BaEV	baboon endogenous virus
BAAM	Beck airway airflow monitor		
		BAG	buccoaxiogingival
Bab	Babinski	BAHA	bone-anchored hearing aid
BAC	Bacterial Artficial Chromosome	BAI	blunt abdominal injury
			breath-actuated inhalers
	benzalkonium chloride		Brief Assessment Interview
	blood-alcohol concentration	BAIQ	below average intelligence quotient
	bronchioloalveolar carcinoma	BAK cage	an interbody fusion system used to stabilize the spine
	buccoaxiocervical		
BACCA	basal cell cancer	BAL	balance
BACE	beta-site APP (amyloid precursor protein)-cleaving enzyme		blood-alcohol level
			British antilewisite (dimercaprol)
			bronchoalveolar lavage
BACI	bovine anti-cryptosporidium immunoglobulin	BALB	binaural alternate loudness balance
BACM	blocking agent corticosteroid myopathy	BALF	bronchoalveolar lavage fluid
BACON	bleomycin, doxorubicin, lomustine, vincristine, and mechlorethamine	B-ALL	B cell acute lymphoblastic leukemia
		BALT	bronchus-associated lymphoid tissue
BACOP	bleomycin, doxorubicin (Adriamycin), cyclophosphamide, vincristine, and prednisone	BAM	bony acetabular morphology
			Brain Acoustic Monitor
		BaM	barium meal
BACPAC	Bulk Activities Post Approval Change	BAN	British Approved Name
		BAND	band neutrophil (stab)
BACs	bacterial artificial chromosomes	BANS	back, arm, neck and scalp
		BAO	basal acid output
BACT	bacteria	BAoV	bicuspid aortic valve
	base-activated clotting time	BAP	blood agar plate
		BAPS	balance activation proprioceptive system
BAD	Benadryl, Ativan, and Decadron		
			biomechanical ankle platform system
	bipolar affective disorder		
	blunt aortic disruption	BAPT	Baptist
BADL	basic activities of daily living	BAR	biofragmentable anastomotic ring
BADLS	Bristol Activities of Daily Living Scale	Barb	barbiturate
		BARN	bilateral acute retinal necrosis
BaE	barium enema		
BAE	bronchial artery embolization	BAR Troche	Benadryl, Ativan, and Reglan troche

BAS	balloon atrial septostomy	B&B	bismuth and bourbon
	Barnes Akathisia Scale		bowel and bladder
	behavioral activation system	B/B	backward bending
		BBA	born before arrival
	bile acid sequestrants	BBAS	blade and balloon atrial septostomy
	boric acid solution		
	bronchial asthma (in) status	BBB	baseball bat beating
			blood-brain barrier
BaS	barium swallow		bundle branch block
BASA	baby aspirin (81 mg chewable tablets of aspirin)	BBBB	bilateral bundle branch block
		BBC	bilateral breast cancer
BASIS	Basic Achievement Skills Individual Screener		Brown-Buerger cystoscope
		BBD	baby born dead
BASK	basket cells		before bronchodilator
BASMI	Bath Ankylosing Spondylitis Metrology Index		benign breast disease
		BBE	biofield breast examination
baso.	basophil		
BASO STIP	basophilic stippling	BBFA	both bones forearm
		BBFF	both bone foreman fracture
BAT	Behavioral Avoidance Test		
	blunt abdominal trauma	BBFP	blood and body fluid precautions
	borreliacidal-antibody test		
	brightness acuity tester	BBI	Bowman Birk inhibitor
BATF	Bureau of Alcohol, Tobacco and Firearms	BBIC	Bowman Birk inhibitor concentrate
		BBL	bottle blood loss
BATO	boronic acid adduct of technetium oxime	BBM	banked breast milk
		BBOW	bulging bag of water
batt	battery	BBP	blood-borne pathogen
BAVP	balloon aortic valvuloplasty		butyl benzyl phthalate
		BBR	bibasilar rales
BAU	bioequivalent allergy units	BBS	Berg Balance Scale
			bilateral breath sounds
BAV	bicuspid aortic valve	BBSE	bilateral breath sounds equal
BAW	bronchoalveolar washing		
BB	baby boy	BBSI	Brigance Basic Skills Inventory
	backboard		
	back to back	BBT	basal body temperature
	bad breath		Buteyko breathing technique
	bed bath		
	bed board	BB to MM	belly button to medial malleolus
	beta-blocker		
	blanket bath	B Bx	breast biopsy
	blood bank	BC	back care
	blow bottle		basket catheter
	blue bloaters		battered child
	body belts		bed and chair
	both bones		beta carotene
	breakthrough bleeding		bicycle
	breast biopsy		birth control
	brush biopsy		bladder cancer
	buffer base		

	blood culture	B cell	B lymphocyte
	Blue Cross	BCETS	Board Certified Expert in Traumatic Stress
	bone conduction		
	Bourn control	BCF	basic conditioning factor
	breast cancer		Baylor core formula
	buccocervical	BCG	bacille Calmette-Guérin vaccine
	buffalo cap (cap for intravenous line)		bicolor guaiac
B/C	because	BCH	benign coital headache
	blood urea nitrogen/creatinine ratio	BCHA	bone-conduction hearing aid
B&C	bed and chair	BChE	butyrylcholinesterase
	biopsy and curettage	BCI	blunt carotid injury
	board and care	BCIR	Barnett continent intestinal reservoir
	breathed and cried		
BCA	balloon catheter angioplasty	BCL	basic cycle length
			bio-chemoluminescence
	basal cell atypia	B/C/L	BUN,(blood urea nitrogen),creatinine, lytes (electrolytes)
	bichloracetic acid		
	bicinchoninic acid		
	brachiocephalic artery	B-CLL	B-cell chronic lymphocytic leukemia
BCAA	branched-chain amino acids		
		BCLP	bilateral cleft lip and palate
BC < AC	bone conduction less than air conduction		
		BCLS	basic cardiac life support
BC > AC	bone conduction greater than air conduction	BCM	below costal margin
			birth control medication
B. cat	*Branhamella catarrhalis*		birth control method
B-CAVe	bleomycin, lomustine (CCNU), doxorubicin (Adriamycin), and vinblastine (Velban)		body cell mass
		BCMA	bar-code medication administration
		BCME	bis (chloromethyl) ether
BCB	Brilliant cresyl blue (stain)	BCNP	Board Certified Nuclear Pharmacist
BCBR	bilateral carotid body resection		
		BCNU	bacteria-controlled nursing unit
BC/BS	Blue Cross/Blue Shield		
BCC	basal cell carcinoma		carmustine (BiCNU; Gliadel)
	birth control clinic		
BCCa	basal cell carcinoma	BCOC	bowel care of choice
BCD	basal cell dysplasia		bowel cathartic of choice
	bleomycin, cyclophosphamide, and dactinomycin	BCP	biochemical profile
			birth control pills
	borderline of cardiac dullness		blood cell profile
			carmustine, cyclophos-phamide, and prednisone
BCDCSW	Board Certified Diplomate in Clinical Social Work		
		BCPAP	Broun continuous positive airway pressure
BCDH	bilateral congenital dislocated hip		
		BCPNN	Bayesian Confidence Propagation Neural Network
BCE	basal cell epithelioma		
	beneficial clinical event	BCQ	breast central quadrantectomy
BCEDP	breast cancer early detection program		

BCR	bicaudate ratio	BDAS	balloon dilation atrial septostomy
	breakpoint cluster region (gene)	BDBS	Bonnet-Dechaume-Blanc syndrome
	bulbocavernosus reflex	BDC	burn-dressing change
BCRE	black cohosh root extract	BDCM	bromodichloromethane
BCRS	Brief Cognitive Rate Scale	BDD	body dysmorphic disorder
BCRT	breast-conservation followed by radiation therapy		bronchodilator drugs
		BDE	bile duct exploration
BCS	battered child syndrome	BDF	bilateral distal femoral
	breast-conserving surgery		black divorced female
	Budd-Chiari syndrome	BDI	Beck Depression Inventory
BCSF	bone cell stimulating factor		bile duct incision
			bile duct injury
BCSS	bone cell stimulating substance	BDI SF	Beck Depression Inventory-Short Form
BCT	Bag Carrying Test	BDL	below detectable limits
	breast-conserving therapy		bile duct ligation
	broad complex tachycardias	B-DLCL	diffuse large B-cell lymphoma
BCTP	bi-component triton tri-n-butyl phosphate	BDM	black divorced male
		BDNF	brain-derived neurotrophic factor
BCU	burn care unit		
BCUG	bilateral cystourethrogram	BDOD	brain-dead organ donor
BCVA	best corrected visual acuity	B-DOPA	bleomycin, dacarbazine, vincristine (Oncovin), prednisone, and doxorubicin (Adriamycin)
BCVI	blunt cerebrovascular injury		
BD	band neutrophil		
	base deficit	BDP	beclomethasone dipropionate (Beconase AQ; QVAR)
	base down		
	behavior disorder		best demonstrated practice
	Behçet disease	BDR	background diabetic retinopathy
	bile duct		
	bipolar disorder(s)		black dot ringworm
	birth date		bronchodilator response
	birth defect		bulk dose regimen
	blood donor	BDS	bile duct stone(s)
	brain dead	BDV	Borna disease virus
	bronchial drainage	BE	bacterial endocarditis
	bronchodilator		barium enema
	buccodistal		Barrett esophagus
	1,4-butanediol		base excess
	twice daily (in the United Kingdom, Australia, and elsewhere)		below elbow
			bioequivalence
			bread equivalent
bd	twice daily (in the United Kingdom, Australia, and elsewhere)		breast examination
		B ↑ E	both upper extremities
		B ↓ E	both lower extremities
B-D	Becton Dickinson and Company	B & E	brisk and equal
BDAE	Boston Diagnostic Aphasia Examination	BEA	below-elbow amputation

BEAC carmustine (BiCNU), etoposide, cytarabine (ara-C), and cyclophosphamide

BEACOPP bleomycin, etoposide, doxorubicin (Adriamycin), cyclophosphamide, vincristine (Oncovin), procarbazine, and prednisone

BEAM brain electrical activity mapping
carmustine BCNU), etoposide, cytarabine (ara-C), and methotrexate

BEAR Bourn electronic adult respirator

BEC bacterial endocarditis

BECs bronchial epithelial cells

BED binge-eating disorder
biochemical evidence of disease
biological effective dose
biological equivalent dose

BEE basal energy expenditure

BEF bronchoesophageal fistula

BEGA best estimate of gestational age

BEH behavior
benign essential hypertension

Beh Sp behavior specialist

BEI bioelectric impedance
butanol-extractable iodine

BEL blood ethanol level

BEP bleomycin, etoposide, and cisplatin (Platinol)
brain stem evoked potentials

BE-PEG balanced electrolyte with polyethylene glycol

BET bacterial endotoxins test

BEV billion electron volts
bleeding esophageal varices

BF biofeedback
black female
bone fragment
boyfriend
breakfast fed
breast-feed

B/F bound-to-free ratio

B & F back and forth

%BF percentage of body fat

BFA baby for adoption
basilic forearm
bifemoral arteriogram

BFC benign febrile convulsion

BFEC benign focal epilepsy of childhood

bFGF basic fibroblast growth factor

BFI Brief Fatigue Inventory

BFL breast firm and lactating

B-FLY butterfly

BFM Berlin-Frankfurt-Munster (cancer study group)
black married female
body fat mass
bright field microscope

BFNC benign familial neonatal convulsions

BFP biologic false positive
blue fluorescent protein

BFR blood filtration rate
blood flow rate

B. frag *Bacillus fragilis*

BFT bentonite flocculation test
biofeedback training

BFU_e erythroid burst-forming unit

BG baby girl
basal ganglia
blood glucose
bone graft

B-G Bender-Gestalt (test)

BGA Bundesgesundheitsamt (German drug regulatory agency)

B-GA-LACTO beta galactosidase

BGC basal-ganglion calcification

BGCT benign glandular cell tumor

BGDC Bartholin gland duct cyst

BGDR background diabetic retinopathy

BGL blood glucose level

BGM blood glucose monitoring

bGS biopsy Gleason score

BGT Bender-Gestalt test
blood glucose testing

BGTT	borderline glucose tolerance test	BICU	burn intensive care unit
		BID	brought in dead
BH	bowel habits	*BID*	twice daily (b.i.d. preferred)
	breath holding		
BHA	butylated hydroxyanisole	*b.i.d.*	twice daily
BHC	benzene hexachloride	BIDA	amonafide
	Braxton Hicks contractions	BIDS	bedtime insulin, daytime sulfonylurea
bHCG	beta human chorionic gonadotropin	BIF	bifocal
		BIG	botulism immune globulin
BHD	carmustine, hydroxyurea, and dacarbazine		Breast International Group
		BIGEM	bigeminal
BHDS	Birt-Hogg-Dube syndrome	BIH	benign intracranial hypertension
B-HEXOS-A-LK	beta hexosaminidase A leukocytes		bilateral inguinal hernia
BHI	biosynthetic human insulin	BIL	bilateral
			brother-in-law
	brain-heart infusion	BILAT SLC	bilateral short leg case
BHMCO	behavioral health managed care organization	BILAT SXO	bilateral salpingo-oophorectomy
BHN	bridging hepatic necrosis	Bili	bilirubin
BHR	bronchial hyperrespon-siveness (hyperactivity)	BILI-C	conjugated bilirubin
		BIL MRY	bilateral myringotomy
BHP	boarding home placement	BIMA	bilateral internal mammary arteries
	British Herbal Pharmacopeia		
		BIN	twice a night (this is a dangerous abbreviation)
BHS	Beck Hopelessness Scale		
	beta-hemolytic streptococci	BIND	Biological Investigational New Drug
	breath-holding spell	BIO	binocular indirect ophthalmoscopy
BHT	borderline hypertensive		
	breath hydrogen test	BIOF	biofeedback
	butylated hydroxytoluene	BIP	bipolar affective disorder
BI	Barthel Index		bleomycin, ifosfamide, and cisplatin (Platinol)
	base in		
	Boehringer Ingelheim Pharmaceuticals, Inc.		brain injury program
		BIPA	Benefits Improvement and Protection Act
	bowel impaction		
	brain injury	BiPAP	bilevel (biphasic) positive airway pressure
Bi	bismuth		
BIA	bioelectrical impedance analysis	BiPD	biparietal diameter
		BIPP	bismuth iodoform paraffin paste
	biospecific interaction analysis	BIR	back internal rotation
BIB	brought in by	BIRB	Biomedical Institutional Review Board
BIBA	brought in by ambulance		
BIC	brain injury center	BIS	behavioral inhibition system
BICAP	bipolar electrocoagulation therapy		
			Bispectral Index
bicarb	bicarbonate	Bi-SLT	bilateral, sequential single lung transplantation
BiCNU®	carmustine		
BICROS	bilateral contralateral routing of signals	bisp	bispinous diameter

BIT	behavioral inattention test	BL = BS	bilateral equal breath sounds
BIVAD	bilateral ventricular (biventricular) assist device	bl cult	blood culture
BIW	twice a week (this is a dangerous abbreviation)	B-L-D	breakfast, lunch, and dinner
		bldg	bleeding
BIZ-PLT	bizarre platelets	bld tm	bleeding time
BJ	Bence Jones (protein)	BLE	both lower extremities
	biceps jerk	BLEED	ongoing *bleeding*, *low* blood pressure, *elevated* prothrombin time, *erratic* mental status, and unstable comorbid *disease* (risk factors for continued gastrointestinal bleeding)
	body jacket		
	bone and joint		
BJE	bone and joint examination		
	bones, joints, and extremities		
BJI	bone and joint infection		
BJLO	Benton Judgment Line Orientation (test)		
BJM	bones, joints, and muscles	BLEO	bleomycin sulfate
		BLESS	bath, laxative, enema, shampoo, and shower
BJOA	basal joint osteoarthritis	BLG	bovine beta-lactoglobulin
BJP	Bence Jones protein	BLIC	beta-lactamase inhibitor combination
BK	below knee (amputation)		
	bradykinin	BLIP	beta-lactamase inhibiting protein
	bullous keratopathy		
BKA	below-knee-amputation	BLL	bilateral lower lobe
BKC	blepharokerato-conjunctivitis		blood lead level
			brows, lids, and lashes
bkft	breakfast	BLLS	bilateral leg strength
Bkg	background	BLM	bleomycin sulfate
BKTT	below-knee to toe (cast)	BLN	bronchial lymph nodes
BKWC	below-knee walking cast	BLOBS	bladder obstruction
BKWP	below-knee walking plaster (cast)	BLOC	brief loss of consciousness
BL	baseline (fetal heart rate)	BLPB	beta-lactamase-producing bacteria
	bioluminescence		
	bland	BLPO	beta-lactamase-producing organism
	blast cells		
	blood level	BLQ	both lower quadrants
	blood loss	BLR	blood flow rate
	blue	BLS	basic life support
	bronchial lavage		Bureau of Labor Statistics
	Burkitt lymphoma	BLT	bilateral lung transplantation
B/L	brother-in-law		
BLA	Biological License Application		blood-clot lysis time
			brow left transverse
BLB	Boothby-Lovelace-Bulbulian (oxygen mask)	B.L. unit	Bessey-Lowry units
		BLV	bovine leukemia virus
		BM	bacterial meningitis
	bronchoscopic lung biopsy		black male
			bone marrow
BLBK	blood bank		bone metastases
BLBS	bilateral breath sounds		bowel movement

	breast milk	BMPs	bone-morphogenic proteins
	bullous myringitis	BMR	basal metabolic rate
BMA	biomedical application		best motor response
	bismuth subsalicylate, metronidazole, and amoxicillin	BMRM	bilateral modified radical mastectomy
		BMS	bare-metal stents
	bone marrow aspirate		Bristol-Myers Squibb Company
	British Medical Association		burning mouth syndrome
BMAT	basic motor ability test(s)	BMT	bilateral myringotomy and tubes
BMB	bone marrow biopsy		
BMBF	German Ministry of Education and Research		bismuth subsalicylate, metronidazole, and tetracycline
BMC	bone marrow cells		bone marrow transplant
	bone marrow culture	BMTH	bismuth, metronidazole, tetracycline, and a histamine H_2-receptor antagonist
	bone mineral content		
BMD	Becker muscular dystrophy		
	benchmark dose	BMTN	bone marrow transplant neutropenia
	bone marrow depression		
	bone mineral density	BMTT	bilateral myringotomy with tympanic tubes
BME	basal medium Eagle (diploid cell culture)		
		BMTU	bone marrow transplant unit
	biomedical engineering		
	brief maximal effort	BMU	basic multicellular unit
BMET	basic metabolic panel (see page 392)	BMY	Bristol-Myers Squibb
		BN	battalions
BMF	between meal feedings		bladder neck
	black married female		bulimia nervosa
BMFDS	Burke-Marsden-Fahn dystonia rating scale	BNBAS	Brazelton Neonatal Behavioral Assessment
BMG	benign monoclonal gammopathy	BNC	binasal cannula
			bladder neck contracture
BMI	body mass index	BNCT	boron neutron capture therapy
BMJ	bones, muscles, joints		
BMK	birthmark	BNE	but not exceeding
BMM	black married male	BNF	British National Formulary
	bone marrow micrometastases		
		BNI	blind nasal intubation
BMMC	bone marrow mononuclear T cells	BNL	below normal limits
			breast needle localization
BMMM	bone marrow micrometastases	Bn M	bone marrow
		BNO	bladder neck obstruction
B-MODE	brightness modulation		bowels not open
BMP	basic metabolic profile (panel) (see page 392)	BNP	brain natriuretic peptide
			B-type natriuretic peptide (nesiritide [Natrecor])
	behavior management plan		
		BNPA	binasal pharyngeal airway
	bone morphogenetic protein	BNR	bladder neck retraction
		BNS	benign nephrosclerosis
BMPC	bone marrow plasmacytosis	BNT	back to normal
			Boston Naming Test

BO	base out	BOT	base of tongue
	because of		borderline ovarian tumors
	behavior objective	BOU	burning on urination
	body odor	BOUGIE	bougienage
	bowel obstruction	BOVR	Bureau of Vocational
	bowel open		Rehabilitation
	bucco-occlusal	BOW	bag of water
B & O	belladonna & opium	BOW-I	bag of water–intact
	(suppositories)	BOW-R	bag of water–ruptured
BOA	behavioral observation	BP	bathroom privileges
	audiometry		bed pan
	born on arrival		bench press
	born out of asepsis		benzoyl peroxide
BOB	ball-on-back		bipolar
BOC	beats of clonus		birthplace
BOD	bilateral orbital		blood pressure
	decompression		bodily pain
	burden of disease		body powder
Bod Units	Bodansky units		British Pharmacopeia
BOE	bilateral otitis externa		bullous pemphigoid
BOH	Board of Health		bypass
	bundle of His	BP-200	Bourn Infant Pressure
BOLD	bleomycin, vincristine		Ventilator
	(Oncovin®), lomustine,	BPA	birch pollen allergy
	and dacarbazine	BPAD	bipolar affective disorder
	blood oxygenation level-	BPAR	biopsy-proven actue
	dependent		rejection
BOM	benign ovarian mass	BPb	whole blood lead
	bilateral otitis media		concentration
BOMA	bilateral otitis media, acute	BPCF	bronchopleural cutaneous
BOME	bilateral otitis media with		fistula
	effusion	BPI	bipolar disorder, Type I
BOMP	bleomycin, vincristine	BPII	bipolar type II disorder
	(Oncovin), mitomycin,	BPD	benzoporphyrin derivative
	and cisplatin (Platinol		biparietal diameter
	AQ)		borderline personality
BOO	bladder outlet obstruction		disorder
BOOP	bronchitis obliterans-		bronchopulmonary
	organized pneumonia		dysplasia
BOP	bleeding on probing	BPd	diastolic blood pressure
BOR	bowels open regularly	BPD/DS	biliopancreatic diversion
	bronchia-oto-renal		with a duodenal switch
	(syndrome)		(surgery for obesity)
BORN	State Board of	BPE	benign enlargement of the
	Registration in Nursing		prostate
BORospA	borreliosis (Lyme disease,	BPF	Brazilian purpuric fever
	Borrelia sp.) vaccine,		bronchopleural fistula
	outer surface protein A	BPH	benign prostatic
BOS	base of support		hypertrophy
	bronchiolitis obliterans	BPG	bypass graft
	syndrome		penicillin G benzathine
BOSS	Becker orthopedic spinal		(Bicillin L-A; Permapen)
	system		for IM use only

BPI	bactericidal/permeability increasing (protein)		Benzing retrograde
			birthing room
	Brief Pain Inventory		blink rate
BPIG	bacterial polysaccharide immune globulin		blink reflex
			bowel rest
BPL	benzylpenicilloylpolylysine		brachioradialis
BPLA	blood pressure, left arm		breast reconstruction
BPLND	bilateral pelvic lymph node dissection		breech
			bridge
BPM	beats per minute		bright red
	breaths per minute		brown
BPN	bacitracin, polymyxin B, and neomycin sulfate	Br	bromide
			bromine
BPO	benign prostatic obstruction	BRA	bananas, rice (rice cereal), and applesauce
	benzoyl peroxide		brain
	bilateral partial oophorectomy	BRCA1	breast cancer gene 1
		BRCA2	breast cancer gene 2
BPOP	bizarre parosteal osteochondromatous proliferation (Nora's Lesion)	BRADY	bradycardia
		BRANCH	branch chain amino acids
		BRAO	branch retinal artery occlusion
BPP	biophysical profile	BRAS	bilateral renal artery stenosis
BPPP	bilateral pedal pulses present		
		BRAT	bananas, rice (rice cereal), applesauce, and toast
BP,P,R,T,	blood pressure, pulse, respiration, and temperature		Baylor rapid autologous transfuser
			blunt thoracic abdominal trauma
BPPV	benign paroxysmal positional vertigo		
		BRATT	bananas, rice (rice cereal), applesauce, tea, and toast
BPR	beeper		
	blood per rectum		
	blood pressure recorder	BRB	blood-retinal barrier
			bright red blood
BPRS	Brief Psychiatric Rating Scale	BRBR	bright red blood per rectum
BPS	bilateral partial salpingectomy		
		BRBPR	bright red blood per rectum
	blood pump speed		
BPs	systolic blood pressure	BRC	bladder reconstruction
BPSD	behavioral and psychological symptoms of dementia	BRCM	below right costal margin
		BrdU	bromodeoxyuridine
		BRex	breathing exercise
	bronchopulmonary segmental drainage	Br Fdg	breast-feeding
BPT	BioPort Corporation	BRFS	biochemical relapse-free survival
BPV	benign paroxysmal vertigo		
	benign positional vertigo	BRFSS	Behavioral Risk Factor Surveillance System
	bovine papilloma virus		
Bq	becquerel	BRJ	brachial radialis jerk
BQL	below quantifiable levels	BRM	biological response modifiers
BQR	brequinar sodium		
BR	bathroom	BRN	brown
	bedrest	BRO	brother

BROM	back range of motion		burn scar contracture
BRONK	bronchoscopy	BSCC	bedside commode chair
BRP	bathroom privileges		Bjork-Shiley convexo-
BR RAO	branch retinal artery		concave (valves)
	occlusion	BSCVA	best spectacle-corrected
BR RVO	branch retinal vein		visual acuity
	occlusion	BSD	baby soft diet
BRS	baroreceptor reflex		bedside drainage
	sensitivity	BSE	bovine spongiform
BrS	breath sounds		encephalopathy
BRSV	bovine respiratory		breast self-examination
	syncytial virus	BSEC	bedside easy chair
BRU	basic remodeling unit	BSepF	black separated female
	(osteon)	BSepM	black separated male
	brucellosis (*Brucella*	BSER	brain stem evoked
	melitensis) vaccine		responses
BRVO	branch retinal vein	BSF	black single female
	occlusion		busulfan (Myleran)
BS	barium swallow	BSG	Bagolini striated glasses
	bedside		brain stem gliomas
	before sleep	BSGA	beta streptococcus group
	Behçet syndrome		A
	Bennett seal	BSI	bloodstream infection
	blind spot		body substance isolation
	blood sugar		brain stem injury
	Blue Shield		Brief Symptom Inventory
	bone scan	BSL	baseline
	bowel sounds		Biological Safety Level
	breath sounds		blood sugar level
B & S	Bartholin and Skene	BSL-1	Biosafety Level 1
	(glands)	BS L	breath sounds diminished,
	bending and stooping	base	left base
	Brown and Sharp (suture	BSM	black single male
	sizes)		blood safety module
BS×4	bowel sounds in all four	BSN	Bachelor of Science in
	quadrants		Nursing
BSA	body surface area		bowel sounds normal
	bowel sounds active	BSNA	bowel sounds normal and
	Brief Scale of Anxiety		active
BSAB	Balthazar Scales of	BSNMT	Bachelor of Science in
	Adaptive Behavior		Nuclear Medicine
BSAb	broad-spectrum antibiotics		Technology
BSAP	bone-specific alkaline	BSNT	breast soft and nontender
	phosphatase	BSNUTD	baby shots not up to date
BSB	bedside bag	BSO	bilateral salpingo-
	body surface burned		oophorectomy
BSC	basosquamous (cell)		l-buthionine sulfoximine
	carcinoma	bSOD	bovine superoxide
	bedside care		dismutase
	bedside commode	BSOM	bilateral serous otitis
	best supportive care		media
	biological safety cabinet	BSP	body substance
	Biomedical Science Corps		precautions

	bone sialoprotein		bladder tumor-associated
	Bromsulphalein®		analytes
BSPA	bowel sounds present and		botulinum toxic type A
	active		(Botox)
BSPM	body surface potential	BTA-A	botulinum toxin type A
	mapping		(Botox)
BSR	body stereotactic	BTB	back to bed
	radiosurgery		beat-to-beat (variability)
	bowels sounds regular		breakthrough bleeding
BSRI	Bem Sex Role Inventory	BTBV	beat-to-beat variability
BSRT (R)	Bachelor of Science in	BTC	bilateral tubal cautery
	Radiologic Technology		biliary tree cancer
	(Registered)		bladder tumor check
BSS	Baltimore Sepsis Scale		by the clock
	bedside scale	BTE	Baltimore Therapeutic
	bismuth subsalicylate		Equipment
	black silk sutures		behind-the-ear (hearing
BSS®	balanced salt solution		aid)
BSSG	sitogluside		bisected, totally
BSSO	bilateral sagittal split		embedded
	osteotomy	BTF	blenderized tube
BSSS	benign sporadic sleep		feeding
	spikes	BTFS	breast tumor frozen
BSST	breast self-stimulation test		section
BST	bedside testing	BTG	beta thromboglobulin
	bovine somatotropin	B-Thal	beta thalassemia
	brief stimulus therapy	BTHOOM	beats the hell out of me
BSU	Bartholin, Skene, urethra		(better stated as
	(glands)		"differed diagnosis")
	behavioral science unit	BTI	biliary tract infection
BSu	blood sugar		bitubal interruption
BSUTD	baby shots up to date	BTKA	bilateral total knee
	Base Service Unit		arthroplasty
BSW	Bachelor of Social Work	BTL	bilateral tubal ligation
	bedscale weight	BTM	bilateral tympanic
BT	bedtime		membranes
	behavioral therapy		bismuth subcitrate,
	bituberous		tetracycline, and
	bladder tumor		metronidazole
	Blalock-Taussig (shunt)	BTMEAL	between meals
	bleeding time	BTO	bilateral tubal occlusion
	blood transfusion	BTP	bismuth
	blood type		tribromophenate
	blunt trauma		breakthrough pain
	brain tumor	BTPABA	bentiromide
	breast tumor	BTPS	body temperature pressure
	bowel tones		saturated
Bt	*Bacillus thuringiensis*	BTR	bladder tumor recheck
B-T	Blalock-Taussig (shunt)	BTS	Blalock-Taussig shunt
B/T	between	BTSH	bovine thyrotropin
Bt#	bottle number	BTU	behavior therapy unit
BTA	below the ankle	BTW	back to work
	bladder tumor antigen		between

BTW M	between meals	BVO	branch vein occlusion
BTX	Botulinum toxin type A (Botox)	BVR	Bureau of Vocational Rehabilitation
BtxA	botulinum toxin type A (Botox)	BVRO	bilateral vertical ramus osteotomy
BU	base up (prism) below umbilicus Bodansky units burn unit busulfan (Myleran)	BVRT	Benton Visual Retention Test
		BVT	bilateral ventilation tubes
		BVZ	bevacizumab (Avastin)
BUA	broadband ultrasound attenuation	BW	bandwidth (radiology) birth weight bite-wing (radiograph) body water body weight
BUCAT	busulfan, carboplatin, and thiotepa		
BuCy	busulfan and cyclophosphamide	B & W	Black and White (milk of magnesia & aromatic cascara fluidextract)
BUD	budesonide (Rhinocort)		
BUdR	bromodeoxyuridine	BWA	bed-wetter admission
BUE	both upper extremities	BWC	bladder-wash cytology
BUFA	baby up for adoption	BWCS	bagged white cell study
BULB	bilateral upper lid blepharoplasty	BWF	Blackwater fever
		BWFI	bacteriostatic water for injection
BUN	blood urea nitrogen bunion	BWidF	black widowed female
BUO	bleeding of undetermined origin	BWidM	black widowed male
		BWS	battered woman syndrome Beckwith-Wiedemann syndrome
BUR	back-up rate (ventilator)		
Burd	Burdick suction		
BUS	Bartholin, urethral, and Skene glands bladder ultrasound bulbourethral sling	BWs	bite-wing (x-rays)
		BWSTT	body weight-supported treadmill training
BUSV	Bartholin urethral Skeins vagina	BWT	bowel wall thickness
BUT	biopsy urease test break up time	BWX	bite-wing x-ray
		Bx	behavior biopsy
BV	bacterial vaginitis bevacizumab (Avastin) biological value blood volume	B × B	back-to-back
		BX BS	Blue Cross and Blue Shield
		BXM	B-cell crossmatch
BVAD	biventricular assist device	ΦBZ	phenylbutazone
		BZD	benzodiazepine
BVD	bovine viral diarrhea	BZDZ	benzodiazepine
BVDU	bromovinlydeoxyuridine (brivudin)		
BVE	blood volume expander		
BVF	bulboventricular foramen		
BVH	biventricular hypertrophy		
BVL	bilateral vas ligation		
BVM	bag valve mask		
BVMG	Bender Visual-Motor Gestalt (test)		

C

C	ascorbic acid (Vitamin C)
	carbohydrate
	Catholic
	Caucasian
	Celsius
	centigrade
	*C*hlamydia
	clubbing
	conjunctiva
	constricted
	cyanosis
	cytosine
	hundred
c	with
C′	cervical spine
C+	with contrast
C−	without contrast
C 1	cyclopentolate 1% ophthalmic solution (Cyclogyl)
C_1–C_7	cervical vertebra 1 through 7
C_1–C_8	cervical nerves 1 through 8
C_1–C_9	precursor molecules of the complement system
C_1–C_{12}	cranial nerves 1 to 12
C3	complement C3
C4	complement C4
CI-CV	Drug Enforcement Agency scheduled substances class one through five
C_{II}	second cranial nerve
CA	cancelled appointment
	Candida albicans
	carcinoma
	cardiac arrest
	carotid artery
	celiac artery
	cellulose acetate (filter)
	Certified Acupuncturist
	chronologic age
	Cocaine Anonymous
	community-acquired
	compressed air
	continuous aerosol
	coronary angioplasty
	coronary artery
Ca	calcium

C/A	conscious, alert
Ca++	calcification
	calcium
CA 125	cancer antigen 125
C&A	Clinitest® and Acetest®
CAA	cerebral amyloid angiopathy
	coloanal anastamosis
	crystalline amino acids
CAAP-1	Certified Associate Addiction Professional Level 1
CAB	catheter-associated bacteriuria
	cellulose acetate butyrate
	combined androgen blockade
	complete atrioventricular block
	coronary artery bypass
CAB-BAGE	coronary artery bypass graft
CABG	coronary artery bypass graft
CaBI	calcium bone index
CaBP	calcium-binding protein
CABS	coronary artery bypass surgery
CAC	cardioacceleratory center
	Certified Alcohol Counselor
	Community Action Center
	computerized autocoding
	coronary artery calcification
CACI	computer-assisted continuous infusion
$CaCl_2$	calcium chloride
$CaCO_3$	calcium carbonate
CACP	cisplatin
CACS	cancer-related anorexia/cachexia
CAD	cadaver (kidney donor)
	calcium alginate dressing
	computer-aided diagnosis
	computer-aided dispatch
	coronary artery disease
CADAC	Certified Alcohol and Drug Abuse Counselor
CADASIL	cerebral autosomal dominant arteriopathy with subcortical infarcts and leukoencephalopathy

C

CADD®	Computerized Ambulatory Drug Delivery (pump)	CAH	chronic active hepatitis
			chronic aggressive hepatitis
CADL	communication activities of daily living (speech/ cognitive test)		congenital adrenal hyperplasia
CADP	computer-assisted design of prosthesis	CAHB	chronic active hepatitis B
		CAI	carbonic anhydrase inhibitors
CADRF	coronary artery disease risk factors		carboxyamide aminoimidazoles
CADXPL	cadaver transplant		carotid artery injury
CAE	cellulose acetate electrophoresis		computer-assisted instructions
	coronary artery endarterectomy	'caid	Medicaid
	cyclophosphamide, doxorubicin (Adriamycin), and etoposide	CAIV	cold-adapted influenza virus vaccine
		CAL	callus
			calories (cal)
CAEC	cardiac arrhythmia evaluation center		chronic airflow limitation
			clinical attachment level (dental)
	Cook airway exchange catheter	C_{alb}	albumin clearance
CaEDTA	calcium disodium edetate	cal ct	calorie count
CAF	chronic atrial fibrillation	CALD	chronic active liver disease
	controlled atrial flutter/fibrillation	CALGB	Cancer and Leukemia Group B
	cyclophosphamide, doxorubicin (Adriamycin), and fluorouracil	CALI	chromophore-assisted laser inactivation
		CALLA	common acute lympho- blastic leukemia antigen
CAFF	controlled atrial fibrillation/flutter	CAM	campylobacter vaccine
CAFT	Clinitron® air fluidized therapy		Caucasian adult male
			cell adhesion molecules
CAG	chronic atrophic gastritis		child abuse management
	closed angle glaucoma		complementary and alternative medicine
	continuous ambulatory gamma globin (infusion)		confusion assessment method
	coronary arteriography		controlled ankle motion
CaG	calcium gluconate		cystic adenomatoid malformation
CAGE	a questionnaire for alcoholism evaluation <u>C</u> Have you ever felt the need to <u>c</u>ut down on your drinking? <u>A</u> Have you ever felt <u>a</u>nnoyed by criticism of your drinking? <u>G</u> Have you ever felt <u>g</u>uilty abut your drinking? <u>E</u> Have you ever taken a drink (<u>e</u>ye opener) first thing in the morning?	CAMA	corrected-arm-muscle area
		CAMCOG	Cambridge Cognitive Examination
		CAMD	computer-aided molecular design
		CAMF	cyclophosphamide, Adriamycin, methotrexate, and fluorouracil

CAMP	cyclophosphamide, doxorubicin (Adriamycin), methotrexate, and procarbazine	CaP	cancer of the prostate
		Ca/P	calcium to phosphorus ratio
cAMP	cyclic adenosine monophosphate	CA4P	combretastatin A4 prodrug
		CAPA	Corrective and Preventive Action (related to FDA)
CA-MRSA	community-associated methicillin-resistant *Staphylococcus aureus*	CAPB	central auditory processing battery
		CAPD	central auditory processing disorder
CAMs	cell adhesion molecules		continuous ambulatory peritoneal dialysis
CAN	cardiovascular autonomic neuropathy		
		CAPLA	computer-assisted product license application
	chronic allograft nephropathy		
		CaPPS	calcium pentosan polysulfate
	contrast-associated nephropathy		
		CAPS	aspects of **c**ognition, **a**ffective state, **p**hysical condition, and **s**ocial factors (patient assessment; parameters)
	cord around neck		
CA/N	child abuse and neglect		
CANC	cancelled		
c-ANCA	antineutrophil cytoplasmic antibody		caffeine, alcohol, pepper, and spicy food (dietary restrictions)
CANDA	computer-assisted new drug application		
		CAPWA	computerized arterial pulse waveform analysis
CAN-KLB	*Candida albicans, Klebsiella pneumoniae* vaccine		
		CAR	cancer-associated retinopathy
CANP	Certified Adult Nurse Practitioner		cardiac ambulation routine
CAO	chronic airway (airflow) obstruction		carotid artery repair
			carotid artery rupture
CaO₂	arterial oxygen concentration		coronary artery revascularization
CAOS	computer-assisted orthopedic surgery		Coxsackie adenovirus receptor
CaOx	calcium oxalate	CA-RA	common adductor-rectus abdominis
CAP	cancer of the prostate		
	capsule	CARB	carbohydrate
	cellulose acetate phthalate	CARBO	Carbocaine®
	Certified Addiction Professional		carboplatin (Paraplatin)
		CARD	Cardiac Automatic Resuscitative Device
	cervical acid phosphatase		
	chaotic atrial tachycardia	CARES	Cancer Rehabilitation Evaluation System
	chemistry admission profile		
		CARF	Commission on Accreditation of Rehabilitation Facilities
	chloramphenicol		
	community-acquired pneumonia		
		CARM	Centre for Adverse Reactions Monitoring (New Zealand)
	compound action potentials		
	cyclophosphamide, doxorubicin (Adriamycin), and cisplatin		
		C-arm	fluoroscopy image intensifier

C

75

CARN	Certified Addiction Registered Nurse	CATT	card agglutination test with stained trypanosomes
CARS	Childhood Autism Rating Scale	CAU	Caucasian
CART	classification and regression tree	CAUTI	catheter-associated urinary tract infection
CARTI	community-acquired respiratory tract infection(s)	CAV	computer-aided ventilation congenital absence of vagina cyclophosphamide, doxorubicin (Adriamycin), and vincristine
CAS	carotid artery stenosis cerebral arteriosclerosis Chemical Abstracts Service		
		CAV-1	canine adenovirus type 1
	Clinical Asthma Score combined androgen suppression	CAVB	complete atrioventricular block
		CAVC	common artrioventricular canal
	computer-assisted surgery coronary artery stenosis		
CASA	cancer-associated serum antigen Center on Addiction and Substance Abuse computer-assisted semen analysis	CAVE	Content Analysis of Verbatim Explanation cyclophosphamide, doxorubicin, (Adriamycin) vincristine, and etoposide
		CAVH	continuous arteriovenous hemofiltration
CaSC	carcinoma of the sigmoid colon	CAVHD	continuous arteriovenous hemodialysis
CASHD	coronary arteriosclerotic heart disease	CAVM	cerebral arteriovenous malformation
CASL	continuous arterial spin labeled	CAV-P-VP	cyclophosphamide, doxorubicin (Adriamycin), vincristine, cisplatin, and etoposide
CASP	Child Analytic Study Program		
CASS	computer-aided sleep system		
CAST®	color allergy screening test	CAVR	continuous arteriovenous rewarming
CASWCM	Certified Advanced Social Work Case Manager	CAVS	calcific valve stenosis
		CAVU	continuous arteriovenous ultrafiltration
CAT	Cardiac Arrest Team carnitine acetyl transferase cataract Children's Apperception Test coital alignment technique computed axial tomography methcatinone	CAW	carbonaceous-activated water (Willard Water)
		CAX	central axis
		Ca x P	calcium times phosphorus product
		CB	cesarean birth chronic bronchitis code blue conjugated bilirubin (direct) (umbilical) cord blood
CATH	catheter catheterization Catholic		
CATS	catecholamines	c/b	complicated by

C & B	chair and bed		collected by nurse
	crown and bridge	CBP	chronic benign pain
CB1	cannabinoid receptor, type 1		copper-binding protein
		CBPP	contagious bovine pleuropneumonia
CBA	chronic bronchitis and asthma	CBPS	congential bilateral perisylvian syndrome
	cost-benefit analysis		coronary bypass surgery
	County Board of Assistance	CBR	carotid bodies resected
CBAPF	Certified Board of Addiction Professionals		chronic bedrest
			clinical benefit rate
CBASP	Cognitive Behavioral Analysis System of Psychotherapy		clinical benefit responders
			complete bedrest
		CBRAM	controlled partial rebreathing-anesthesia method
CBAVD	congenital bilateral absence of the vas deferens		
		CBRN	chemical, biological, radiological, or nuclear (agents)
CBC	carbenicillin		
	complete blood count	CB RRR s	cardiac beat, regular
	contralateral breast cancer	M/R/G	rhythm and rate without
CBCDA	carboplatin		murmurs, rubs, or gallops
CBCL	Child Behavior Checklist		
CBCT	community based clinical trials	CBrS	clear breath sounds
		CBS	Caregiver Burden Screen
CBD	closed bladder drainage		Charles Bonnet syndrome
	common bile duct		
	corticobasal degeneration		chronic brain syndrome
CBDE	common bile duct exploration		coarse breath sounds
			Cruveilhier-Baumgarten syndrome
CBDS	common bile duct stone(s)		
CBE	charting by exception	CBT	cognitive behavioral therapy
	child birth education		
	clinical breast examination	CBU	cumulative breath units
		CBV	central blood volume
CBER	Center for Biologics Evaluation and Research (FDA)		cyclophosphamide, carmustine (BiCNu), and etoposide (VePesid)
CBF	cerebral blood flow		
CBFS	cerebral blood flow studies	CBZ	carbamazepine (Tegretol)
		CBZE	carbamazepine epoxide
CBFV	cerebral blood flow velocity	CC	cardiac catheterization
			Catholic
CBG	capillary blood glucose		cerebral concussion
CBGM	capillary blood glucose monitor		chart check (as in 24 hour CC)
CBH	collimated beam handpiece (for laser)		chief complaint
			choriocarcinoma
CBI	Caregiver Burden Index		chronic complainer
	continuous bladder irrigation		circulatory collapse
			clean catch (urine)
CBM	cryopreserved bone marrow		comfort care
			complications and comorbidity
CBN	chronic benign neutropenia		

	coracoclavicular		child care clinic
	cord compression		Comprehensive Cancer
	corpus callosum		Center
	creatinine clearance	C/cc	colonies per cubic
	critical condition		centimeter
	cubic centimeter (cc),	CC & C	colony count and culture
	(mL); Note, mL is	CCC-A	Certificate of Clinical
	preferred as a poorly		Competence in
	written cc looks like the		Audiology
	dangerous abbreviation	CCCE	Clinical Center
	for unit, "u"		Coordinator Educator
	with correction (with	CCC-SP	Certificate of Clinical
	glasses)		Competence in Speech-
C_c	concentration of drug in		Language Pathology
	the central compartment	CCD	charged-coupled device
C/C	cholecystectomy and		childhood celiac disease
	operative cholangiogram		chin-chest distance
	complete upper and lower		clinical cardiovascular
	dentures		disease
CCII	Clinical Clerk–2nd year	CCDC	Certified Chemical
C & C	cold and clammy		Dependency Counselor
CCA	calcium-channel	CCDC-1	Certified Chemical
	antagonist		Dependency Counselor,
	Certified Coding Associate		Level One
	cholangiocarcinoma	CCDS	color-coded duplex
	circumflex coronary artery		sonography
	common carotid artery	CCE	clubbing, cyanosis, and
	concentrated care area		edema
	countercurrent		countercurrent
	chromatography		electrophoresis
	critical care area	CCF	cephalin cholesterol
CCAM	congenital cystic		flocculation
	adenomatoid mal-		Cleveland Clinic
	formation (of the lung)		Foundation
CCAP	capsule cartilage articular		compound comminuted
	preservation		fracture
CCAT	common carotid artery		congestive cardiac
	thrombosis		failure
C-	Certified Clinical Alcohol,		crystal-induced
CATODSW	Tobacco and Other		chemotactic factor
	Drugs Social Worker	CCFE	cyclophosphamide,
CCAVC	complete common		cisplatin, fluorouracil,
	atrioventricular canal		and estramustine
CCB	calcium channel blocker(s)	CCFs	chronic-care facilities
	Community Care Board	CCG	Children's Cancer Group
	corn, callus, and bunion	CCH	community care home
CCBT	Certified Cognitive		Cook County Hospital
	Behavioral Therapist	CCHD	complex congenital heart
CCC	Cancer Care Center		disease
	central corneal clouding		cyanotic congenital heart
	(Grade 0+ to 4+)		disease
	Certificate of Clinical	CCHF	Congo-Crimean
	Competency		hemorrhagic fever

CCHS	congenital central hypoventilation syndrome
CCI	chronic coronary insufficiency
	Correct Coding Initiative
	corrected count increment
CCJAP	Certified Criminal Justice Addiction Professional
CCJAS	Certified Criminal Justice Addiction Specialist
CCK	cholecystokinin
CCK-OP	cholecystokinin octapeptide
CCK-PZ	cholecystokinin pancreozymin
CCL	cardiac catheterization laboratory
	critical condition list
CCl_4	carbon tetrachloride
CCLE	chronic cutaneous lupus erythematosus
CCM	calcium citrate malate
	cerebral cavernous malformation
	Certified Care Manager
	children's case management
	country coordinating mechanism
	cyclophosphamide, lomustine (CCNU; CeeNU), and methotrexate
CCMHC	Certified Clinical Mental Health Counselor
CCMSU	clean catch midstream urine
CCMU	critical care medicine unit
CCN	continuing care nursery
	cyr61, ctfg, nov (family of proteins)
CCNS	cell cycle-nonspecific
CCNU	lomustine (CeeNu)
CCO	continuous cardiac output
	Corporate Compliance Officer
CCOHTA	Canadian Coordinating Office for Health Technology Assessment
C-collar	cervical collar
CCP	crystalloid cardioplegia

CCPD	continuous cycling (cyclical) peritoneal dialysis
CCPs	Corporate Compliance Programs
CCR	California Cancer Registry
	cardiac catheterization recovery
	Continuity of Care Record
	continuous complete remission
	counterclockwise rotation
C_{cr}	creatinine clearance
cCR	complete clinical remission
CCRC	Certified Clinical Research Coordinator
	continuing care residential community
CC-RCC	clear-cell renal-cell carcinoma
CCRN	Certified Critical Care Registered Nurse
CCRT	combined chemo-radiotherapy
CCRU	critical care recovery unit
CCS	cell cycle-specific
	certified coding specialist
	color contrast sensitivity
CC & S	cornea, conjunctiva, and sclera
CCSA	Canadian Cardiovascular Society Angina (score)
CCSK	clear cell sarcoma of the kidney
CCSP	Certified Chiropractic Sports Physician
	Clara cell secretory protein
CCS-P	Certified Coding Specialist, Physician-Based
CCSS	Childhood Cancer Survivor Study
CCT	calcitriol
	carotid compression tomography
	central corneal thickness
	Certified Cardiographic Technician
	closed cerebral trauma
	closed cranial trauma

C

collision cell technology
congenitally corrected transposition (of the great vessels)
Critical Care Technician
crude coal tar

CCTGA congenitally corrected transposition of the great arteries

CCT in PET crude coal tar in petroleum

CCTV closed circuit television

CCU coronary care unit
critical care unit

CCUA clean catch urinalysis

CCUP colpocystourethropexy

CCV Critical Care Ventilator (Ohio)
critical closing volume

CCW childcare worker
counterclockwise

CCWR counterclockwise rotation

CCX complications

CCY cholecystectomy

CD cadaver donor
candela
Castleman disease
celiac disease
cervical dystonia
cesarean delivery
character disorder
chemical dependency
childhood disease
chlorproguanil-dapsone (Lapdap)
chronic dialysis
circular dichroism
closed drainage
clusters of differentiation
common duct
communication disorders
complementarity-determining
complicated delivery
conjugate diameter
contact dermatitis
continuous drainage
conventional denture
convulsive disorder
cortical dysplasia
Crohn disease
cumulative doses
cyclodextran

cytarabine and daunorubicin

Cd cadmium
concentration of drug
cigarettes per day
cup-to-disk ratio

CD4 antigenic marker on helper/inducer T cells (also called OKT 4, T4, and Leu3)

CD8 antigenic marker on suppressor/cytotoxic T cells (also called OKT 8, T8, and Leu 8)

C&D curettage and desiccation
cystectomy and diversion
cytoscopy and dilatation

CDA Certified Dental Assistant
chenodeoxycholic acid (chenodiol)
congenital dyserythropoietic anemia

2-CDA cladribine (Leustatin; chlorodeoxyadenosine)

CDAD *Clostridium difficile*-associated diarrhea

CDAI Crohn Disease Activity Index

CDAK Cordis Dow Artificial Kidney

CDAP continuous distended airway pressure

CDB cough and deep breath

CDC calculated day of confinement
cancer detection center
carboplatin, doxorubicin, and cyclophosphamide
Centers for Disease Control and Prevention
Certified Drug Counselor
chenodeoxycholic acid (chenodiol)
Clostridium difficile colitis

CDCA chenodeoxycholic acid (chenodiol)

CDCP Centers for Disease Control and Prevention (CDC is official abbreviation)

CDCR conjunctivo-dacryocystorhinostomy

CDD	Certificate of Disability for Discharge	CDLE	chronic discoid lupus erythematosus
	Clostridium difficile disease	CdLS	Cornelia de Lange syndrome
	cytidine deaminase	CDM	charge description master
CDDP	cisplatin (Platinol AQ)		clinical development monitor
CDE	canine distemper encephalitis	CDMS	clinically definite multiple sclerosis
	Certified Diabetes Educator	CDP	cancer detection program
	common data element		chemical dependence profile
	common duct exploration		Chemical Dependency Professional
CDER	Center for Drug Evaluation and Research (FDA)		Child Development Program
CDFI	color Doppler flow imaging		clinical development plan
CDG	carbohydrate-deficient glycoprotein		complete decongestive physiotherapy
	congenital disorders of glycosylation		crystalline degradation product
CDGE	constant denaturant gel electrophoresis	CDQ	cytidine diphosphate corrected development quotient
CDGP	constitutional delay of growth and puberty	CDR	clinical data repository
CDH	chronic daily headache		Clinical Dementia Rating
	congenital diaphragmatic hernia		continuing disability review
	congenital dislocation of hip	CDRH	Center for Devices and Radiological Health
	congenital dysplasia of the hip	CDR(H)	cup-to-disk ratio horizontal
CDHP	5-chloro-2 4-dihydroxypyridine	CDRs	complementary determining regions
CDI	Children's Depression Inventory	CDR(V)	cup-to-disk ratio vertical
	clean, dry, and intact	CDS	Chemical Dependency Specialist
	color Doppler imaging		Chronic Disease Score
	Cotrel Duobosset Instrumentation		closed-door seclusion
CDIC	*Clostridium difficile*-induced colitis		color Doppler sonography
		CDSC	Communicable Disease Surveillance Centre (United Kingdom)
C Dif	*Clostridium difficile*	CDSPIES	congestive heart failure, drugs, spasm, pneumothorax, infection, embolism, and secretions (differential diagnosis mnemonic)
C Diff	*Clostridium difficile*		
CDJ	choledochojejunostomy		
CDK	climatic droplet keratopathy		
	cyclin-dependent kinase		
CDKI	cyclin-dependent kinase inhibitor	CDSR	Cochrane Database of Systematic Reviews
CDK2	cyclin-depenent kinases 2		
CDLC	continuous double-loop closure	CDSSs	clinical decision support systems

C

CDT	carbohydrate-deficient transferrin	CEB	calcium entry blocker
			carboplatin, etoposide, and bleomycin
	Chemical Dependency Technician	CEBV	chronic Epstein-Barr virus
	clinical development team	CEC	capillary electrochromatography
	complete decongestive therapy (for lymphedema)		Council for Exceptional Children
	connecting discourse tracking (measure of speech perception)	CECA	Childhood Experience of Care and Abuse (interview)
	cystic dysplasia of the testis	CECD	congenital endothelial corneal dystrophy
CDTA	cyclohexane-1,2-diaminetetraacetic acid	CEc̄/IOL	cataract extraction with intraocular lens
CDTM	collaborative drug therapy management	CECT	contrast-enhanced computed tomography
CDU	chemical dependency unit	CED	Camurati-Engelmann disease
	color-coded duplex ultrasonography		clinically effective dose
CDV	canine distemper virus		cystoscopy-endoscopy dilation
	cardiovascular		
	cyclophosphamide, doxorubicin, and vincristine	CEDS	Certified Eating Disorders Specialist
CDX	chlordiazepoxide (Librim)	CEE	Central European encephalitis
cdyn	dynamic compliance		conjugated equine estrogen (Premarin; conjugated estrogen)
CE	California encephalitis		
	capillary electrophoresis		
	carboplatin and etoposide	CEF	chick embryo fibroblast
	cardiac enlargement		cyclophosphamide, epirubicin, and fluorouracil
	cardiac enzymes		
	cardioesophageal		
	Carpentier-Edwards (heart-valve prosthesis)	CEFM	continuous external fetal monitoring
	cataract extraction	CEFOT	cefotaxime (Claforan)
	central episiotomy	CEFOX	cefoxitin (Mefoxtin)
	chemoembolization	CEFTAZ	ceftazidime
	chest expansion	CEFUR	cefuroxime
	cholesterol ester	CEI	continuous extravascular infusion
	community education		
	consultative examination		converting enzyme inhibitor
	continuing education		
	contrast echocardiology	CEL	cardiac exercise laboratory
	cystic echinococcosis	CELIP	Claims Expansion Line-item Processing
C&E	consultation and examination	CELP	chronic erosive lichen planus
	cough and exercise		
	curettage and electrodesiccation	CEM	Clinical Event Manager
CEA	carcinoembryonic antigen	CEMD	consultative examination by physician
	carotid endarterectomy	ceMRI	contrast-enhanced magnetic resonance imaging
	cost-effectiveness analysis		

CEN	Certified (Nurse)– Emergency Room	CES-D	Center for Epidemiologic Studies – Depression
CENOG	computerized electroneuro- ophthalmogram	CESI	cervical epidural steroid injection
CEO	chief executive officer	CET	common extensor tendon
CEOT	calcifying epithelial odontogenic tumor	CETP	cholesterol ester transfer protein
CEP	cardiac enzyme panel	CEV	cyclophosphamide, etoposide, and vincristine
	chronic eosinophilic pneumonia		
	cognitive evoked potential	CE w/IOL	cataract extraction with intraocular lens
	congenital erythropoietic porphyria	CF	calcium leucovorin (citrovorum factor)
	countercurrent electrophoresis		cancer-free
			cardiac failure
	cyclophosphamide, etoposide, and cisplatin (Platinol AQ)		Caucasian female
			Christmas factor
			cisplatin and fluorouracil
CEPE	cataract extraction by phacoemulsification		complement fixation
CEPH	cephalic		contractile force
	cephalosporin		count fingers
CEPH FLOC	cephalin flocculation		cystic fibrosis
		C&F	cell and flare
CEPP (B)	cyclophosphamide, etopside, procarbazine, prednisone, and bleomycin		chills and fever
		CFA	common femoral artery
			complete Freund adjuvant
CER	conditioned emotional response		cryptogenic fibrosing alveolitis
			cystic fibrosis anthropathy
CE&R	central episiotomy and repair	CFAC	complement-fixing antibody consumption
CERA	cortical evoked response audiometry	C-factor	cleverness factor
		CFCF	carbon fiber composite frame cage
CERAD	Consortium to Establish a Registry for Alzheimer Disease	CFCs	chlorofluorocarbons
		CFD	color-flow Doppler
CERD	chronic end-stage renal disease		computational fluid dynamics
CERULO	ceruloplasmin	CFF	critical fusion (flicker) frequency
CERV	cervical		
CES	Cauda equina syndrome	CFFT	critical flicker fusion threshold
	central excitatory state	CFH	chemical fume hood
	cognitive environmental stimulation	CFI	confrontation fields intact
		CFIDS	chronic fatigue immune dysfunction syndrome
	estrogen, conjugated (conjugated estrogen substance)	CFL	cadaveric fascia lata
			calcaneofibular ligament
CESB	chronic electrical stimulation of the brain		cisplatin, fluorouracil, and leucovorin calcium

C

CFLX	ciprofloxacin (Cipro)	CFVR	coronary flow velocity reserve
	circumflex	CFX	circumflex artery
CFM	cerebral function monitor	CG	cardiogreen (dye)
	close fitting mask		caregiver
	craniofacial microsomia		cholecystogram
	cyclophosphamide, fluorouracil, and mitoxantrone		contact guarding contralateral groin
CFNS	chills, fever, and night sweats	CGA	clonal group A comprehensive geriatric assessment
CFP	cystic fibrosis protein		contact guard assist
CFPT	cyclophosphamide, fluorouracil, prednisone, and tamoxifen	CGB	chronic gastrointestinal (tract) bleeding
		CGCG	central giant-cell granuloma
CFR	case-fatality rates	CGD	chronic glycogen deficit
	Code of Federal Regulations		chronic granulomatous disease
	coronary flow reserve		cobalt gray equivalent
CFRB	critical findings read back	CGF	continuous gavage feeding (infant feeding)
CFS	cancer family syndrome		
	Child and Family Service	CGI	Clinical Global Impressions (scale)
	childhood febrile seizures		
	chronic fatigue syndrome	CGIC	Clinical Global Impression of Change
	congenital fibrosarcoma		
	craniofacial surgery	CGI-S	Clinical Global Impressions, Severity of Illness
CFSAN	Center for Food Safety and Applied Nutrition (FDA)		
		CGL	chronic granulocytic leukemia
CFT	capillary filling time		
	chronic follicular tonsillitis		with correction/with glasses
	complement fixation test	CGM	central gray matter
CFTR	cystic fibrosis transmembrane (conductance) regulator	CGMP	Current Good Manufacturing Practices
		cGMP	cyclic guanine monophosphate
	cystic fibrosis transmembrane receptor	CGN	chronic glomerulonephritis
CFU	colony-forming units	cGN	crescentic glomerulonephritis
CFU-E	colony-forming unit–erythroid	C-GRD	coffee-ground
CFU-G	colony-forming unit–granulocyte	CGRP	calcitonin gene-related peptide
CFU-G/M	colony-forming unit–granulocyte/macrophage	CGS	cardiogenic shock catgut suture centimeter-gram-second system
CFU-M	colony-forming unit–macrophage		
CFU-S	colony-forming unit–spleen	CGTT	cortisol glucose tolerance test
CFV	common femoral vein	cGy	centigray

CH	Caribbean Hispanic	
	chest	
	chief	
	child (children)	
	chronic	
	cluster headache	
	concentric hypertrophy	
	congenital	
	hypothyroidism	
	convalescent hospital	
	crown-heal	
C_h	hepatic clearance	
ch^1	Christ Church	
	chromosone	
CH_{50}	total hemolytic	
	complement	
C&H	cocaine and heroin	
CHA	compound hypermetropic	
	astigmatism	
	congenital hypoplastic	
	anemia	
CHAD	cyclophosphamide,	
	altretamine,	
	(hexamethylmelamine),	
	doxorubicin	
	(Adriamycin), and	
	cisplatin (DDP)	
CHADS	an index that quantifies	
	baseline risk of stroke	
	for individuals with	
	atrial fibrillation	
	(congestive heart	
	failure, hypertension,	
	age greater than 75,	
	diabetic, and history of	
	stroke)	
CHAI	Commission for	
	Healthcare Audit and	
	Inspection (United	
	Kingdom)	
	continuous hepatic artery	
	infusion	
CHAM-OCA	cyclophosphamide,	
	hydroxyurea,	
	dactinomycin,	
	methotrexate,	
	vincristine, leucovorin,	
	and doxorubicin	
CHAM-PUS	Civilian Health and	
	Medical Program of the	
	Uniformed Services	
CHAP	child health associate	
	practitioner	

C

	cyclophosphamide, altretamine, (hexamethylmelamine), doxorubicin (Adriamycin), and cisplatin (Platinol AQ)
CHAQ	childhood health assessment questionnaire
CHARGE	coloboma (of eyes), hearing deficit, choanal atresia, retardation of growth, genital defects (males only), and endo-cardial cushion defect
CHART	complaint, history, assessment, Rx (treatment), transport continuous hyperfractionated accelerated radiotherapy Craig Handicap Assessment and Reporting Technique
CHB	chronic hepatitis B complete heart block congenital heart block
CHBHA	congenital Heinz body hemolytic anemia
CHC	concentric hypertrophic cardiomyopathy
CH_3- CCNU	semustine
CHCT	caffeine-halothane contracture test
cHct	central hematocrit
CHD	center hemodialysis changed diaper childhood diseases chronic hemodialysis common hepatic duct congenital heart disease coordinate home care
CHE	chronic hepatic encephalopathy comprehensive health examination
CHEDDAR	Chief Compliant; History: social and physical as well as contributing factors; Examination; Details of problems and complaints; Drugs and

	dosage—list current meds; Assessment, diagnostic process, total impression; Return visit information or referral (format of documentation)	CHM	complete hydatidiform mole
		CHN	central hemorrhagic necrosis
			Chinese herb nephropathy
			Community Health Nurse
			community nursing home
CHEF	clamped homogeneous electric field	CHO	carbohydrate
			Chemical Hygiene Officer
ChEI	cholinesterase inhibitor		Chinese hamster ovary
CHEM 7	see page 392	C_{H_2O}	free-water clearance
CHEMO	chemotherapy	CHO_a	cholera vaccine, attenuated live (oral)
ChemoRx	chemotherapy		
CHEOPS	Children's Hospital of Eastern Ontario Pain Scale	CHO_{cn}-LPS	cholera vaccine, lipopolysaccharide-toxin conjugate
CHESS	chemical shift suppression	$C_2 H_5 OH$	alcohol (ethyl alcohol)
		$CHO_{i\text{-}w}$	cholera vaccine, inactivated whole cell
CHF	congestive heart failure		
	Crimean hemorrhagic fever	$CHO_{i\text{-}w\text{-}BS}$	cholera vaccine, inactivated whole cell, B subunit
CHFV	combined high-frequency of ventilation	chol	cholesterol
		c̄ hold	withhold
CHG	change	CHO_o	cholera, oral vaccine
	chlorhexidine gluconate	CHOP	cyclophosphamide, doxorubicin (hydroxy-daunorubicin), vincristine (Oncovin), prednisone
CHI	chikungunya virus vaccine		
	closed head injury		
	Consolidated Health Informatics		
	contrast harmonic imaging	CHOP-Bleo	cyclophosphamide, doxorubicin (hydroxydaunorubicin), vincristine (Oncovin), prednisone, and bleomycin
	creatinine-height index		
CHIK	Chikungunya (virus)		
CHILD	congenital hemidysplasia with ichthyosiform nevus and limb defects (syndrome)		
		CHO_{tox}	cholera toxin/toxoid vaccine
CHIN	community health information network	CHPB	Canadian Health Protection Branch (the equivalent of the U.S. Food and Drug Administration)
CHIP	comprehensive health insurance plan		
	iproplatin		
CHIR	Chiron Corporation		
Chix	chickenpox	CHPX	chickenpox
CHL	conductive hearing loss	CHR	Cercaria-Hullen reaction
CHLC	Cooperative Human Linkage Center		chronic
			complete hematological response
ChloMP	chlorambucil, mitoxantrone, and prednisolone	CHRPE	congenital hypertrophy of the retinal pigment epithelium
ChlVPP	chlorambucil, vinblastine, procarbazine, and prednisone	CHRS	congenital hereditary retinoschisis

CHS	Chediak-Higashi syndrome contact hypersensitivity	CIB	Carnation Instant Breakfast®
CHT	Certified Hand Therapist Certified Hyperbaric Technician Certified Hypnotherapist chemotherapy closed head trauma		crying-induced bronchospasm cytomegalic inclusion bodies
		CIBD	chronic inflammatory bowel disease
ChT	chemotherapy	CIBI	Clinician Interview-Based
CHTN	chronic hypertension		Impression (of change)
CHU	closed head unit	CIBIC	Clinician Interview-Based
CHUC	Certified Health Unit Coordinator	CIBIC- plus	Impression of Change Clinician Interview-
CHVP	cyclophosphamide, doxorubicin (hydroxydaunorubicin), teniposide (VM26), and prednisone		Based Impression of Change with Caregiver Input
		CIBP	chronic intractable benign pain
CHW	community health workers	C-IBS	constipated predominant
CHWG	chewing gum		irritable bowel syndrome
CHX	chlorhexidine (Peridex; Periogard)	CIC	cardioinhibitory center circulating immune
CI	cardiac index cerebral infarction cesium implant Clinical Instructor cochlear implant cognitively impaired colon inertia commercial insurance complete iridectomy confidence interval continuous infusion contraindications convergence insufficiency core imprint (cytology) coronary insufficiency		complexes clean intermittent catheterization completely in-the-canal (hearing aid) coronary intensive care
		CICE	combined intracapsular cataract extraction
		CICU	cardiac intensive care unit
		CICVC	centrally inserted central venous catheter
		CID	Center for Infectious Diseases (CDC) Central Institute for the Deaf cervical immobilization device chemotherapy-induced diarrhea combined immunodeficiency cytomegalic inclusion disease
Ci	curie(s)		
CI30	cumulative incidence at 30 years		
CIA	calcaneal insufficiency avulsion chemotherapy-induced amenorrhea chemotherapy-induced anemia chronic idiopathic anhidrosis		
		CIDP	chronic inflammatory demyelinating polyradiculoneuropathy (polyneuropathy)
CIAA	competitive insulin autoantibodies	CIDS	cellular immunodeficiency syndrome
CIAED	collagen-induced autoimmune ear disease		continuous insulin delivery system

C

CIE	capillary immunoelectrophoresis	C_{IN}	insulin clearance
	chemotherapy-induced emesis	CIND	cognitive impairment, no dementia
	congenital ichthyosiform erythroderma	CINE	chemotherapy-induced nausea and emesis
	counterimmuno-electrophoresis		cineangiogram
	crossed immunoelectrophoresis	CINV	chemotherapy-induced nausea and vomiting
CIEA	continuous infusion epidural analgesia	CIO	corticosteroid-induced osteoporosis
CIEP	counterimmuno-electrophoresis	CIOMS	The Council for International Organization of Medical Sciences
	crossed immunoelectrophoresis	CIP	Cardiac Injury Panel critical illness polyneuropathy
CIFN	chemotherapy-induced fever and neutropenia	CIPD	chronic intermittent peritoneal dialysis
CIG	cigarettes	CipRGC	ciprofloxacin-resistant *Neisseria gonorrhoeae*
CIH	Certified in Industrial Health	CIR	continent intestinal reservoir
	continuous infusion haloperidol	CIRB	central institutional review board
CIHD	chronic ischemic heart disease	Circ	circulation circumcision
CIHR	Canadian Institutes of Health Research		circumference
CII	continuous insulin infusion	circ. &	circulation and sensation
CIIA	common internal iliac artery	sen.	
CIL	carbamazepine-induced lupus	CIRF	cocaine-induced respiratory failure
CIM	change in menses	CIRT	carbon ion radiotherapy
	chemotherapy-induced mucositis	CIS	Cancer Information Service (National Cancer Institute)
	constraint-induced movement		carcinoma in situ
	convective interaction media		clinically isolated syndrome
	corticosteroid-induced myopathy		Commonwealth of Independent States
	critical illness myopathy		continuous interleaved sampling
CIMCU	cardiac intermediate care unit	CI&S	conjunctival irritation and swelling
CIMT	carotid (artery) intima-media thickness	CISC	clean intermittent self-catheterization
	constraint-induced movement therapy	CISCA	cisplatin, cyclophos-phamide, and doxo-rubicin (Adriamycin)
CIN	cervical intraepithelial neoplasia	CISCOM	The Centralized Information Service for Complementary Medicine
	chemotherapy-induced neutropenia		
	chronic interstitial nephritis		

CISD	critical incident stress debriefing (used by EMTs)	CK MM	creatine kinase MM fraction (primarily in skeletal muscle)
Cis-DDP	cisplatin (Platinol AQ)	CKW	clockwise
CISH	chromogen in situ hybridization	Cl	chloride
		CL	central line
CISM	critical incident stress management (debriefing used by EMTs)		chemoluminescence
			clear liquid
			cleft lip
CIS-R	Clinical Interview Schedule, Revised		cloudy
			confidence limits
CI-Stim	cochlear implant stimulation		contact lens
			critical list
CIT	chemotherapy-induced toxicities		cutaneous leishmaniasis
			cycle length
	constraint-induced therapy (protocol)		lung compliance
		C_L	compliance of the lungs
	conventional immunosuppressive therapy	C-L	consultation-liaison
		CLA	community living arrangements
	conventional insulin therapy		congenital lactic acidosis
			congenital laryngeal atresia
CIT IDS	citation identifiers (National Library of Medicine)		conjugated linoleic acid
		C lam	cervical laminectomy
		CLAMSS	cleavage- and ligation-associated mutation-specific sequencing
CITP	capillary isotachophoresis		
CIU	chronic idiopathic urticaria		
		CLAP	contact laser ablation of prostate
CIV	common iliac vein		
	continuous intravenous (infusion)	CLARE	contact lens-associated acute red eye
CIVI	continuous intravenous infusion	CLAS	Cancer Linear Analogue Scale
CIXU	constant infusion excretory urogram		congenital localized absence of skin
CIWA-Ar	Clinical Institute Withdrawal Assessment for Alcohol–revised	CLASS	computer laser-assisted surgical system
		CLASS I	congestive heart failure with no limitation with ordinary activity (New York Heart Association Classification)
CJD	Creutzfeldt-Jakob disease		
cJET	congenital junctional ectopic tachycardia		
CJR	centric jaw relation		
CK	check	CLASS II	congestive heart failure with slight limitation of physical activity
	conductive keratoplasty		
	creatine kinase		
CK-BB	creatine kinase BB band (primarily in brain)	CLASS III	congestive heart failure with marked limitation of physical activity
CKC	cold-knife conization		
CKD	chronic kidney disease	CLASS IV	congestive heart failure with inability to engage in any physical activity without symptoms
CK-ISO	creatine kinase isoenzyme		
CK-MB	creatine kinase MB fraction (primarily in cardiac muscle)		
		Clav	clavicle

C

CLB	chlorambucil (Leukeran)		close
	coccidian-like body		cod liver oil
CLB_atx	*Clostridium botulinum* antitoxin	CLOX	clock-drawing task (cognitive impairment test)
CLBBB	complete left bundle branch block	CL & P	cleft lip and palate
CLBD	cortical Lewy body disease	CL PSY	closed psychiatry
		CLPU	contact lens-induced peripheral ulceration
CLBP	chronic low back pain		
CLB_tox	*Clostridium botulinum* toxoid vaccine	Cl_r	renal clearance
		CLRB	clinical laboratory (results) read back
CLC	cork leather and celastic (orthotic)		
		Cl Red	closed reduction
CL/CP	cleft lip and cleft palate	CLRO	community leave for reorientation
CLD	central lung distance		
	chronic liver disease	CLS	capillary leak syndrome
	chronic lung disease		community living skills
	Clostridium difficile vaccine	CLSE	calf-lung surfactant extract (Infasurf)
Cl_d	dialysis clearance	CLSM	confocal laser scanning microscopy
CLE	centrilobular emphysema		
	congenital lobar emphysema	CLT	chronic lymphocytic thyroiditis
	constant-load exercise		complex lymphedema therapy
	continuous lumbar epidural (anesthetic)		
			cool lace tent
CLED	cysteine lactose electrolyte-deficient (agar)	Cl_T	total body clearance
		CLV	cutaneous leukocytoclastic vasculitis
CLEIA	chemiluminescent enzyme immunoassay	CL VOID	clean voided specimen
		CLW_c	*Clostridium welchii* type C (Pigbel) toxoid vaccine
CLEP	college level examination program		
		clysis	hypodermoclysis
CLF	cholesterol-lecithin flocculation	CLZ	clozapine (Clozaril)
		cm	centimeter (2.54 cm = 1 inch)
CLG	clorgyline		
CLH	chronic lobular hepatitis	CM	capreomycin (Capastat)
C_h	hepatic clearance		CarboMedics (heart valve prosthesis)
CLI	central lymphatic irradiation		cardiac monitor
	clomipramine (Anafranil)		case management
	critical leg (limb) ischemia		case manager
CLIA	Clinical Laboratory Improvement Act		Caucasian male
			centimeter (cm)
Cl_{int}	intrinsic clearance		chondromalacia
CLL	chronic lymphocytic leukemia		cochlear microphonics
			common migraine
CLLE	columnar-lined lower esophagus		continuous microwave
			continuous murmur
cl liq	clear liquid		contrast media
Cl_{nr}	nonrenal clearance		costal margin
CLO	Campylobacter-like organism		cow's milk
			culture media

cutaneous melanoma

cystic mesothelioma

tomorrow morning (this is a dangerous abbreviation)

cM   centimorgan (one one-hundredth of a morgan; the unit of distance on a linkage map)

cm1   circumflex marginal 1

cm2   circumflex marginal 2

cm^2 square centimeters

cm^3 cubic centimeter

CMA   Certified Medical Assistant

Certified Movement Analyst

compound myopic astigmatism

cost-minimization analysis

cow's milk allergy

CMAF   centrifuged microaggregate filter

CMAI   Cohen-Mansfield Agitation inventory

CMAP   compound muscle action potential

CMAPs   compound muscle action potentials

C_{max} maximum concentration of drug

CMB   carbolic methylene blue

CMBBT   cervical mucous basal body temperature

CMC   carboxymethylcellulose

carpal metacarpal (joint)

chloramphenicol

chronic mucocutaneous candidiasis

clinically meaningful change

closed mitral commissurotomy

CMD   congenital muscular dystrophy

cytomegalic disease

CMDRH   Center for Medical Devices and Radiological Health (of the Food and Drug Administration)

CME   cervicomediastinal exploration (examination)

continuing medical education

cystoid macular edema

CMER   current medical evidence of record

CMF   cyclophosphamide, methotrexate and fluorouracil

CMFP   cyclophosphamide, methotrexate, fluorouracil, and prednisone

CMFT   cyclophosphamide, methotrexate, fluorouracil, and tamoxifen

CMFVP   cyclophosphamide, methotrexate, fluorouracil, vincristine, and prednisone

CMG   cystometrogram

CMGM   chronic megakaryocytic granulocytic myelosis

CMGN   chronic membranous glomerulonephritis

CMH   Cochran Mantel Haenszel

current medical history

CMHC   Certified Mental Health Counselor

community mental health center

C/MHC   Community/Migrant Health Center

CMHN   Community Mental Health Nurse

CMI   case mix index

cell-mediated immunity

clomipramine (Anafranil)

Cornell Medical Index

CMID   cytomegalic inclusion disease

C_{min} minimum concentration of drug

CMIR   cell-mediated immune response

CMJ   carpometacarpal joint

cervicomedullary junction

CMK   congenital multicystic kidney

CML   cell-mediated lympholysis

chronic myelogenous leukemia

chronic myeloid leukemia

C

CML-BP	blastic phase chronic myeloid leukemia	CMRI	cardiac magnetic resonance imaging
CMM	Comprehensive Major Medical (insurance)	CMRIT	combined modality radioimmunotherapy
	continuous metabolic monitor	CMRNG	chromosomally mediated resistant *Neisseria gonorrhoeae*
	cutaneous malignant melanoma		
CMME	chloromethyl methyl ether	CMRO	chronic multifocal recurrent osteomyelitis
CMML	chronic myelomacrocytic leukemia	$CMRO_2$	cerebral metabolic rate for oxygen
CMMS	Columbia Mental Maturity Scale	CMS	Centers for Medicare and Medicaid Services (replaces Health Care Financing Administration [HCFA])
CMN	Certificate of Medical Necessity		
	congenital melanocytic nevi		
	congenital mesoblastic nephroma		children's medical services
CMO	cardiac minute output		circulation motion sensation
	cetyl myristoleate		chocolate milkshake
	Chief Medical Officer		constant moderate suction
	comfort measures only (resuscitation order)		continuous motion syndrome
	consult made out	CMSC	Certified Medical Staff Coordinator
CMO 1	corticosterone methyl oxidase type 1	CMSUA	clean midstream urinalysis
CMOP	cardiomyopathy	CMT	carpometatarsal (joint)
C-MOPP	cyclophosphamide, mechlorethamine, vincristine (Oncovin), procarbazine, and prednisone		Certified Massage Therapist
			Certified Medication Technician
			Certified Medical Transcriptionist
CMP	cardiomyopathy		Certified Music Therapist
	chondromalacia patellae		cervical motion tenderness
	comprehensive (complete) metabolic profile (see page 392)		Charot-Marie-Tooth (phenotype) (disease)
	cushion mouthpiece		Chiropractic manipulative treatment
CMPA	cow's milk protein allergy		choline magnesium trisalicylate (Trilisate)
CMPF	cow's milk, protein-free		combined modality therapy
CMPS	chronic myofascial pain syndrome		continuing medication and treatment
CMPT	cervical mucous penetration test		cutis marmorata telangiectasia
CMR	cardiovascular magnetic resonance	CMTX	chemotherapy treatment
	cerebral metabolic rate	CMUA	continuous motor unit activity
	chief medical resident		
	child (1-4 years) mortality rates	CMV	cisplatin, methotrexate, and vinblastine
	crude mortality rate		

	controlled mechanical ventilation	C-NES	conversion nonepileptic seizures
	conventional mechanical ventilation	CNF	cyclophosphamide, mitoxantrone (Novatantrone), and fluorouracil
	cool mist vaporizer		
	cytomegalovirus		
	cytomegalovirus vaccine	CNH	central neurogenic hypernea
CMVIG	cytomegalovirus immune globulin		
			contract nursing home
CMVS	culture midvoid specimen	CNHC	chronodermatitis nodularis helicis chronicus
CN	charge nurse		community nursing home care
	congenital nystagmus		
	cranial nerve	CNI	calcineurin inhibitors
	tomorrow night (this is a dangerous abbreviation)	CNL	chemonucleolysis
			chronic neutrophilic leukemia
Cn	cyanide		
C/N	contrast-to-noise ratio		Connaught Laboratories
CN II–XII	cranial nerves 2 through 12	CNLD	chronic neonatal lung disease
CNA	Certified Nurse Aide	CNLSD	condensation nucleation light scattering detection
	chart not available		
C_{Na}	sodium clearance		
CNAG	chronic narrow angle glaucoma	CNM	certified nurse midwife
		CNMP	chronic nonmalignant pain
CNAP	continuous negative airway pressure	CNMT	Certified Nuclear Medicine Technologist
CNB	core-needle biopsy	CNN	congenital nevocytic nevus
CNC	clinical nurse coordinator	CNO	Chief Nursing Officer
	Community Nursing Center		community nursing organization
	Consonant-Vowel Nucleus-Consonant (Maryland CNC word list)	CNOP	cyclophosphamide, mitoxantrone (Novantrone), vincristine (Oncovin), and prednisone
CNCbl	cyanocobalamin (vitamin B_{12})	CNOR	Certified Nurse, Operating Room
CND	canned	CNP	capillary nonprofusion
	cannot determine	CNPB	continuous negative pressure breathing
	chronic nausea and dyspepsia		
CNDC	chronic nonspecific diarrhea of childhood	CNPS	cardiac nuclear probe scan
		CNR	contrast-to-noise ratio (radiology)
CNE	Chief Nurse Executive		
	chronic nervous exhaustion	CNRN	Certified Neurosurgical Registered Nurse
	continuing nursing education	CNS	central nervous system
	could not establish		Certified Nutrition Specialist
	culture-negative endocarditis		Clinical Nurse Specialist
			coagulase-negative staphylococci
CNEP	continuous negative extrathoracic pressure		Crigler-Najjar syndrome

C

CNSD	Certified Nutrition Support Dietitian
CNSHA	congenital nonspherocytic hemolytic anemia
CNT	could not tell
	could not test
CNTA	combined neurosurgical and transfacial approach
CNTF	ciliary neurotrophic factor
CNV	choroidal neovascularization
CNVM	choroidal neovascular membrane
CO	carbon monoxide
	cardiac output
	castor oil
	centric occlusion
	Certified Orthoptist
	cervical orthosis
	corneal opacity
	corn oil
	court order
Co	cobalt
C/O	check out
	complained of
	complaints
	under care of
^{60}Co	radioactive isotope of cobalt
CO_2	carbon dioxide
CO_3	carbonate
COA	children of alcoholic
	coenzyme A
	condition on admission
CoA	coarctation of the aorta
COAD	chronic obstructive airway disease
	chronic obstructive arterial disease
COAG	chronic open angle glaucoma
COAGSC	coagulation screen
COAP	cyclophosphamide, vincristine (Oncovin), cytarabine (ara-C), and prednisone
COAR	coarctation
COARCT	coarctation
COB	cisplatin, vincristine (Oncovin), and bleomycin
	coordination of benefits

COBE	chronic obstructive bullous emphysema
COBRA	Consolidated Omnibus Budget Reconciliation Act of 1985
COBS	chronic organic brain syndrome
COBT	chronic obstruction of biliary tract
COC	calcifying odontogenic cyst
	chain of custody
	combination oral contraceptive
	continuity of care
COCCIO	coccidioidomycosis
COCM	congestive cardiomyopathy
COD	carotid occlusive disease
	cataract, right eye
	cause of death
	chronic oxygen dependency
	codeine
	coefficient of oxygen delivery
	condition on discharge
CODAS	chronotherapeutic oral drug absorption system
CODE 99	patient in cardiac or respiratory arrest
COD-MD	cerebro-oculardysplasia muscular dystrophy
CODO	codocytes
COE	court-ordered examination
COEPS	cortically originating extrapyramidal symptoms
COER-24	24-hour controlled-onset, extended-release (dosage form)
COFS	cerebro-oculo-facio-skeletal
COG	center of gravity
	Central Oncology Group
	Children's Oncology Group
	cognitive function tests
COGN	cognition
COGTT	cortisone-primed oral glucose tolerance test

COH	carbohydrate	conc.	concentrated
	controlled ovarian	CONG	congenital
	hyperstimulation		gallon
COHb	carboxyhemoglobin	CONJ	conjunctiva
Coke	Coca-Cola®	CONPA-	cyclophosphamide,
	cocaine	DRI I	vincristine, doxorubicin,
COL	colonoscopy		and melphalan
COLD	chronic obstructive lung	CONPA-	conpadri I plus high-dose
	disease	DRI II	methotrexate
	Computer Output to Laser	CONPA-	conpadri I plus intensified
	Disk	DRI III	doxorubicin
COLD A	cold agglutin titer	CoNS	coagulase-negative
Collyr	eye wash		staphylococci
col/ml	colonies per milliliter	CONT	continuous
colp	colporrhaphy		contusions
COLTRU	*colletotrichum truncatum*	CON-	contralateral
COM	calcium oxalate	TRAL	
	monohydrate	CONTU	contusion
	center of mass	CONV	conversation
	chronic otitis media	Conv. ex.	convergence excess
COMBO	combination ultrasound	ConvRX	conventional therapy
	with electrical	CO-Ox	Co-oximetry
	stimulation	COP	center of pressure
COMF	comfortable		change of plaster
COMLA	cyclophosphamide,		cicatricial ocular
	vincristine (Oncovin),		pemphigoid
	methotrexate, calcium		*Colibacilosis porcina*
	leucovorin, and		vaccine
	cytarabine (ara-C)		colloid osmotic pressure
COMM E	Committee E, a German		complaint of pain
	Federal Health Agency		cycophosphamide,
	committee for the		vincristine (Oncovin),
	evaluation of herbal		and prednisone
	remedies	CoP	Communities of Practice
COMP	compensation		Conditions of
	complications		Participation
	composite	COP 1	copolymer 1
	compound	COPA	cuffed oropharyngeal
	compress		airway
	cyclophosphamide,	COP-	cyclophosphamide,
	vincristine (Oncovin),	BLAM	vincristine (Oncovin),
	methotrexate, and		prednisone, bleomycin,
	prednisone		doxorubicin
COMS	clinical outcomes		(Adriamycin), and
	management system		procarbazine
COMT	catechol-*O*-methyl-		(Matulane)
	transferase	COPD	chronic obstructive
COMTA	Commission on Message		pulmonary disease
	Therapy Accreditation	COPE	chronic obstructive
CON	catheter over a needle		pulmonary emphysema
	certificate of need	COPP	cyclophosphamide, vin-
	conservatorship		cristine, procarbazine,
CON A	concanavalin A		and prednisone

C

95

COPS	community outpatient service		cytochrome C oxidase
		COX-2	cyclo-oxygenase-2
COPT	circumoval precipitin test	CP	centric position
CoQ10	coenzyme Q_{10}		cerebral palsy
COR	coefficient of reproducibility		Certified Paramedic
			chemical peel
	conditioned orientation response		chemistry profiles
			chest pain
	coronary		chloroquine-primaquine
CoR	custodian of records		chondromalacia patella
CORA	conditioned orientation reflex audiometry		chronic pain
			chronic pancreatitis
CORBA	Common-Object Request Broker Architecture		cleft palate
			clinical pathway
CORE	cardiac or respiratory emergency		closing pressure
			cold pack
CORF	Comprehensive Outpatient Rehabilitation Facility		convenience package
			cor pulmonale
COR P	cor pulmonale		creatine phosphokinase
CORT	Certified Operating Room Technician		cyclophosphamide and cisplatin (Platinol)
COS	cataract, left eye		cystopanendoscopy
	change of shift		process capability
	Chief of Staff	C_p	concentration of drug plasma
	clinically observed seizure		
	controlled ovarian stimulation		phosphate clearance
		Cp	*Chlamydia pneumoniae*
	Crisis Outpatient Services	C/P	carbohydrate-to-protein ratio
C_{osm}	osmolal clearance		
COSTART	Coding symbols for a thesaurus of adverse reaction terms	C&P	compensation and pension
			complete and pain-free (range of motion)
COT	content of thought		complete and pushing
	court-ordered treatment		cystoscopy and pyelography
COTA	Certified Occupational Therapy Assistant	CPA	cardiopulmonary arrest
			carotid photoangiography
COTE	comprehensive occupational therapy evaluation		cerebellar pontile angle
			chest pain alert
COTT CH	cottage cheese		color power angiography
COTX	cast-off, to x-ray		conditioned play audiometry
COU	cardiac observation unit		costophrenic angle
	cataracts, both eyes		cyclophosphamide (Cytoxan)
COV	coefficient of variation		cyproterone acetate (Androcur)
COW	circle of Willis		
COWA	controlled oral word association		
COWAT	Controlled Oral Word Association Test	CPAF	chlorpropamide-alcohol flush
COWS	cold to the opposite and warm to the same	C_{PAH}	para-amino hippurate clearance
COX	Coxsackie virus	CPAP	continuous positive airway pressure
	cyclo-oxygenase		

CPB	cardiopulmonary bypass	CPE-C	cyclopentenylcytosine
	cisplatin, cyclophosphamide, and carmustine (BiCNU)	CPEFM	Clear-Plan Easy Fertility Monitor
	competitive protein binding	CPEO	chronic progressive external ophthalmoplegia
CPBA	competitive protein-binding assay	CPER	chest pain emergency room
CPBP	cardiopulmonary bypass	CPET	cardiopulmonary exercise testing
CPC	cancer prevention clinic		
	cerebral palsy clinic	CPETU	chest pain evaluation and treatment unit
	Certified Procedural Coder	CPF	cerebral perfusion pressure
	chronic passive congestion		chlorpyrifos (an insecticide)
	clinicopathologic conference	CPFT	Certified Pulmonary Function Technologist
	coil planet centrifuge	CPG	clinical practice guidelines
	continue plan of care	CPG2	carboxypeptidase G2
CPC-H	Certified Procedural Coder, Hospital-Based	CPGN	chronic progressive glomerulonephritis
CPCR	cardiopulmonary-cerebral resuscitation	CPH	chronic persistent hepatitis
CPCS	clinical pharmacokinetics consulting service	CPhT	Certified Pharmacy Technician
CPD	cephalopelvic disproportion	CPI	chronic public inebriate
	chorioretinopathy and pituitary dysfunction		constitutionally psychopathia inferior
	chronic peritoneal dialysis	CPID	chronic pelvic inflammatory disease
	citrate-phosphate-dextrose		
CPDA-1	citrate-phosphate-dextrose-adenine-one	CPIP	chronic pulmonary insufficiency of prematurity
CPDA-2	citrate-phosphate-dextrose-adenine-two	CPK	creatine phosphokinase (BB, MB, MM are isoenzymes)
CPDD	calcium pyrophosphate deposition disease	CPK-1	creatine phosphokinase MM fraction
CPDG2	carboxypeptidase-G2		
CPDR	Center for Prostate Disease Research (Department of Defense)	CPK-2	creatine phosphokinase MB fraction
		CPK-BB	creatine phosphokinase BB fraction
CPE	cardiogenic pulmonary edema	CPKD	childhood polycystic kidney disease
	chronic pulmonary emphysema	CPK-MB	creatine phosphokinase of muscle band
	Clinical Pastoral Education		
	clubbing, pitting, or edema	CPL	criminal procedure law
	complete physical examination	CPM	cancer pain management
	cytopathic effect		central pontine myelinolysis
CPEB	cytoplasmic polyadenylation element binding (protein)		chlorpheniramine maleate
			chronic progressive myelopathy

C

97

	Clinical Practice Model		computerized patient record
	continue present management		tablet (French)
	continuous passive motion	CPR-1	all measures except cardiopulmonary resuscitation
	counts per minute		
	cycles per minute		
	cyclophosphamide (Cytoxan)	CPR-2	no extraordinary measures (to resuscitate)
CPmax	peak serum concentration	CPR-3	comfort measures only
CPMDI	computerized pharmacokinetic model-driven drug infusion	CPRAM	controlled partial rebreathing anesthesia method
CPmin	trough serum concentration	CP/ROMI	chest pain, rule out myocardial infarction
CPMM	constant passive motion machine	CPRS	Categorical Pain Relief Scale
CPMP	Committee for Proprietary Medicinal Products (of the European Union)	CPRS-OCS	Comprehensive Psychiatric Rating Scale, Obsessive-Compulsive Subscale
CPN	chronic pyelonephritis	CPS	carbamyl phosphate synthetase
	common peroneal nerve		cardiopulmonary support
CPNI	common peroneal nerve injury		Center for Prevention Services (CDC)
CPO	chief privacy officer		cervical pedicle screw
	continue present orders		chest pain syndrome
CPOE	computerized physician (prescriber) order entry		child protective services
			Chinese paralytic syndrome
CPOM	continuous pulse oximeter monitoring		chloroquine-pyrimethamine sulfadoxine
CPOX	chicken pox		chronic paranoid schizophrenia
CPP	central precocious puberty		clinical performance score
	cerebral perfusion pressure		clinical pharmacokinetic service
	chronic pelvic pain		CoaguChek® Plus System
	coronary perfusion pressure		coagulase-positive staphylococci
	cryo-poor plasma		complex partial seizures
CPPB	continuous positive pressure breathing		counts per second
CPPD	calcium pyrophosphate dihydrate		cumulative probability of success
	cisplatin	CPs	clinical pathways
CP & PD	chest percussion and postural drainage	CPS I	carbamyl phosphate synthetase I
CPPS	chronic pelvice pain syndrome	cPSA	complexed prostate-specific antigen
CPPV	continuous positive pressure ventilation	CPSC	Consumer Product Safety Commission
CPQ	Conner Parent Questionnaire	CPSI	Chronic Prostatitis Symptom Index
CPR	cardiopulmonary resuscitation		
	computer-based patient records		

CPSP	central post-stroke pain		chorioretinal
CPT	camptothecin		clockwise rotation
	carnitine palmitoyl transferase		closed reduction
	chest physiotherapy		colon resection
	child protection team		complete remission
	chromo-perturbation		contact record
	chronic paranoid type		controlled release
	cold pressor test		cosmetic rhinoplasty
	Continuous Performance Test		creamed
			credentialing
	corticosteroid pulse treatment	Cr	crutches
			cycloplegia retinoscopy
	current perception threshold		caloric restrictions
			chromium
	Current Procedural Terminology (coding system)		creatinine
		C/R	conscious, rational
		C & R	convalescence and rehabilitation
CPT-2000	Current Procedural Terminology, 2000 Edition		cystoscopy and retrograde
		CR_1	first cranial nerve
		CRA	central retinal artery
CPT-11	irinotecan hydrochloride (Camptosar)		chronic rheumatoid arthritis
CPTA	Certified Physical Therapy Assistant		cis-retinoic acid (isotretinin, Accutane®)
CPT/C	current perception threshold, computerized		Clinical Research Associate
CPTH	chronic post-traumatic headache		colorectal anastomosis
CPU	children's psychiatric unit		Contract Research Assistant
	clinical pharmacology unit		corticosteroid-resistant asthma
CPUE	chest pain of unknown etiology		
CPUM	Certified Professional in Utilization Management	CRABP	cellular retinoic acid binding protein
CPV	cowpox virus	CRAbs	chelating recombinant antibodies
CPX	complete physical examination	CRADA	Cooperative Research and Development Agreement (with NIH)
CPZ	chlorpromazine Compazine® (CPZ is a dangerous abbreviation as it could be either)		
		CRAG	cerebral radionuclide angiography
CQ	chloroquine	CrAg	cryptococcal antigen
CQDS	cumulative quality disruption score	CRAMS	circulation, respiration, abdomen, motor, and speech
CQI	continuous quality improvement		
		CRAN	craniotomy
CR	caloric restrictions	CRAO	central retinal artery occlusion
	capillary refill		
	cardiac rehabilitation	CRAX	crackers
	cardiorespiratory	CRB	Clinical Review Board
	case reports	CRBBB	complete right bundle branch block
	chief resident		

C

CRBIs	catheter-related bloodstream infections
CRBP	cellular retinol-binding protein
CRBSI	catheter-related bloodstream infections
CRC	case review committee
	child-resistant container
	clinical research center
	Clinical Research Coordinator
	colorectal cancer
CRCLM	colorectal cancer liver metastases
CR & C	closed reduction and cast
CrCl	creatinine clearance
CRD	childhood rheumatic disease
	chronic renal disease
	chronic respiratory disease
	colorectal distension
	cone-rod dystrophy
	congenital rubella deafness
	crown-rump distance
CRE	cumulative radiation effect
CREAT	serum creatinine
CREC	ciprofloxacin-resistant *Escherichia coli*
CREF	cycloplegic refraction
CRELM	screening tests for Congo-Crimean, Rift Valley, Ebola, Lassa, and Marburg fevers
CREP	crepitation
CREST	calcinosis, Raynaud disease, esophageal dysmotility, sclerodactyly, and telangiectasia
CRF	cardiac risk factors
	case report form
	chronic renal failure factor
CRG-L2	Cancer related gene-Liver 2
CRH	corticotropic-releasing hormone
CRFZ	closed reduction of fractured zygoma
CRH	corticotropin-releasing hormone

CRHCa	cancer-related hypercalcemia
CRI	Cardiac Risk Index
	catheter-related infection
	chronic renal insufficiency
CRIB	Clinical Risk Index for Babies
CRIE	crossed radioimmuno-electrophoresis
CRIF	closed reduction and internal fixation
CRIMF	closed reduction/intermaxillary fixation
CRIS	controlled-release infusion system
crit	hematocrit
CRKL	crackles
CRL	crown rump length
CRM	circumferential resection margins
	continual reassessment method
	cream
	cross-reacting mutant
CRM +	cross-reacting material positive
CRMD	children with retarded mental development
CRN	crown
CRNA	Certified Registered Nurse Anesthetist
CRNFA	Certified Registered Nurse, First Assistant
CRNH	Certified Registered Nurse in Hospice
CRNI	Certified Registered Nurse Intravenous
CRNP	Certified Registered Nurse Practitioner
CRO	cathode ray oscilloscope
	contract research organization(s)
CROM	cervical range of motion
	chronic refractory osteomyelitis
CROMY	chronic refractory osteomyelitis
CROS	contralateral routing of signals
CRP	canalith repositioning procedure

	chronic relapsing pancreatitis		chemoradiotherapy
	coronary rehabilitation program		choice reaction time
			circuit resistance training
	C-reactive protein		copper reduction test
C&RP	curettage and root planning		cranial radiation therapy
CRPA	C-reactive protein agglutinins	Cr Tr	crutch training
		CRTs	case report tabulations
CRPD	chronic restrictive pulmonary disease	CRTT	Certified Respiratory Therapy Technician
CRPF	chloroquine-resistant *Plasmodium falciparum*	CRTX	cast removed take x-ray
		CRU	cardiac rehabilitation unit
CRPP	closed reduction and percutaneous pinning		catheterization recovery unit
CRPS I	complex regional pain syndrome type I		clinical research unit
		CRV	central retinal vein
CRQ	Chronic Respiratory (Disease) Questionnaire	CRVF	congestive right ventricular failure
CRR	community rehabilitation residence	CRVO	central retinal vein occlusion
		CRx	chemotherapy
CRRT	continuous renal replacement therapy	CIIRx	Century II Bicarbonate Dialysis Machine
CRS	Carroll Self-Rating Scale	CRYO	cryoablation
	catheter-related sepsis		cryosurgery
	Center for Scientific Review (NIH)	CRYST	crystals
		CS	cardiogenic shock
	Chemical Reference Substances		cardioplegia solution
			cat scratch
	child restraint system(s)		cervical spine
	Chinese restaurant syndrome		cesarean section
			chest strap
	chronic rhinosinusitis		cholesterol stone
	cocaine-related seizure(s)		chlorobenzylidene malononitrile
	colon-rectal surgery		
	congenital rubella syndrome		cigarette smoker
			clinically significant
	continuous running suture		clinical stage
	cryoreductive surgery		close supervision
	cytokine-release syndrome		conditionally susceptible
CRST	calcification, Raynaud phenomenom, scleroderma, and telangiectasia		congenital syphilis
			conjunctiva-sclera
			consciousness
			conscious sedation
CRT	cadaver renal transplant		consultation
	capillary refill time		consultation service
	Cardiac Rescue Technician		coronary sinus
	cardiac resynchronization therapy		corticosteroid(s)
			cranial setting
	cartilage roof triangle		Cushing syndrome
	cathode ray tube		cycloserine
	central reaction time		*o*-chlorobenzylidene malononitrile
	Certified Rehabilitation Therapist	C&S	conjunctiva and sclera

C

	cough and sneeze	C sect.	cesarean section
	culture and sensitivity	CSF	cerebrospinal fluid
C/S	cesarean section		colony-stimulating
	consultation		factors
	culture and sensitivity	CSFELP	cerebrospinal fluid
CSA	central sleep apnea		electrophoresis
	compressed spectral	CSFP	cerebrospinal fluid
	activity		pressure
	Controlled Substances	CSGIT	continuous-suture graft-
	Act		inclusion technique
	controlled substance	C-Sh	chair shower
	analogue	CSH	carotid sinus
	corticosteroid-sensitive		hypersensitivity
	asthma		chronic subdural
CsA	cyclosporine (cyclosporin		hematoma
	A)	CSHQ	Children's Sleep Habits
CsA-ME	cyclosporine		Questionnaire
	microemulsion (Neoral)	CSI	chemical shift imaging
CSAP	cryosurgical ablation of		Computerized Severity
	the prostate		Index
CSB	caffeine sodium benzoate		continuous subcutaneous
	Cheyne-Stokes breathing		infusion
	Children's Services Board		coronary stent
CSBF	coronary sinus blood flow		implantation
CSBO	complete small bowel		corticosteroid injection
	obstruction		craniospinal irradiation
CSC	central serous	CsI	cesium iodide
	chorioretinopathy	CSICU	cardiac surgery intensive
	cornea, sclera, and		care unit
	conjunctiva	CSID	congenital sucrase-
	cryogen spray cooling		isomaitase deficiency
	cryopreserved stem cells	CSII	continuous subcutaneous
CSCI	continuous subcutaneous		insulin infusion
	infusion	CSIO	continuous subcutaneous
CSCR	central serous		infusion of opiates
	chorioretinopathy	CS IV	clinical stage 4
CSD	cat scratch disease	CSL	chemical safety level
	celiac sprue disease	CSLO	confocal scanning laser
	cortical spreading		ophthalmoscopy
	depression	CSLU	chronic status leg ulcer
C S&D	cleaned, sutured, and	CSM	carotid sinus massage
	dressed		cerebrospinal meningitis
CSDD	Center for the Study of		cervical spondylotic
	Drug Development		myelopathy
CSDH	chronic subdural		circulation, sensation, and
	hematoma		movement
	combined systolic and		Committee on Safety of
	diastolic hypertension		Medicines (United
CSE	combined spinal/epidurals		Kingdom)
	cross-section	CSME	cotton-spot macular
	echocardiography		edema
CSEA	combined spinal-epidural	CSMN	chronic sensorimotor
	anesthesia		neuropathy

C

CSN	cystic suppurative necrosis		contraction stress test
CSNB	congenital stationary night blindness		convulsive shock therapy
			cosyntropin stimulation test
CSNRT	corrected sinus node recovery time		static compliance
CSNS	carotid sinus nerve stimulation	C_{STAT}	static lung compliance
		CSTE	Council of State and Territorial Epidemiologists
CSO	Chief Security Officer		
	Consumer Safety Officer (FDA)	CSU	cardiac surgery unit
	copied standing orders		cardiac surveillance unit
CSOM	chronic serous otitis media		cardiovascular surgery unit
			casualty staging unit
	chronic suppurative otitis media		catheter specimen of urine
		CSVD	cerebral small-vessel disease
CSP	cellulose sodium phosphate	CSW	cerebral salt-wasting (syndrome)
	cervical spine pain		
	chiral stationary phase		Clinical Social Worker
C-spine	cervical spine		commercial sex worker
CSR	central supply room	CSWCM	Certified Social Work Case Manager
	Cheyne-Stokes respiration		
	clinical statistical report	CSWs	commercial sex workers
	corrected sedimentation rate	CSWSS	continuous spike-waves during slow sleep
	corrective septorhinoplasty	CT	calcitonin
C-S RT	craniospinal radiotherapy		calf tenderness
CSS	Canadian Stroke Scale (score)		cardiothoracic
			carpal tunnel
	carotid sinus stimulation		cellulose triacetate (filter)
	Central Sterile Services		cervical traction
	chemical sensitivity syndrome		chemotherapy
			chest tube
	chewing, sucking, and swallowing		*Chlamydia trachomatis*
			circulation time
	child safety seats		client
	Churg-Strauss syndrome		clinical trial
C_{SS}	concentration of drug at steady-state		clotting time
			coagulation time
			coated tablet
CSSD	closed system sterile drainage		compressed tablet
			computed tomography
CSSU	cardiac short-stay unit		Coomb test
CST	cardiac stress test		corneal thickness
	castration		corneal transplant
	central sensory conducting time		corrective therapy
			cytarabine and thioguanine
	cerebroside sulfotransferase		
			cytoxic drug
	Certified Surgical Technologist	C_t	concentration of drug in tissue
	cesarean section prior to labor at term	C/T	compared to
		CTA	catamenia (menses)

103

	clear to auscultation	CTHA	computed tomography hepatic arteriography
	computed tomography angiography	CTI	certification of terminal illness
C-TAB	cyanide tablet		
CTAP	clear to auscultation and percussion	CTICU	cardiothoracic intensive care unit
	computed tomography during arterial portography	CTID	chemotherapy-induced diarrhea
CTB	ceased to breathe	CTL	cervical, thoracic, and lumbar
	cholera toxin B		chronic tonsillitis
CTC	Cancer Treatment Center		control (subjects)
	circular tear capsulotomy		cytotoxic T-lymphocytes
	circulating tumor cells	CTLSO	cervicothoracic-lumbosacral orthosis
	Clinical Trial Certificate (United Kingdom's equivalent to the Investigational New Drug Application)	CTM	Chlor-Trimeton
			clinical trials materials
			computed tomographic myelography
	Common Toxicity Criteria	CT/MPR	computed tomography with multiplanar reconstructions
	computed tomographic colonography		
	cyclophosphamide, thiotepa, and carboplatin	CTN	calcitonin
		C & T N, BLE	color and temperature normal, both lower extremities
CTCL	cutaneous T-cell lymphoma (mycosis fungoides)	cTnC	cardiac troponin C
		cTnI	cardiac troponin I
CT & DB	cough, turn & deep breath	cTNM	clinical-diagnostic staging of cancer
CTD	carpal tunnel decompression	CTnT	cardiac troponin T
	chest tube drainage	CTO	chronic total (coronary) occlusion
	connective tissue disease		
	corneal thickness depth	CTP	comprehensive treatment plan
	cumulative trauma disorder	CTPA	clear to percussion and auscultation
CTDW	continues to do well		
CTEP	Cancer Therapy Evaluation Program	CTPN	central total parenteral nutrition
	Center for Therapy Evaluation Programs (National Cancer Institute)	CTR	carpal tunnel release
			carpal tunnel repair
			Certified Tumor Registrar
			cosmetic transdermal reconstruction
CTF	Colorado tick fever		
	continuous tube feeding	CTRB	Clinical Trial Review Board
CTG	cardiotocography		
C/TG	cholesterol to triglyceride ratio		critical tests read back
		CTRS	Certified Therapeutic Recreation Specialist
CTGA	complete transposition of the great arteries		
			Conners Teachers Rating Scale
	corrected transposition of the great arteries	CT-RT	chemo-radiotherapy
CTH	clot to hold	CTS	cardiothoracic surgeon

	carpal tunnel syndrome	CUSA	Cavitron ultrasonic suction aspirator
	closed-tube sampling		
CTSP	called to see patient	CUT	chronic undifferentiated type (schizophrenia)
CTT	cotton-thread test		
CTU	computed tomographic urography	CUTA	congenital urinary tract anomaly
CTW	central terminal of Wilson	CV	cardiovascular
CTX	cerebrotendinous xanthomatosis		cell volume
			cisplatin and etoposide (VePesid)
	cervical traction		coefficient of variation
	chemotherapy		color vision
	cyclophosphamide (Cytoxan)		common ventricle
			consonant vowel
CTXN	contraction		contrast venography
CTZ	chemoreceptor trigger zone		curriculum vitae
		C/V	cervical/vaginal
	co-trimoxazole (sulfamethoxazole and trimethoprin)	CVA	cerebrovascular accident
			costovertebral angle
			cough-variant asthma
CU	cause undetermined	CVAAS	cold vapor atomic absorption spectrometry
	cause unknown		
	chronic undifferentiated	CVAD	central venous access device
	clinical units		
	color unit	CVAH	congenital virilizing adrenal hyperplasia
	convalescent unit		
	Cuprophan (filter)	CVAT	costovertebral angle tenderness
Cu	copper		
C$_u$	urea clear clearance	CVB	chronic villi biopsy
C/U	checkup		group B coxsackievirus
	creatinine/urea ratio	CVC	central venous catheter
CUA	clean urinalysis		chief visual complaint
	cost-utility analysis		consonant-vowel-consonant
CUC	chronic ulcerative colitis		
	Clinical Unit Clerk	CVD	cardiovascular disease
CUD	cause undetermined		collagen vascular disease
	controlled unsterile delivery		
		CVDU	chronic ventilator-dependent unit
CUFCM	Century Ultrafiltration Control Machine		
		CVEB	cisplatin, vinblastine, etoposide, and bleomycin
CUG	cystourethrogram		
Cu-IUD	copper intrauterine device	CVENT	controlled ventilation
CUP	carcinoma of unknown primary (site)	CVF	cardiovascular failure
			central visual field
CUPS	carcinoma of unknown primary site		cervicovaginal fluid
		CVG	coronary vein graft
CUR	curettage		cutis verticis gyrata
	cystourethrorectocele	CVHD	chronic valvular heart disease
CUS	carotid ultrasound		
	chronic undifferentiated schizophrenia	CVI	carboplatin, etoposide, ifosfamide, and mesna uroprotection
	compression ultrasonography		
	contact urticaria syndrome		

C

	cerebrovascular insufficiency	CVS	cardiovascular surgery
	chronic venous insufficiency		cardiovascular system
			challenge virus standard
	common variable immunodeficiency (disease)		chorionic villi sampling
			clean voided specimen
			continuing vegetative state
	continuous venous infusion	CVSCU	cardiovascular special care unit
CVICU	cardiovascular intensive care unit	CVSD	congenital ventricular septal defecct
CVID	common variable immune deficiency	CVST	cardiovascular stress test
CVINT	cardiovascular intermediate		cerebral venous sinus thrombosis
CVL	central venous line	CVSU	cardiovascular specialty unit
	cervicovaginal lavage		
	clinical vascular laboratory	CVT	calf vein thrombosis
CVLP	chimeric virus-like particles	CVTC	central venous tunneled catheter
CVLT	California Verbal Learning Test	CVU	clean voided urine
		CVUG	cysto-void urethrogram
CVM	Center for Veterinary Medicine (NIH)	CVVH	continuous venovenous hemofiltration
CVMT	cervical-vaginal, motion tenderness	CVVHDF	continuous venovenous hemodiafiltration
CVN	central venous nutrient	CW	careful watch
CVNSR	cardiovascular normal sinus rhythm		case worker
			chest wall
CVO	central vein occlusion		clockwise
	conjugate diameter of pelvic inlet		compare with
		C/W	consistent with
CvO$_2$	mixed venous oxygen content		crutch walking
		CWA	chemical warfare agents
CVOD	cerebrovascular obstructive disease	CWAF	Chemical Withdrawal Assessment Flowsheet
CVOR	cardiovascular operating room	CWAP	continuous wave arthroscopy pump
CVP	central venous pressure	CWD	canal-wall down
	cyclophosphamide, vincristine, and prednisone		cell-wall defective
			change wet dressing
			chronic wasting disease
CVPP	lomustine, vinblastine, procarbazine, and prednisone	CWE	cotton-wool exudates
		CWL	Caldwell-Luc
		CWM	comprehensive weight management
CVR	cerebral vascular resistance		
	cerebrovascular resuscitation	CWMS	color, warmth, movement, and sensation
	coronary vascular reserve	CWP	centimeters of water pressure
CVRI	coronary vascular resistance index		childbirth without pain
CVRS	Cardiovascular-Respiratory Score		coal worker's pneumoconiosis
			cold wet packs

cWPW	concealed Wolff-Parkinson-White syndrome
CWR	clockwise rotation
CWS	Certified Wound Care Specialist
	comfortable walking speed
	cotton-wool spots
CWT	compensated work training
CWV	closed wound vacuum
CX	cancel
	cervix
	chronic
	circumflex
	circumflex artery
	culture
	cylinder axis
	cystectomy
Cx	consultation
CXA	circumflex artery
CxBx	cervical biopsy
CxMT	cervical motion tenderness
CXR	chest x-ray
CXTX	cervical traction
CY	calendar year
	cyclophosphamide (Cytoxan)
C&Y	Children with Youth (program)
CYA	cover your ass
CyA	cyclosporine
CyADIC	cyclophosphamide, doxorubicin (Adriamycin), and dacarbazine
CYC	cyclophosphamide
Cyclo C	cyclocytidine HCl
CYL	cylinder
CYP	cytochrome P-450 system
CYP450	cytochrome P450 system
CYRO	cryoprecipitate
CYSTA	cystathionine
CYSTO	cystogram
	cystoscopy
CYT	cyclophosphamide (Cytoxan)
CYTA	cytotoxic agent
CYVA DIC	cyclophosphamide, vincristine, Adriamycin, and dacarbazine
CZE	capillary zone electrophoresis
CZI	crystalline zinc insulin (regular insulin)
CZP	clonazepam (Klonopin

D	daughter
	day
	dead
	decay
	dependent
	depression
	dextrose
	dextro
	diarrhea
	diastole
	dictated
	dilated
	diminished
	Dinamap (blood pressure monitor)
	diopter
	distal
	distance
	divorced
$D+$	note has been dictated/ look for report
$D-$	note not dictated, save chart for doctor
$D_{0(2/7/00)}$	Day zero (the day treatment begins, February 7th, 2000)
D_1	day one (first day of treatment)
	first diagonal branch (coronary artery)
D-1	dorsal vertebrae 1 to 12
D-12	dorsal nerves 1-12
D_2	second diagonal branch (coronary artery)
	ergocalciferol
2/d	twice a day (this is a dangerous abbreviation)
2-D	two-dimensional
3-D	three-dimensional
D_3	cholecalciferol
D-3+7	cytarabine and daunorubicin
4D	4 prism diopters
4-D	four-dimensional
D5	dextrose 5% injection
5xD	five times a day (this is a dangerous abbreviation)
D-15	Farnsworth panel D-15 color vision test

D50	50% dextrose injection	DAF	decay-accelerating factor
D_{5/.45}	dextrose 5% in 0.45%		delayed auditory feedback
	sodium chloride	DAFE	Dial-A-Flow Extension®
	injection	DAFM	double-aerosol face mask
DA	darbepoetin alfa (Aranesp)	DAFNE	dose adjustment for
	dark adaptation (test)		normal eating
	Debtors Anonymous	DAG	diacylglyerol
	degenerative arthritis		dianhydrogalactitol
	delivery awareness	DAH	diffuse alveolar
	Dental Assistant		hemorrhage
	diagnostic arthroscopy		disordered action of the
	diastolic augmentation		heart
	direct admission	DAI	diffuse axonal injury
	direct agglutination	DAIDS	Division of AIDS (of the
	disk areas		National Institute of
	diversional activity		Allergy and Infectious
	dopamine		Diseases, NIH)
	drug addict	DAL	diffuse aggressive
	drug aerosol		lymphomas
Da	daltons		drug analysis laboratory
D/A	discharge and advise	DALE	disability-adjusted life
DAA	dead after arrival		expectancy
	dissection aortic	DALM	dysplasia-associated
	aneurysm		lesion or mass
DA/A	drug/alcohol addiction	DALY	disability-adjusted life
DAB	days after birth		year(s)
	diamino benzidine	DAM	diacetylmonoxine
DABA	Diplomate of the	DAMA	discharged against
	American Board of		medical advice
	Anesthesiology	DAMP	deficits in attention, motor
DAC	day activity center		control, and perception
	disabled adult child	DAN	diabetic autonomic
	Division of Ambulatory		neuropathy
	Care	DANA	drug-induced antinuclear
DACL	Depression Adjective		antibodies
	Checklists	DAo	descending aorta
DACS	density-adjusted cell	DAOM	depressor anguli oris
	sorting		muscle
DACT	dactinomycin (Cosmegen)	DAP	dapsone
DAD	diffuse alveolar damage		diabetes-associated
	diode array detector		peptide
	Disability Assessment of		diastolic augmentation
	Dementia		pressure
	dispense as directed		distending airway
	drug administration device		pressure
	father		Draw-A-Person
DADS	distal acquired	DAPT	Draw-A-Person Test
	demyelinating	DAR	daily affective rhythm
	symmetrical		data, action, response
	(neuropathy)	DARE	data, action, response, and
DAE	diving air embolism		evaluation
DAEC	diffuse-adherence	DARP	drug abuse rehabilitation
	Entamoeba coli		program

	drug abuse reporting program		deep breathe
D/ART	depression/awareness, recognition and treatment		demonstration bath
			dermabrasion
			diaphragmatic breathing
			difficulty breathing
DAS	day of admission surgery		direct bilirubin
	developmental apraxia of speech		double blind
		DBA	Diamond-Blackfan anemia
	died at scene		
	distractive auditory stimuli	DB & C	deep breathing and coughing
	dynamometer anchoring station		
		DBD	milolactol (dibromodulicitol)
DAs	daily activities		
DASE	dobutamine-atropine stress echocardiography	DBDS	Dementia Behavior Disturbance Scale
DASH	Dietary Approaches to Stop Hypertension (diet)	DBE	deep breathing exercise
		DBED	penicillin G benzathine (for IM use only; Bicillin L-A)
	Disabilities of the Arm, Shoulder and Hand (rating)		
		dBEMCL	decibel effective masking contralateral
DASI	Duke Activity Status Index	D₅BES	dextrose in balanced electrolyte solution
DAST	Drug Abuse Screening Test		
		DBI	documented by initials
DAT	daunorubicin, cytarabine, (ara-C), and thioguanine	DBI®	phenformin HCl
		DBIL	direct bilirubin
	definitely abnormal tracing (electrocardiogram)	DBKT	Diabetes: Basic Knowledge Test
	dementia of the Alzheimer type	DBL	double beta-lactam
		DBM	dibenzoylmethane
	diet as tolerated	DBMT	displacement bone marrow transplantation
	diphtheria antitoxin		
	direct agglutination test	DBP	D-binding protein
	direct amplification test		diastolic blood pressure
	direct antiglobulin test		dibutyl phthalate
DAU	daughter	DBPCFC	double-blind, placebo-controlled food challenge
	drug abuse urine		
DAUNO	daunorubicin		
DAVA	vindesine sulfate (Eldisine; desacetyl vinblastine amide sulfate)	DBPT	dacarbazine (DTIC), carmustine (BCNU), cisplatin (Platinol), and tamoxifen
DAVE	The Data Assessment and Verification program	DBQ	debrisoquin
		DBS	deep brain stimulation
DAVM	dural arteriovenous malformation		desirable body weight
			diminished breath sounds
DAV SEP	deviated septum		dried blood stain
DAW	dispense as written	DBT	dialectical behavior therapy
DAWN	Drug Abuse Warning Network		
		DBW	dry body weight
dB	decibel	DBZ	dibenzamine
DB	database	DC	daunorubicin and cytarabine
	date of birth		

D

	daycare		designated compensable event
	decrease		detection-controlled estimation
	dendritic cells		
	dextrocardia		
	diagonal conjugate	DCF	data collection form
	direct Coombs (test)		Denomination Commune Francaise (French-approved nonproprietary name)
	direct current		
	discharge (This is a dangerous abbreviation as it is read as discontinue)		
			docetaxel, cisplatin, and fluorouracil
	discomfort		pentostatin (Nipent; 2′ deoxycoformycin)
	Doctor of Chiropractic		
D&C	dilatation and curettage		
	direct and consensual	DCFS	Department of Children and Family Services
D/C	disconnect		
	discontinue	DCG	diagnostic cardiogram
DCA	directional coronary atherectomy	DCH	delayed cutaneous hypersensitivity
	disk/condyle adhesion	DCIA	deep circumflex iliac artery (flap)
	double-cup arthroplasty		
	sodium dichloroacetate	DCIS	ductal carcinoma *in situ*
DCAG	double-coronary artery graft	DCL	diffuse cutaneous leishmaniasis
DCAP-BTLS	deformities, contusions, abrasions, and punctures/penetrations, burns, tenderness, lacerations, and swelling (an assessment mnemonic used by EMTs)	DCLHb	diaspirin cross-linked hemoglobin
		DCM	dementia care mapping
			dilated cardiomyopathy
		DCMP	dilated cardiomyopathy
		DCMXT	dichloromethotrexate
		DCN	Darvocet N
		DCNU	chlorozotocin
DC-ART	disease controlling anti-rheumatic therapy	DCO	diffusing capacity of carbon monoxide
DC&B	dilation, currettage, and biopsy	DCP	dynamic compression plate
DCBE	double-contrast barium enema	DCP®	calcium phosphate, dibasic
DCC	day care center(s)	DCPM	daunorubicin, cytarabine, prednisolone, and mercaptopurine
	diabetes care clinic		
	direct current cardioversion	DCPN	direction-changing positional nystagmus
DCCF	dural carotid-cavernous fistula	DCR	dacryocystorhinostomy
			delayed cutaneous reaction
DCCs	day care centers		
DCCT	Diabetes Control and Complications Trial (questionnaire)	DCRC	disseminated colorectal cancer
		DCRF	data case report forms
DCD	developmental coordination disorder	3DCRT	three-dimensional conformal radiation therapy
DC'd	discontinued		
DCE	delayed contrast-enhancement	DCS	damage-control surgery

	decompression sickness	DDAVP®	desmopressin acetate
	dorsal column stimulator	DDC	zalcitabine (dideoxy-cytidine; Hivid)
DCSA	double-contrast shoulder arthrography	DDD	defined daily doses
DCSW	Diplomate in Clinical Social Work		degenerative disk disease
			dense deposit disease
DCT	daunorubicin, cytarabine, and thioguanine		fully automatic pacing
		DDDR	pacemaker code (D =
	decisional conflict theory		chamber paced-**d**ual,
	deep chest therapy		D = chamber sensed-**d**ual, D = response to
	direct (antiglobulin) Coombs test		sensing-**d**ual, R =
	dynamic contour tonometry		programmability-**r**ate modulation)
DCTM	delay computer tomographic myelography	DDE	dichlorodiphenylethylene
		DDGB	double-dose gallbladder (test)
DCU	day care unit	DDH	developmental dysplasia of the hip
DCUS	duplex-color ultrasonography		
		DDHT	double-dissociated hypertropia
DCW	direct care worker		
DCYS	Department of Children and Youth Services	DDI	didanosine (dideoxyinosine; Videx)
			dressing dry, intact
DD	delayed diarrhea	DDIs	drug-drug interactions
	delivery date	DDis	developmental disorder
	dependent drainage	DDiv	Doctor of Divinity
	Descemet detachment	DDMC	diabetes disease management clinic
	detrusor dyssynergia		
	developmentally delayed	DDNS	digestive disease and nutrition service
	developmental disabilities		
	developmentally disabled	DDP	cisplatin (Platinol AQ)
	dialysis dementia	DDRA	dead despite resuscitation attempt
	died of the disease		
	differential diagnosis	DDRE	Division of Drug Risk Evaluation (FDA)
	discharge diagnosis		
	disk diameter	DDS	dialysis disequilibrium syndrome
	Doctor of Divinity		
	double dose (used by Radiology)		Doctor of Dental Surgery
			double-decidual sac (sign)
	down drain		4, 4-diaminodiphenyl-sulfone (dapsone)
	dry dressing		
	dual disorder	DDST	Denver Development Screening Test
	Duchenne dystrophy		
	due date	DDT	chlorophenothane
	dysthymic disorder	DDTP	drug dependence treatment program
D/D	diarrhea/dehydration		
D → D	discharge to duty	DDx	differential diagnosis
D & D	debridement and dressing	DE	dermal epidermal (junction)
	diarrhea and dehydration		
	drilling and drainage		digitalis effect
DDA	dideoxyadenosine	D_5E_{48}	5% Dextrose and Electrolyte 48
DDAH	dimethylarginine dimethylaminohydrolase		

D₅E₇₅	5% Dextrose and Electrolyte 75	DEL	delivered
			delivery
2-DE	two-dimensional echocardiography		deltoid
		DEM	drug evaluation matrix
	two-dimentional gel electrophoresis	DEMRI	dynamic enhanced magnetic resonance imaging
3-DE	three-dimensional echocardiography		
		DEPs	diesel exhaust particles
D&E	dilation and evacuation	DEP ST SEG	depressed ST segment
DEA#	Drug Enforcement Administration number (physician's federal narcotic number)		
		DER	disulfiram-ethanol reaction
		DERM	dermatology
DEAE	diethylaminoethyl	DES	desflurane (Supreme)
DEB	diepoxybutane (test)		diethylstilbestrol
	dystrophic epidermolysis bullosa		diffuse esophageal spasm
			disequilibrium syndrome
DEC	deciduous (primary teeth)		Dissociative Experience Scale
	decrease		
	diethylcarbamazine (Hetrazan)		drug eluting stent
			dry-eye syndrome
	Drug Evaluation and Classification (a standardized curriculum to train police officers)		dysfunctional elimination syndrome (urology)
		DESAT	desaturation
		DESF	desflurane (Suprane)
DECA	nandrolone decanoate (Deca-Durabolin)	DESI	Drug Efficacy Study Implementation
DECAFS	Department of Children and Family Services	DET	diethyltryptamine
			dipyridamole echocardiography test
DECEL	deceleration		
decub	decubitus	DETOX	detoxification
DED	diabetic eye disease	DEV	deviation
	died in emergency department		duck embryo vaccine
		DEVR	dominant exudative vitreoretinopathy
DEEDS	drugs, exercise, education, diet, and self-monitoring		
		DEX	dexamethasone
DEEG	depth electroencephalogram		dexrazoxane (Zinecard)
			dexter (right)
	deteriorating electroencephalogram		dexverapamil
		DEXA	dual-energy x-ray absorptiometry
DEET	diethyltoluamide		
DEF	decayed, extracted, or filled	DF	day frequency (of voiding)
	defecation		decayed and filled
	deficiency		deferred
2-DEF	two-dimensional echo-derived ejection fraction		defibrotide
			degree of freedom
DEFT	defendant		dengue fever
	driven equilibrium Fourier transform (technique)		dexfenfluramine
			diabetic father
DEG	diethylene glycol		diastolic filling
degen	degenerative		dietary fiber
DEHP	diethylhexyl phthalate		dorsiflexion

	drug-free		disseminated granuloma annulare
	dye-free	DGC	dystrophin-glycoprotein complex
DFA	delayed feedback audiometry		
	diet for age	DGE	delayed gastric emptying
	difficulty falling asleep	DGF	delayed graft function
	direct fluorescent antibody	DGGE	denaturing gradient gel electrophoresis
	distal forearm		
DFD	defined formula diets	DGI	disseminated gonococcal infection
	degenerative facet disease		
DFE	dilated fundus examination	DGL	deglycyrrhizinated licorice
		DGR	duodenogastric reflux
	distal femoral epiphysis	DGM	ductal glandular mastectomy
DFG	direct forward gaze		
DFI	disease-free interval	DGs	documentation guidelines
DFLE	disability-free life expectancy	DGT	decaffeinated green tea
		DH	delayed hypersensitivity
DFM	decreased fetal movement		Dental Hygienist
	deep finger massage		dermatitis herpetiformis
	deep friction massage		developmental history
DFMC	daily fetal movement count		diaphragmatic hernia
		D+H	delusions and hallucinations
DFMR	daily fetal movement record		
		D-H	Dimon-Hughston (intertrochanteric osteotomy technique)
DFO	deferoxamine (Desferal)		
DFOM	deferoxamine (Desferal)		
DFP	diastolic filling period	DHA	dihydroxyacetone
	isoflurophate (diisopropyl flurophosphate)		docosahexaenoic acid
		DHAC	dihydro-5-azacytidine
DFR	diabetic floor routine	DHAD	mitoxanthrone HCl (Novantrone)
DFRC	deglycerolized frozen red cells		
		DHANP	Diplomate of the Homeopathic Academy of Naturopathic Physicians
DFS	disease-free survival		
	Division of Family Services		
	Doppler flow studies	DHAP	dexamethasone, high-dose cytarabine, (ara-A) cisplatin (Platinol AQ)
DFSP	dermatofibrosarcoma protuberans		
		DHA-TP	dihydroartemisinin, trimethoprim, and piperaquine
DFT	defibrillation threshold (testing)		
DFU	dead fetus in uterus	DHBV	duck hepatitis B virus
	diabetic foot ulcer	DHCA	deep hypothermia circulatory arrest
DFV	D'Aoust Fineman virus		
	dengue fever vaccine	DHCC	dihydroxycholecalciferol
	diarrhea, fever, and vomiting	DHD	dissociated horizontal deviation
DFW	Dexide face wash	DHE	dental health education
DFWO	dorsiflexory wedge osteotomy	DHE 45®	dihydroergotamine mesylate
DG	diagnosis	DHEA	dehydroepiandrosterone
	dorsal glides	DHEAS	dehydroepiandrosterone sulfate
	downward gaze		
DGA	DiGeorge anomaly		

D

DHF	dengue hemorrhagic fever	diag.	diagnosis
		DIAM	drug-induced aseptic meningitis
	diastolic heart failure		
DHFR	dihydrofolate reductase	DIAP-PERS	(causes of transient incontinence)
DHHS	Department of Health and Human Services		**d**elirium/confusion, **i**nfection, (urinary),
DHI	Dizziness Handicap Inventory		**a**trophic urethritis/vaginitis, **p**harmaceuticals, **p**sychological,
	dynamic hyperinflation		
DHIC	detrusor hyperactivity with impaired contractility		**e**xcessive excretion (e.g., CHF, hyperglycemia)
			restricted mobility, and
DHL	diffuse histocytic lymphoma		**s**tool impaction
		DIAS	diastolic
DHP	dihydropyridine		
DHP-1	dehydropeptidase-1	DIAS BP	diastolic blood pressure
DHPG	ganciclovir	Diath SW	diathermy short wave
DHPLC	denaturing high-performance liquid chromatography	DIAZ	diazepam (Valium)
		DIB	disability insurance benefits
DHPR	dihydropteridine reductase		
DHPS	dihydropteroate synthase	DIBC	drug-induced blood cytopenias
DHR	delayed hypersensitivity reaction	DIBD	drug-induced behavioral disinhibition
DHS	Department of Human Services	DIB-R	Diagnostic Interview for Borderlines (personality disorders)-Revised
	duration of hospital stay		
	dynamic hip screw	DIBS	dead-in-bed syndrome
DHST	delayed hypersensitivity test	DIC	dacarbazine (DTIC-Dome)
			diagnostic imaging center
DHT	dihydrotachysterol (Hytakeral; DHT®)		differential interference contrast
	dihydrotestosterone		disseminated intravascular coagulation
	dissociated hypertropia		
	Dobhoff tube		drug information center
DHTF	Dobhoff tube feeding	DICC	dynamic infusion cavernosometry and cavernosography
DI	(Beck) Depression Inventory		
	date of injury	DICE	dexamethasone, ifosfamide, cisplatin, and etopside, with mesna
	Debrix Index		
	detrusor instability	DICLOX	dicloxacillin (Dynapen)
	diabetes insipidus	DICP	demyelinated inflammatory chronic polyneuropathy
	diagnostic imaging		
	Disability Index		
	dorsal interossei	DICT	dose-intensive chemotherapy
	drug interactions		
D&I	debridement and irrigation	DID	death(s) from intercurrent disease
	dry and intact		
DIA	drug-induced agranulocytosis		delayed ischemia deficit
	drug-induced amenorrhea		dissociative identity disorder
	Drug Information Association		

	drug-induced disease		diplopia
di,di	dichorionic, diamniotic		distal interphalangeal
DIE	died in emergency department		drip infusion pyelogram drug-induced parkinsonism
	drug-induced esophagitis	DIP$_{ant}$	diphtheria antitoxin
DIED	died in emergency department	DIPC	dynamic infusion pharmacocavemosometry
DIEP	deep inferior epigastric perforator	DIPJ	distal interphalangeal joint
DIF	differentiation-inducing factor	DIR	directions
DIFF	differential blood count	DIRD	drug-induced renal disease
DIG	digoxin (this is a dangerous abbreviation)	DIS	Diagnostic Interview Schedule (questionnaire)
DIH	died in hospital		digital imaging spectrophotometer
DIHS	drug-induced hypersensitivity syndrome		dislocation
DIJOA	dominantly inherited juvenile optic atrophy	DISC	disabled infectious single cycle (virus)
DIL	daughter-in-law		dynamic integrated stabilization chair
	dilute		
	drug-induced lupus	disch.	discharge
	drug information leaflet	DISCUS	Dyskinesia Indentification System Condensed User Scale
DILC	dose-intensity limiting criterium		
DILD	diffuse infiltrative lung disease	DISH	diffuse idiopathic skeletal hyperostosis
	drug-induced liver disease	DISI	dorsal intercalated segmental (segment) instability
DILE	drug-induced lupus erythematosus		
DILS	drug-induced lupus syndrome	DISIDA	diisopropyl iminodiacetic acid
DIM	diminish	D$_5$ISOM	5% Dextrose and Isolyte M
D$_5$IMB	Ionosol MB with 5% dextrose injection	D$_5$ISOP	5% Dextrose and Isolyte P
DIMD	drug-induced movement disorders	DISR	drug-induced skin reactions
DIMOAD	diabetes insipidus, diabetes mellitus, optic atrophy, and deafness	DIST	distal
			distilled
DIMS	disorders of initiating and maintaining sleep	DIT	diiodotyrosine
			drug-induced thrombocytopenia
DIND	delayed ischemic neurologic deficit	DIU	death in utero
DIOS	distal ileal obstruction syndrome		diuretic(s)
		DIV	double-inlet ventricle
	distal intestinal obstruction syndrome	DIVA	digital intravenous angiography
DIP	desquamative interstitial pneumonia	Div ex	divergence excess
		DIVP	dilute intravenous Pitocin
	diphtheria toxoid vaccine	DJD	degenerative joint disease

D

DK	dark	DLNMP	date of last normal menstrual period
	diabetic ketoacidosis		
	diseased kidney	DLNs	distant lymph nodes
DKA	diabetic ketoacidosis	DLP	dislocation of patella
	didn't keep appointment		double-limb progression
DKB	deep knee bends	DLPD	diffuse lymphocytic poorly differentiated
DKC	double knee to chest		
	dyskeratosis congenita	DLPFC	dorsolateral prefrontal cortex
D-K-S	Damus-Kaye-Stansel (operation/procedure)	D5LR	dextrose 5% in lactated Ringer injection
DL	danger list		
	deciliter (dL)	DLROW	a test used in mental status examinations (patient is asked to spell WORLD backwards)
	diagnostic laparoscopy		
	direct laryngoscopy		
	drug level		
	dual lumen		
dL	deciliter (100 mL)	DLS	daily living skills
D_L	maximal diffusing capacity		digitalis-like substances
			dynamic light scattering
DLB	dementia with Lewy bodies	DLSC	double-lumen subclavian catheter
	direct laryngoscopy and bronchoscopy	DLST	drug-induced lymphocyte stimulation test
DLBCL	diffuse large B-cell lymphoma	DLT	dose-limiting toxicity
			double-lung transplant
DLBD	diffuse Lewy body disease	DLU	diffused lung uptake
DLBL	diffuse large B-cell lymphoma	DLV	delavirdine (Rescriptor)
		DLW	doubly labeled water
DLC	double lumen catheter	DM	dehydrated and malnourished
DLCL	diffuse large cell lymphoma		dermatomyositis
			dextromethorphan
DLCO sb	diffusion capacity of carbon monoxide, single breath		diabetes mellitus
			diabetic mother
			diastolic murmur
DLD	date of last drink		disease management
DLE	decrement-load exercise		
	discoid lupus erythematosus	DM-1	diabetes mellitus type 1
		DM-2	diabetes mellitus type 2
	disseminated lupus erythematosis	DMA	Director of Medical Affairs
DLF	digitalis-like factor	DMAC	disseminated *Mycobacterium avium* complex
	ductal lavage fluid		
DLI	donor leukocyte infusions	DMAD	disease-modifying antirheumatic drug
DLIF	digoxin-like immunoreactive factors	DMAE	dimethylaminoethanol
		DMAIC	disseminated *Mycobacterium avium-intracellulare* complex
DLIS	digoxin-like immunoreactive substance		
		DMARD	disease modifying antirheumatic drug
DLMP	date of last menstrual period	DMAS	Drug Management and Authorization Section
DLNG	dl-norgestrel		

DMAT	disaster medical assistance team	DM Isch	diaphragmatic myocardial ischemia
DMB	data monitoring board	DMKA	diabetes mellitus ketoacidosis
DMBA	dimethylbenzanthracene		
DMC	dactinomycin, methotrexate, and cyclophosphamide	DMN	dysplastic melanocytic nevus
		DMO	dimethadone
	diabetes management center	DMOADs	disease-modifying osteoarthritis drugs
DMD	Descemet membrane detachment	DMOOC	diabetes mellitus out of control
	disciform macular degeneration	DMORTs	Disaster Mortuary Operational Response Teams
	Doctor of Dental Medicine	DMP	data monitoring plan
	drowsiness monitoring device		dimethyl phthalate
		DMPA	depot-medroxypro-gesterone acetate
	Duchenne muscular dystrophy	DMPC	dimyristoylphosphatidyl choline
DMD w/ SRNM	disciform macular degeneration with subretinal neovascular membrane	DMPG	dimyristoylphosphatidyl glycerol
		DMPS	dimercaptopropane-sulfonic acid
DME	diabetic macular edema	D-MRI	dynamic magnetic resonance imaging
	Director of Medical Education	DMS	dimethylsulfide
	durable medical equipment	DMSA	succimer (dimercaptosuc-cinic acid; Chemet)
DMEC	data-monitoring and ethics committee	DMSO	dimethyl sulfoxide
DMEM	Dulbecco Modified Eagle Medium	DMT	dimethyltryptamine
		DMTU	dimethylthiourea
DMEPOS	durable medical equipment, prosthetics, orthotics, and supplies	DMV	disk, macula, and vessels
			Doctor of Veterinary Medicine
DMERC	Durable Medical Equipment Regional Carrier	DMVP	disk, macula, vessel, periphery
		DMX	diathermy, massage, and exercise
DMEs	drug-metabolizing enzymes	DN	denuded
			diabetic nephropathy
DMETS	Division of Medication Errors and Technical Support (FDA)		dicrotic notch
			down
			dysplastic nevus (nevi)
DMF	decayed, missing, or filled	D & N	distance and near (vision)
	dimethylformamide	DNA	deoxyribonucleic acid
	Drug Master File		did not answer
DMFS	decayed, missing, or filled surfaces		did not attend
			does not apply
DMH	Department of Mental Health	DNA ds	deoxyribonucleic acid double-stranded
DMI	desipramine (Norpramin)	DNA ss	deoxyribonucleic acid single-stranded
	diaphragmatic myocardial infarction		

D

DNCB	dinitrochlorobenzene	DOA	date of admission
DNC	did not come		dead on arrival
	dilatation and curettage		dominant optic atrophy
	(usually written as		driver of automobile
	D&C)		duration of action
DND	died a natural death	DOA-DRA	dead on arrival despite
DNE	diabetes nurse educator		resuscitative attempts
DNEPTE	did not exist prior to	DOB	dangle out of bed
	enlistment		date of birth
DNET	dysembryoplastic		Dobrava hantavirus
	neuroepithelial tumor		dobutamine
DNFC	does not follow		doctor's order book
	commands	DOC	date of conception
DNI	do not intubate		diabetes out of control
DNIC	diffuse noxious inhibitory		died of other causes
	control		diet of choice
DNIF	duties not including flying		docetaxel (Taxotere)
DNKA	did not keep appointment		drug of choice
DNN	did not nurse	DOCA	desoxycorticosterone
DNP	did not pay		acetate
	dinitrophenylhydrazine	DOCP	desoxycorticosterone
	do not publish		pivalate
DNR	daunorubicin	DOD	date of death
	did not respond		dead of disease
	do not report		Department of Defense
	do not resuscitate		drug overdose
	dorsal nerve root	DODD	demand oxygen delivery
DNS	deviated nasal septum		device
	Director of Nursing	DOE	date of examination
	Services		disease-oriented evidence
	doctor did not see patient		dyspnea on exertion
	do not show	DOES	disorders of excessive
	dysplastic nevus syndrome		somnolence
D₅ 1/4 NS	dextrose 5% in 1/4 normal	DOH	Department of Health
	saline (0.225% sodium	DOI	date of implant
	chloride) injection		(pacemaker)
D₅ 1/2NS	dextrose 5% in 0.45%		date of injury
	sodium chloride	DO₂I	oxygen delivery index
	injection	DOJ	Department of Justice
D₅NS	5% dextrose in normal	DOL	days of life
	saline (0.9% sodium	DOL #2	second day of life
	chloride) injection	DOLV	double-outlet left
DNT	did not test		ventricle
	dysembryoplastic	DOM	Doctor of Oriental
	neuroepithelial tumor		Medicine
DO	diet order		domiciliary
	dissolved oxygen		domiciliary care
	distocclusal	DOMS	delayed-onset muscle
	Doctor of Osteopathy		soreness
	doctor's order	DON	Director of Nursing
D/O	disorder		donepezil HCl (Aricept)
✓DO	check doctor's order	DOOC	diabetes out of control
DO₂	oxygen delivery	DOP	dopamine

DOPS	diffuse obstructive	
	pulmonary syndrome	
	dihydroxyphenylserine	
	Director of Pharmacy	
	Service(s)	
DOR	date of release	
DORV	double-outlet right	
	ventricle	
DORx	date of treatment	
DOS	date of surgery	
	dead on scene	
	doctor's order sheet	
DOSA	day of surgery admission	
DOSAK	Central Tumor Registry	
	operated by the	
	German-Austrian-Swiss	
	Association for Head	
	and Neck Tumors	
DOSS	docusate sodium (dioctyl	
	sodium sulfosuccinate)	
DOT	date of transcription	
	date of transfer	
	died on table	
	directly observed	
	therapy	
	Directory of Occupational	
	Titles	
	Doppler ophthalmic test	
DOTS	directly observed	
	treatment, short course	
DOV	date of visit	
	distribution of ventilation	
DOX	doxepin	
	doxorubicin (Adriamycin)	
doz	dozen	
DP	dental prosthesis	
	diastolic pressure	
	disability pension	
	discharge planning	
	dorsalis pedis (pulse)	
D/P	dialysate-to-plasma ratio	
DPA	Department of Public	
	Assistance	
	dipropylacetic acid	
	D-penicillamine	
	(penicillamine;	
	Cuprimine)	
	dual photon	
	absorptiometry	
	durable power of attorney	
DPAP	diastolic pulmonary artery	
	pressure	
DPB	days postburn	

D

	diffuse panbronchiolitis
DPBS	Dulbecco phosphate-buffered saline
DPC	delayed primary closure
	discharge planning coordinator
	distal palmar crease
DPCP	diphenylcyclopropenone (diphencyprone)
DPD	dihydropyrimidine dehydrogenase
DPDL	diffuse poorly differentiated lymphocytic lymphoma
2,3-DPG	2,3-diphosphoglyceric acid
DPH	Department of Public Health
	diphenhydramine (Benadryl)
	Doctor of Public Health
	phenytoin (diphenylhydantoin; Dilantin)
DPI	dietary protein intake
	Doppler perfusion index
	dry powder inhaler
DPIL	dextrose (percentage), protein (grams per kilogram) Intralipid® (grams per kilogram)
DPL	diagnostic peritoneal lavage
D5PLM	dextrose 5% and Plasmalyte M® injection
DPM	distintegrations per minute (dpm)
	Doctor of Podiatric Medicine
	drops per minute
DPN	^{11}C-diprenorphine
	deep peroneal nerve
	diabetic peripheral neuropathy
DPOA	durable power of attorney
DPOAE	distortion-product otoacoustic emission
DPOAHC	durable power of attorney for health care
DPP	dentine phosphoproteins
	dorsalis pedal pulse

	duration of positive pressure	DREAM	downstream regulatory element antagonistic modulator (gene)
DPPC	colfosceril palmitate (dipalmitoylphosphatidylcholine)	DRESS	depth resolved surface coil spectroscopy
DPR	Department of Professional Regulation		drug rash with eosinophilia and systemic symptoms
	diagnostic procedure room		
DPS	disintegration per second	DREZ	dorsal root entry zone
DPSS	Department of Public Social Service	DRG	diagnosis-related groups
			dorsal root ganglia
DPsy	Doctor of Psychology	DRGE	drainage
DPT	Demerol, Phenergan, and Thorazine (this is a dangerous abbreviation)	DRI	defibrillation response interval
			Dietary Reference Intakes
	diphtheria, pertussis, and tetanus (immunization)		Discharge Readiness Index
			dopamine reuptake inhibitor
	Driver Performance Test	DRIL	distal revascularization internal ligation
DPTPM	diphtheria, pertussis, tetanus, poliomyelitis, and measles	DRM	drug-related morbidity
DPU	delayed pressure urticaria	DRN	drug-related neutropenia
DPUD	duodenal peptic ulcer disease	DRP	data review plan
			drug-related problem
DPVSs	dilated perivascular spaces	DRPLA	dentatorubral-pallidolluysian atrophy
DPXA	dual-photon x-ray absorptiometry		
		DRR	drug regimen review
DQ	developmental quotients	DRS	designated record set
D/Q	deep quiet		Disability Rating Scale
D&Q	deep and quiet		disease-related symptoms
DQA	Data Quality Audit		Duane retraction syndrome
DQM	data quality manager	DRSG	dressing
DQOL	diabetes quality of life	DRSI	disease-related symptom improvement
DQOLS	Dermatology Quality of Life Scales	DRSP	drug-resistant *Streptococcus pneumoniae*
Dr	doctor		
DR	delivery room	DRT	drug-related thrombocytopenia
	diabetic retinopathy		
	diagnostic radiology	DrTPar	diphtheria toxoid (reduced antigen quantity for adults), tetanus toxoid, and acellular pertussis (reduced antigen quantity for adults) vaccine, for adult use
	dining room		
	diurnal rhythm		
	drug resistant		
DRA	distal rectal adenocarcinoma		
	drug-related admissions		
DRAPE	drug-related adverse patient event	DRUB	drug screen-blood
DRC	dose-response curve	DRUJ	distal or radial ulnar joint
DRE	digital rectal examination	dRVVT	diluted Russell viper venom time
	Drug Recognition Expert (for detection of impaired drivers)	DS	deep sleep
			Dextrostix®

	discharge summary	DSHS	Department of Social and Health Services
	disoriented		
	distant supervision	DSI	deep shock insulin
	double strength		Depression Status Inventory
	Down syndrome		
	drug screen	DSIAR	double-stapled ileoanal reservoir
D/S	5% dextrose and 0.9% sodium chloride (saline) injection	DSM	disease state management drink skim milk
D&S	diagnostic and surgical dilation and suction	DSM-IV	Diagnostic and Statistical Manual of Mental Disorders, 4th edition
D5S	dextrose 5% in 0.9% sodium chloride (saline) injection	dSMA	distal spinal muscular atrophy
D$_5$-1/2S	5% dextrose in 0.45% sodium chloride (saline) injection	DSMB	Data and Safety Management Board Data and Safety Monitoring Board
DSA	digital subtraction angiography (angiocardiography)	DSMO	Designated Standard Maintenance Organization
DSAP	disseminated superficial actinic porokeratosis	DSO	distal subungual onychomycosis
DSB	drug-seeking behavior	DSP	diabetic sensorimotor polyneuropathy
DSBs	double-strand (DNA) breaks		digital signal processor distal symmetrical polyneuropathy
DSC	differential scanning calorimeter		
	Down syndrome child	DSPC	distearoylphosphatidyl choline
	dynamic susceptibility contrast	DSPD	dangerous severe personality disorder
DSD	degenerative spinal disease	D-SPINE	dorsal spine
	detrusor sphincter dyssynergia	DSPN	distal symmetric polyneuropathy
	digital selenium drum (radiology)	DSPS	delayed sleep phase syndrome
	discharge summary dictated	DSRCT	desmoplastic small round cell tumor
	dry sterile dressing	DSRF	drainage subretinal fluid
DSDB	direct self-destructive behavior	DSS	dengue shock syndrome Department of Social Services
ds DNA	double-stranded desoxyribonucleic acid		Disability Status Scale discharge summary sheet
DSF	doxorubicin, streptozocin, and fluorouracil		disease-specific survival distal splenorenal shunt
DSG	desogestrel dressing		docusate sodium (dioctyl sodium sulfosuccinate)
DSG	deoxyspergualin	DSSLR	double, seated straight leg raise
DSHEA	Dietary Supplement Health and Education Act of 1994		
DSHR	delayed skin hypersensitivity reaction	DSSN	distal symmetric sensory neuropathy

D

121

DSSP	distal symmetric sensory polyneuropathy		direct-to-consumer (advertising)
DSST	Digit-Symbol Substitution Test		diticarb (diethyldiothio-carbamate)
DST	daylight saving time		tubocurarine (D-tubocurarine)
	dexamethasone suppression test	DTCA	direct-to-consumer advertising
	digit substitution test	DTD	diastropic dysplasia
	donor-specific (blood) transfusion	DTD #30	dispense 30 such doses
DSU	day stay unit	DTF	deep transverse friction
	day surgery unit	DTH	delayed-type hypersensitivity
DSUH	direct suggestion under hypnosis	DTI	diffusion-tensor imaging
D/Sum	discharge summary		Doppler tissue imaging
DSV	digital subtraction ventriculography	DTIC	dacarbazine (DTIC-Dome)
DSVP	Dietary Supplement Verification Program (United States Pharmacopeia Purity Compliance)	D TIME	dream time
		DTIs	direct thrombin inhibitors
		DTM	deep tissue massage
			dermatophyte test medium
DSW	Doctorate in Social Work	DTMS	drug therapy management service
DSWI	deep sternal wound infection	DTO	danger to others
	deep surgical wound infection		deodorized tincture of opium (warning: this is NOT paregoric)
DSX	dysmetabolic syndrome X	DTOGV	dextral-transposition of great vessels
DT	delirium tremens	DTP	differential time to positivity
	dietary thermogenesis		
	dietetic technician		diphtheria, tetanus toxoids, pertussis (antigens unspecified) vaccine
	diphtheria and tetanus toxoids, adsorbed, pediatric strength		
	discharge tomorrow		distal tingling on percussion (+Tinel sign)
	docetaxel (Taxotere)		
D/T	date/time	DTPA	pentetic acid (diethylenetriaminepen-taacetic acid)
	due to		
d/t	due to	DTPa	diphtheria, tetanus toxoids, acellular pertussis vaccine, for pediatric use
d4T	stavudine (Zerit)		
D & T	diagnosis and treatment		
	dictated and typed		
DTaP	diphtheria and tetanus toxoids with acellular pertussis vaccine	DTPa-HIB	diphtheria toxoid, tetanus toxoid, acellular pertussis, and Haemophilus influenzae type b conjugate vaccine
DTBC	tubocurarine (D-tubocurarine)		
DTBE	Division of Tuberculosis Elimination		
DTC	day treatment center		
	differentiated thyroid cancer		

DTPa-HIB-IPV	diphtheria toxoid, tetanus toxoid, acellular pertussis, *Haemophilus influenzae* type b conjugate, and poliovirus inactivated vaccine
DTP_w	diphtheria, tetanus toxoids, whole-cell pertussis vaccine
DTR	Dance Therapist, Registered
	deep tendon reflexes
	Dietetic Technician Registered
dtr	daughter
DTs	delirium tremens
DTS	danger to self
	donor specific transfusion
3D TSE	three-dimensional turbo-spin echo (images)
DTT	diphtheria tetanus toxoid
	dithiothreitol
DTUS	diathermy, traction, and ultrasound
DVG	double vein graft
DTV	due to void
DTVP	Developmental Test of Visual Perception
DTwP	diphtheria and tetanus toxoids with whole-cell pertussis vaccine
DTX	detoxification
DU	decubitus ulcer
	depleted uranium
	developmental unit
	diabetic urine
	diagnosis undetermined
	duodenal ulcer
	duroxide uptake
DUB	Dubowitz (score)
	dysfunctional uterine bleeding
DUBI	dysfunctional urinary bladder instability
DUD	dihydrouracil dehydrogenase
DUE	drug use evaluation
D&UE	dilation and uterine evacuation
DUF	Doppler ultrasonic flowmeter

DUI	driving under the influence
DUID	driving under the influence of drugs
DUII	driving under the influence of intoxicants
DUIL	driving under the influence of liquor
DUKM	dialysate urea kinetic modeling
DUM	drug use monitoring
DUN	dialysate urea nitrogen
DUNHL	diffuse undifferentiated non-Hodgkins lymphoma
DUO	Duotube®
DUR	drug utilization review
	duration
DUS	digital ultrasound
	distal urethral stenosis
	Doppler ultrasound stethoscope
	duplex ultrasonography
3DUS	three-dimensional ultrasound
DUSN	diffuse unilateral subacute neuroretinitis
DV	distance vision
	domestic violence
	double vision
D&V	diarrhea and vomiting
	disks and vessels
DVA	Department of Veterans Affairs
	directional vacuum-assisted (biopsy)
	distance visual acuity
	vindesine (Eldisine; desacetyl vinblastine amide sulfate)
DVAB	directional vacuum-assisted biopsy
DVC	direct visualization of vocal cords
D V® Cream	dienestrol vaginal cream
DVD	dissociated vertical deviation
	double-vessel disease
DVH	dose-volume histogram
DVI	atrioventricular sequential pacing

		DWDL	diffuse well-differentiated lymphocytic lymphoma
	digital vascular imaging		
	direct visual inspection		
DVIU	direct vision internal urethrotomy	DWI	diffusion-weighted (magnetic resonance) imaging
DVPX	divalproex sodium (Depakote)		driving while intoxicated
DVM	Doctor of Veterinary Medicine		driving while impaired
DVMP	disks, vessels, and macula periphery	DWI/PI	diffusion-weighted imaging/perfusion imaging
DVP	digital volume pulse	DWMRI	diffusion-weighted magnetic resonance imaging
DVPA	daunorubicin, vincristine, prednisone, and asparaginase		
DVR	Division of Vocational Rehabilitation	DWR	deep water running
	dose-volume relationship	DWRT	delayed work recall test
	double-valve replacement	DWSCL	daily-wear soft contact lens
DVSA	digital venous subtraction angiography	DWV	Dandy-Walker variant (a congenital anomaly)
DVT	deep vein thrombosis	DWW	dynamic wall walk
DVTS	deep venous thromboscintigram	Dx	diagnosis
			disease
DVVC	direct visualization of vocal cords	DXA	dual-energy x-ray absorptiometry
DW	daily weight	DXG	dioxalane guanine
	deionized water	DxLS	diagnosis responsible for length of stay
	detention warrant		
	dextrose in water	DXM	dexamethasone
	diffusion-weighted (imaging)		dextromethorphan
	distilled water	DXR	delayed xenograft rejection
	doing well	DXT	deep x-ray therapy
	double wrap	DXRT	deep x-ray therapy
D/W	dextrose in water	DXS	Dextrostix®
	discussed with	DY	dusky (infant color)
D-W	Dandy-Walker (deformity/malformation)		dysprosium
	Danis-Weber (classification for ankle fractures)	DYF	drag your feet (author's note: see you in court)
		DYFS	Division of Youth and Family Services
		DysD	dysthymic disorder
D₅W	5% dextrose (in water) injection	DYTRO	dynamic tone-reducing orthosis
D10W	10% dextrose (in water) injection	DZ	diazepam (valium)
			disease
D20W	20% dextrose (in water) injection		dizygotic
			dozen
D50W	50% dextrose (in water) injection	DZP	diazepam (Valium)
D70W	70% dextrose (in water) injection	DZT	dizygotic twins
5 DW	5% dextrose (in water) injection	DZX	dexrazoxane (Zinecard)

E

E	East (as in the location e.g., 2E, would be second floor, East wing)
	edema
	effective
	eloper
	enema
	engorged
	eosinophil
	Escherichia
	esophoria for distance
	ethambutol [part of tuberculosis regimen, see RHZ(E/S)/HR]
	evaluation
	evening
	expired
	eye
	methylenedioxy-methamphetamine (MDMA; Ecstasy)
E′	elbow
	esophoria for near
E_1	estrone
E_2	estradiol
E_3	estriol
4E	4 plus edema
E20	Enfamil 20®
E → A	say E,E,E, comes out as A,A,A upon auscultation of lung showing consolidation
EA	early amniocentesis
	elbow aspiration
	electroacoustic analysis
	electroacupuncture
	enteral alimentation
	epidural anesthesia
	episodic ataxia
	esophageal atresia
E/A	ratio of peak mitral early diastolic and atrial contraction velocity
	European-American
E&A	evaluate and advise
EAA	electrothermal atomic absorption
	essential amino acids
	extrinsic allergic alveolitis
EAB	elective abortion
	Ethical Advisory Board
EAC	erythema annulare centrifugum
	esophageal adenocarcinoma
	external auditory canal
EACA	aminocaproic acid (epsilon-aminocaproic acid)
	esophageal adenocarcinoma
EADL	extended activities of daily living
EADs	early after-depolarizations
EAE	experimental allergic encephalomyelitis
	experimental autoimmune encephalomyelitis
EAEC	enteroaggregative *Escherichia coli*
EAggEC	enteroaggregative *Escherichia coli*
EAHF	eczema, allergy, and hay fever
EAL	electronic artificial larynx
EAM	external auditory meatus
EAP	Early Access Program (premarketing use of drug)
	Employment (Employee) Assistance Programs
	erythrocyte acid phosphatase
	etoposide, doxorubicin (Adriamycin), and cisplatin (Platinol)
EAR	estimated average requirement
EARLIES	early decelerations
EART	extended abdominal radiation therapy
EAR OX	ear oximetry
EAS	external anal sphincter
EASC	endoscopic ambulatory surgery center
EAST	external rotation, abduction stress test
EAT	Eating Attitudes Test
	ectopic atrial tachycardia

E

EATL	enteropathy-associated T-cell lymphoma	EBRT	external beam radiation therapy
EAU	experimental autoimmune uveitis	EBS	empiric Bayesian screening epidermolysis bullosa simplex
EB	eosinophilic bronchitis epidermolysis bullosa Epstein-Barr (virus)	EBSB	equal breath sounds bilaterally
EBA	epidermolysis bullosa acquisita	EBT	electron beam tomography erythromycin breath test
EBB	electron beam boosts equal breath bilaterally	EBV	Epstein-Barr virus
EBBS	equal bilateral breath sounds	EBVCA	Epstein-Barr viral capsid antigen
EBC	early (stage) breast cancer endoscopic brush cytology esophageal balloon catheter	EBVEA	Epstein-Barr virus, early antigen
		EBVNA	Epstein-Barr virus, nuclear antigen
EBCPGs	evidence-based clinical practice guidelines	EC	ejection click electrical cardioversion electrocautery emergency contraception endocervical enteric coated *Escherichia coli* etopside and carboplatin European Community extracellular eye care eyes closed
EBCT	electron-beam computed tomography		
EBD	endocardial border delineation endoscopic balloon dilation evidence-based decision (making)		
EBE	equal bilateral expansion		
EBEA	Epstein-Barr (virus) early antigen	E₂C	estradiol cypionate
EBF	erythroblastosis fetalis	E & C	education and counseling
EBL	endoscopic band ligation estimated blood loss	ECA	enteric coated aspirin (tablets) Epidemiological Catchment Area ethacrynic acid external carotid artery
EBL-1	European bat lyssavirus 1		
EBLV	European bat lyssavirus		
EBM	evidence-based medicine expressed breast milk		
EBMT	European Bone Marrow Transplant (registry group)	ECAD	extracorporeal albumin dialysis
		e-CAM	electronic Compilation of Analytical Methods
EBNA	Epstein-Barr (virus) nuclear antigen	ECASA	enteric coated aspirin (tablets)
EBO	evidence-based outcomes	ECBD	exploration of common bile duct
EBOS	early-onset benign occipital seizure	ECBO	enterocytopathogenic bovine orphan (virus)
EBOV	Ebola virus	ECC	early childhood caries edema, clubbing, and cyanosis embryonal cell cancer emergency cardiac care Emergency Communications Center
EBO-Z	Ebola Zaire virus		
EBP	epidural blood patch		
EBR	external beam radiotherapy eye-blink rate		
EBRs	evidence-based recommendations		

E

	endocervical curettage	ECI	extracorporeal irradiation
	estimated creatinine clearance	ECIB	extracorporeal irradiation of blood
	external cardiac compression	ECIC	external carotid and internal carotid
	extracorporeal circulation		extracranial to intracranial (anastamosis)
ECCE	extracapsular cataract extraction	EC/IC	extracranial/intracranial
ECD	endocardial cushion defect	ECID	European Centre for Infectious Disease
	equivalent current dipole		
	Erdheim-Chester disease	ECK1	*Escherichia coli* K1
E-CD	E-cadherin	ECL	electrochemiluminescence
ECDB	encourage to cough and deep breathe		enterochromaffin-like
			extend of cerebral lesion
ECDC	European Centre for Disease Prevention and Control		extracapillary lesions
		ECLA	extracorporeal lung assist
		ECLP	extracorporeal liver perfusion
ECDPC	European Centre for Disease Prevention and Control (EDCD is used)		
		ECM	erythema chronicum migrans
ECE	endothelin-converting enzyme		esophagocardiomyotomy
			extracellular mass
	extracapsular extension		extracellular matrix
ECEMG	evoked compound electromyography	ECM/BCM	extracellular mass, body cell mass ratio
ECF	epirubicin, cisplatin, and fluorouracil	ECMO	enterocytopathogenic monkey orphan (virus)
	extended care facility		extracorporeal circulation membrane oxygenation (oxygenator)
	extracardiac Fontan (procedure)		
	extracellular fluid	ECN	extended care nursery
ECF-A	eosinophil chemotactic factors of anaphylaxis	ecNOS	endothelial constitutive nitric oxide synthetase
ECFV	extracellular fluid volume	ECochG	electrocochleography
ECG	electrocardiogram	ECOG	Eastern Cooperative Oncology Group
ECGE	extracorporeal gas exchange		
		ECoG	electrocochleography
ECHINO	echinocyte		electrocorticogram
ECHO	echocardiogram	E coli	*Escherichia coli*
	enterocytopathogenic human orphan (virus)	ECO$_{tox}$	*Escherichia coli* (heat-labile toxin) vaccine
	etoposide, cyclophosphamide, doxorubicin (hydroxydaunomycin), and vincristine (Oncovin)	ECP	emergency care provider
			emergency contraceptive pills
			eosinophil cationic protein
			extracorporeal photochemotherapy
ECHO (2D)	echocardiogram (2-dimensional)		extracorporeal photopheresis
EChoG	electrocochleography	ECPL	endocavitary pelvic lymphadenectomy
ECHO/ RV	echocardiography/ radionuclide ventriculography	ECPD	external counterpressure device

ECPP	extracorporeal photopheresis	EDAS	encephalodural arteriosynangiosis
ECR	emergency chemical restraint	EDAT	Emergency Department Alert Team
	extensor carpi radialis	EDAX	energy-dispersive analysis of x-rays
ECRB	extensor carpi radialis brevis	EDB	ethylene dibromide
ECRL	extensor carpi radialis longus		extensor digitorum brevis
ECS	elective cosmetic surgery	EDC	effective dynamic compliance
	electrocerebral silence		electrodesiccation and curettage
	endometrial-cancer-specific		
ECT	electroconvulsive therapy		end diastolic counts
	emission computed tomography		estimated date of conception
	enhanced computed tomography		estimated date of confinement
ECTb	Emory Cardiac Toolbox		estramustine, docetaxel, and carboplatin
ECTR	endoscopic carpal tunnel release		extensor digitorum communis
ECU	electrocautery unit	EDCF	endothelium-derived constricting factor
	emergency care unit		
	emotional care units	EDCP	eccentric dynamic compression plates
	environmental control unit		
	extensor carpi ulnaris	EDCTP	European and Developing Countries Clinical Trials Partnership
ECV	emergency center visits		
	external cephalic version (obstetrics)		
		EDD	endothelium-dependent dilation
ECVD	extracellular volume depletion		esophageal detector device
ECVE	extracellular volume expansion		expected date of delivery
ECW	extracellular water	EdD	Doctor of Education
ED	eating disorder(s)	EDENT	edentulous
	education	EDF	elongation, derotation, and flexion
	effective dose		
	elbow disarticulation	EDH	epidural hematoma
	emergency department		extradural hematoma
	emotional disorder	EDHF	endothelium-derived hyperpolarizing factor
	epidural		
	erectile dysfunction	EDI	Eating Disorders Inventory
	ethynodiol diacetate		
	every day (this is a dangerous abbreviation)		electrodeionization
		EDITAR	extended-duration topical arthropod repellent
	extensive disease		
	extensor digitorum	EDL	extensor digitorum longus
ED_{50}	median effective dose	ED/LD	emotionally disturbed and learning disabled
EDA	elbow disarticulation		
EDAM	edatrexate	EDLF	endogenous digitalis-like factors
EDAP	Emergency Department Approved for Pediatrics		
		EDLS	endogenous digitalis-like substance
	etoposide, dexamethasone, cytarabine, (Ara-C and cisplatin (Platinol AQ)	EDM	early diastolic murmur

	esophageal Doppler monitor		expressed emotion external ear
	extensor digiti minimi	E & E	eyes and ears
EDMD-AD	autosomal dominate Emery-Dreifuss muscular dystrophy	EEA	electroencephalic audiometry elemental enteral
EDNO	endothelium-related nitric oxide		alimentation end-to-end anastomosis
ED-OU	emergency department/observation unit		energy expended with activity
EDP	emergency department physician	EEC	ectrodactyly-ectodermal dysplasia (cleft syndrome)
EDQ	end-diastolic pressure extensor digiti quinti (tendon)		endogenous erythroid colony
EDQM	European Directorate for the Quality of Medicines	EECP	enhanced external counter-pulsation
EDQV	extensor digiti quinti five	EEE	eastern equine encephalomyelitis
EDR	edrophonium (Tensilon) escalating dose regimen extreme drug resistance		edema, erythema, and exudate external eye examination
EDRF	endothelium derived relaxing factor (nitric oxide)	EEG EELS	electroencephalogram electron energy loss spectrometry
EDS	Ehlers-Danlos syndrome excessive daytime somnolence	EEN EENT	estimated energy needs eyes, ears, nose, and throat
EDSS	Expanded Disability Status Scale (Score)	EEP EER	end expiratory pressure extended endocardial resection
EDT	exposure duration threshold	EES®	erythromycin ethylsuccinate
EDTA	edetic acid (ethylenedi-aminetetraacetic acid)	EET EEV	early exercise testing encircling endocardial ventriculotomy
EDTU	emergency diagnostic and treatment unit	EF	eccentric fixation ejection fraction
EDU	eating disorder unit		endurance factor
EDV	end-diastolic volume epidermal dysplastic verruciformis		erythroblastosis fetalis extended-field (radiotherapy)
EDW	estimated dry weight		
EDX	edatrexate	EFA	essential fatty acid
EDXRF	energy-dispersive x-ray fluorescence	EFAD	essential fatty acid deficiency
EE	emetic episodes end to end	E-FAP	Emory Functional Ambulation Profile
	energy expenditure	EFBW	estimate fetal body weight
	equine encephalitis	EFD	episode free day
	erosive esophagitis	EFE	endocardial fibroelastosis
	esophageal endoscopy ethinyl estradiol		epidemic fatal encephalopathy
	exchange efficiency (units)	EFF	effacement

EFI	extended-field irradiation	EH	eccentric hypertrophy
EFR	effective filtration rate		educationally handicapped
EFS	event-free survival		enlarged heart
EFHBM	eosinophilic		essential hypertension
	fibrohistiocytic lesion		extramedullary
	of bone marrow		hematopoiesis
EFM	electronic fetal	Eh	*Entamoeba histolytica*
	monitor(ing)	EHB	elevate head of bed
	external fetal monitoring		extensor hallucis brevis
EFMM	external fetal maternal	EHBA	extrahepatic biliary
	monitor		atresia
EFMT	electric field mediated	EHBF	extrahepatic blood flow
	transfer	EHC	enterohepatic circulation
EFN	effusion	EHD	electronic home
EEPIA	European Federation of		detention
	Pharmaceutical	EHDA	etidronate sodium
	Industries and	EHDP	etidronate disodium
	Associations		(Didronel)
EFV	efavirenz (Sustiva)	EHE	epithelioid
EFW	estimated fetal weight		hemangioendothelioma
EF/WM	ejection fraction/wall	EHEC	enterohemorrhagic
	motion		*Escherichia coli*
e.g.	for example	EHF	epidemic hemorrhagic
EGA	esophageal gastric (tube)		fever
	airway		extremely high frequency
	estimated gestational age	EHH	episodic hypothermia with
EGB	endoscopic grasp biopsy		hyperhidrosis
EGb	extract of *Ginkgo biloba*		esophageal hiatal hernia
EGBUS	external genitalia,	EHI	exertional heat illness
	Bartholin, urethral, and	EHL	electrohydraulic
	Skene glands		lithotripsy
EGC	early gastric carcinoma		extensor hallucis longus
EGCG	epigallocatechin gallate	EHN	ethotoin
EGFR	epidermal growth factor	EHO	extrahepatic obstruction
	receptor	EHPH	extrahepatic portal
EGD	esophagogastroduodeno-		hypertension
	scopy	EHR	electronic health record
EGDT	esophagogastric	2EHRZ/	daily ethambutol,
	devascularization and	6HE	isoniazid, rifampicin,
	transection		and pyrazinamide for 2
EGF	epidermal growth factor		months, followed by
EGF-R	epidermal growth factor		isoniazid and
	receptor		ethambutol for 6
EGG	electrogastrography		months
EGJ	esophagogastric junction	2[EHRZ]₃/	the same as 2EHRZ/6HE
EGL	eosinophilic granuloma of	6HE	but given three times
	the lung		weekly in the initial
EGS	ethylene glycol succinate		intensive phase
EGSs	external guide sequences	2EHRZ/	The same as 2EHRZ/6HE,
EGTA	esophageal gastric tube	4HR	followed by 4 months
	airway		of daily isoniazid and
	ethyleneglycoltetracetic		rifampicin
	acid	EHS	employee health service

E

	exertional heat stroke	EISR	expanded international
EHT	electrohydrothermosation		search report
	essential hypertension	EITB	enzyme-linked immuno-
EI	environmental illness		electrotransfer blot
	enzyme immunoassay	EIV	external iliac vein
	extensor indicis	EJ	ejection
E/I	expiratory to inspiratory		elbow jerk
	(ratio)		external jugular
E & I	endocrine and infertility	EJB	ectopic junctional beat
EIA	enzyme immunoassay	EJN	extended jaundice of
	exercise-induced asthma		newborn
EIAB	extracranial-intracranial	EJP	excitatory junction
	arterial bypass		potential
EIAC	enzyme-inducing	EJV	external jugular vein
	anticonvulsants	EK	Ektachem 400 (see page
EIAD	extended-interval		392)
	aminoglycoside dosing		erythrokinase
EIAV	equine infectious anemia	EKC	epidemic
	virus		keratoconjunctivitis
EIB	exercise-induced	EKG	electrocardiogram
	bronchospasm	EKO	echoencephalogram
EIC	early ischemic	EKY	electrokymogram
	change(s)	EL	exercise limit
	electrical impedance		exploratory laparotomy
	cardiography	E-L	external lids
	endometrial intraepithelial	ELA	Establishment License
	carcinoma		Application
	epidermal inclusion cyst	ELAD	extracorporeal liver-assist
	extensive intraductal		device
	component	ELAFF	extended lateral arm free
EICA	extra-intracranial artery		flap
	(bypass)	ELAM	endothelial leukocyte
EID	electroimmunodiffusion		adhesion molecule
	electronic infusion device	ELAMS	Electronic Laboratory
EIDC	extreme intervertebral		Animal Monitoring
	disk collapse		System
EIEC	enteroinvasive	ELB	early light breakfast
	Escherichia coli		elbow
EIL	elective induction of labor	ELBW	extremely low birth weight
eIND	Electronic Investigational		(less than 1000 g)
	New Drug (application)	ELC	earlobe creases
EIOA	excessive intake of	ELCA	excimer laser coronary
	alcohol		angioplasty
EIP	elective interruption of	ELD	end-of-life decision
	pregnancy	ELDU	extralabel drug use
	end-inspiratory pressure	ELEC	elective
	extensor indicis proprius	ELF	elective low forceps
eIPV	enhanced inactivated		endoscopic laser
	polio vaccine		foraminotomy
EIR	entomological inoculation		epithelial lining fluid
	rate		etoposide, leucovorin, and
EIS	endoscopic injection		fluorouracil
	scleropathy		extremely low frequency

ELFA	enzyme-linked fluorescent immunoassay		erythema migrans
			erythema multiforme
ELG	endolumenal		erythromelalgia
	gastroplication		esophageal manometry
	endoluminal graft		estramustine (Emcyt)
ELH	endolymphatic hydrops		extensive metabolizers
ELI	endomyocardial		external monitor
	lymphocytic infiltrates	E & M	Evaluation and
ELIG	eligible		Management (coding
ELISA	enzyme-linked		system)
	immunosorbent assay	EMA	early morning awakening
ELISPOT	enzyme-linked immunospot		endomysial antibody
ELITT	endometrial laser	EMA-CO	etoposide, methotrexate,
	intrauterine thermal		dactinomycin
	therapy		(actinomycin-D),
Elix	elixir		cyclophosphamide,
ELLIP	ellipotocytosis		and vincristine
ELM	epiluminescent		(Oncovin)
	microscopy	EMB	endometrial biopsy
	external laryngeal		endomyocardial biopsy
	manipulation		eosin-methylene blue
ELND	elective lymph node		(agar)
	dissection		ethambutol (Myambutol)
ELOP	estimated length of		Explanation of Medicare
	program		Benefits
ELOS	estimated length of stay	EMBx	endomyocardial biopsy
ELP	electrophoresis	EMC	encephalomyocarditis
	eruptive lingual papillitis		endometrial currettage
ELPS	excessive lateral pressure		essential mixed
	syndrome		cryoglobulinemia
ELR	elevating leg rests		extraskeletal myxoid
	(wheelchair description)		chondrosarcoma
ELS	Eaton-Lambert syndrome	EMD	electromechanical
	endolymphatic sac		dissociation
ELSD	evaporative light	EMDA	electromotive drug
	scattering detection		administration
ELSI	ethical, legal, and social	EMDR	eye movement
	implications		desensitization and
ELSS	emergency life support		reprocessing
	system	EME	extreme medical
ELT	endoscopic laser therapy		emergency
	euglobulin lysis time	EMEA	European Medicines
ELTR	European Liver Transplant		Evaluation Agency
	Registry	EMF	elective midforceps
ELVIS™	Enzyme-Linked Virus		electromagnetic field(s)
	Inducible System		electromagnetic flow
EM	early memory		electromotive forces
	ejection murmur		endomyocardial fibrosis
	electron microscope		erythrocyte maturation
	emergency medicine		factor
	emmetropia		evaporated milk formula
	eosinophilia-myalgia	EMG	electromyograph
	(syndrome)		emergency

132

	essential monoclonal gammopathy	EMSA	electrophoretic mobility shift assay
EMI	educably mentally impaired	EMSU	early morning specimen of urine
	elderly and mentally infirm	EMT	emergency medical technician
	electromagnetic interference		epithelial-mesenchymal transformation
EMIC	emergency maternity and infant care		estramustine (Emcyt)
E-MICR	electron microscopy	EMTA	Emergency Medical Technician, Advanced
EMIT	enzyme-multiplied immunoassay technique (test)	EMTALA	Emergency Medical Treatment and Labor Act
EML	essential medicines lists (World Health Organization)	EMTC	emergency medical trauma center
EMLA®	eutectic mixture of local anesthetics (lidocaine and prilocaine in an emulsion base)	EMT-D	emergency medical technician-defibrillation
		EMTP	Emergency Medical Technician, Paramedic
EMLB	erythromycin lactobionate	EMU	early morning urine
EMMA	eye-movement measuring apparatus		electromagnetic unit
			epilepsy monitoring unit
EMMV	extended mandatory minute ventilation	EMV	equine morbilli virus
			eye, motor, verbal (grading for Glasgow Coma Scale)
EMo	ear mold		
EMP	electromolecular propulsion	EMVC	early mitral valve closure
	estramustine phosphate (Emcyt)	EMW	electromagnetic waves
		EMZL	extranodal marginal-zone (B-cell) lymphoma
EMPD	extramammary Paget disease	EN	enema
EMPI	enterprise master patient index		enteral nutrition
			erythema nodosum
EMR	educable mentally retarded	E/N	eggnog
	electrical muscle stimulation	E 50% N	extension 50% of normal
		ENA	extractable nuclear antigen
	electronic medical record	ENB	esthesioneuroblastoma
	emergency mechanical restraint	ENC	encourage
	empty, measure, and record	eNDA	Electronic New Drug Application
	endoscopic mucosal resection	ENDO	endodontia
			endodontics
	eye-movement recording		endoscopy
EMS	early morning specimen		endotracheal
	early morning stiffness	EndoCAB	plasma antiendotoxin core antibody
	electrical muscle stimulation	ENF	Enfamil
		ENF c Fe	Enfamil with iron
	emergency medical services	ENG	electronystagmogram
	eosinophilia myalgia syndrome		engorged
		ENL	enlarged

E

	erythema nodosum leprosum	EOFAD	early-onset form of familial Alzheimer disease
ENMG	electroneuromyography		
ENMT	ears, nose, mouth, and throat	E of I	evidence of insurability
		EOG	electro-oculogram
ENOG	electroneurography		electro-olfactogram
eNOS	endothelial nitric oxide synthase		Ethrane, oxygen, and gas (nitrous oxide)
ENP	extractable nucleoprotein	EOGBS	early-onset group B streptococcal (sepsis)
ENS	exogenous natural surfactant	EOL	end of file
ENT	ears, nose, throat	EOLC	end-of-life-care
ENTIS	European Network of Teratology Information Services	EOM	error of measurement external otitis media extraocular movement extraocular muscles
ENTV	enzootic nasal tumor virus		
ENVD	elevated new vessels on the disk	EOMB	explanation of Medicare benefits
ENVE	elevated new vessels elsewhere	EOMG	early-onset myasthenia gravis
ENVT	environment	EOMI	extraocular muscles intact
EO	elbow orthosis embolic occlusion	EOO	external oculomotor ophthalmoplegia
	eosinophilia	EOP1	end-of-phase 1
	ethylene oxide	EOP2	end-of-phase 2
	eyes open	EOR	emergency operating room
E & O	errors and omissions		
EOA	erosive osteoarthritis		end of range
	esophageal obturator airway	EORA	elderly onset rheumatoid arthritis
	examine, opinion, and advice	EORTC	European Organization for Research of the Treatment of Cancer
	external oblique aponeurosis	EOS	end of study
EOAE	evoked otoacoustic emissions		eosinophil
		EP	ectopic pregnancy
EOB	edge of bed		electrophysiologic
	end of bed		elopement precaution
	explanation of benefits		endogenous pyrogen
EOC	Emergency Operations Center		Episcopalian esophageal pressure
	enema of choice		etoposide and cisplatin (Platinol AQ)
	epithelial ovarian cancer		
EOD	early-onset disease		evoked potentials
	end of day	E&P	estrogen and progesterone
	end organ damage	EPA	eicosapentaenoic acid
	every other day (this is a dangerous abbreviation)		Environmental Protection Agency
	extent of disease	EPAB	extracorporeal pneumoperititoneal access bubble
EOE	Equal Opportunity Employer		
	extraosseous Ewing sarcoma	E-Panel	electrolyte panel (See page 392)

EPAP	expiratory positive airway pressure	EPN	emphysematous pyelonephritis
EPB	extensor pollicis brevis		estimated protein needs
EPBD	endoscopic papillary balloon dilatation	EPO	epoetin alfa (erythropoietin; Epogen)
EPC	erosive prephloric changes		evening primrose oil
	external pneumatic compression		exclusive provider organization
EPCV	engineering, procurement, construction, and validation	EPOCH	etoposide, prednisone, vincristine (Oncovin), cyclophosphamide,
EPD	electrode placement device		doxorubicin (hydroxydaunorubicin)
	equilibrium peritoneal dialysis	EPP	erythropoietic protoporphyria
EPEC	enteropathogenic *Escherichia coli*		extrapleural pneumonectomy
EPEG	etoposide (VePesid)	EPPK	epidermolytic palmoplantar keratoderma
EPEs	extrapyramidal effects		
EPF	Enfamil Premature Formula®	EPPROM	extremely preterm premature rupture of the membranes (less
EPG	electronic pupillography		than or equal to 24 weeks)
	Episodic Payment Group		
EPHI	electronic protected health information	EPQ	Exercise Participation Questionnaire
EPI	echoplanar imaging	EPQ-R	Eysenck Personality Questionnaire—Revised
	epinephrine		
	epirubicin (Ellence)	EPR	electronic prescription record
	epitheloid cells		
	exercise pressure index		electron paramagnetic (spin) resonance
	exocrine pancreatic insufficiency		
	Expanded Program of Immunizations, (World Health Organization)		electrophrenic respiration
			emergency physical restraint
	Eysenck Personality Inventory		epirubicin (Ellence)
EPIC	etoposide, prednisolone, ifosfamide, and cisplatin		estimated protein requirement
EPID	epidural	EPS	electrolyte-polyethyleneglycol solution
epiDX	epirubicin (4'-epidoxorubicin; Ellence)		
EPIG	epigastric		electrophysiologic study
EPIS	epileptic postictal sleep		expressed prostatic secretions
	episiotomy		extrapulmonary shunt
epith.	epithelial		extrapyramidal syndrome (symptom)
EPL	effective patent life		
	extensor pollicis longus (tendon)	EPSA	evoked potential signal averaging
EPM	electronic pacemaker	EPSCCA	extrapulmonary small cell carcinoma
EPMR	electronic patient medical record		

E

EPSDT	early periodic screening, diagnosis, and treatment
EPSE	extrapyramidal side effects
EPSP	excitatory postsynaptic potential
EPSS	E point septal separation
EPT	electroporation therapy
	endpoint temperature
EPT®	early pregnancy test
EPTE	existed prior to enlistment
EPTS	existed prior to service
EQC	equivalent quality control
ER	emergency room
	end range
	estrogen receptors
	extended release
	extended external rotation
	external resistance
E & R	equal and reactive
	examination and report
ER+	estrogen receptor-positive
ER−	estrogen receptor-negative
ERA	estrogen receptor assay
	evoked response audiometry
%ERAD	eradication rates
ERAS	Electronic Residency Application Service
erbB1	estrogen receptor (tyrosine kinase family) type B1
ERBD	endoscopic retrograde biliary drainage
ER by ICA	estrogen receptor immunocytochemistry assay
ERC	endoscopic retrograde cholangiography
ERCP	endoscopic retrograde cholangiopancreatography
ERCT	emergency room computerized tomography
ERD	early retirement with disability
ERE	external rotation in extension
ERF	external rotation in flexion
ERFC	erythrocyte rosette forming cells
ERG	electroretinogram
ERI	elective replacement indicator

ERIG	equine-rabies immune globulin
ERL	effective refractory length
ERLND	elective regional lymph node dissection
ERM	epiretinal membrane
ERMS	exacerbating-remitting multiple sclerosis
ERNA	equilibrium radionuclide angiocardiography
ERP	effective refractory period
	emergency room physician
	endocardial resection procedure
	endoscopic retrograde pancreatography
	event-related potentials
	estrogen receptor protein
	exposure and ritual prevention
ERPF	effective renal plasma flow
ER/PR	estrogen receptor/ progesterone receptor
ERS	endoscopic retrograde sphincterotomy
	evacuation of retained secundines (afterbirth)
ERSR	Electronic Regulatory Submission and Review
ERT	estrogen replacement therapy
	external radiotherapy
ERTD	emergency room triage documentation
ERUS	endorectal ultrasound
ERV	early revascularization
	expiratory reserve volume
e-Rx	electronic prescription
Er:YAG	Erbium: yttrium aluminum garnet (laser)
ERYTH	erythromycin
ES	electrical stimulation
	Eleutherococcus senticosus (Siberian Ginseng)
	embryonic stem (cells)
	emergency service
	endoscopic sclerotherapy
	endoscopic sphincterotomy

136

	end-to-side	ESLD	end-stage liver disease
	Ewing sarcoma		end-stage lung disease
	ex-smoker	ESM	ejection systolic murmur
	extra strength		endolymphatic stromal
ESA	early systolic acceleration		myosis
	end-to-side anastomosis		ethosuximide (Zarontin)
	ethmoid sinus	ESN	educationally subnormal
	adenocarcinoma	ESN(M)	educationally subnormal-
ESADDI	estimated safe and		moderate
	adequate daily dietary	ESN(S)	educationally subnormal-
	intake		severe
ESAP	evoked sensory (nerve)	ESO	esophagus
	action potential		esotropia
ESAS	Edmonton System	ESO/D	esotropia at distance
	Assessment System	ESO/N	estropia at near
ESAT	extrasystolic atrial	ESP	endometritis, salpingitis,
	tachycardia		and peritonitis
ESBL	extended-spectrum beta-		end-systolic pressure
	lactamases		especially
ESBLKP	extended-spectrum beta-		extrasensory perception
	lactamase-producing	ESPAC	European Study Group for
	Klebsiella pneumoniae		Pancreatic Cancers
ESC	embryonic stem cells	ES/PNET	Ewing sarcomas and
	end systolic counts		peripheral
ESCC	esophageal squamous cell		neuroectodermal tumor
	carcinoma	ESR	early sheath removal
ESCOP	European Scientific		erythrocyte sedimentation
	Cooperative on		rate
	Phytotherapy	ESRD	end-stage renal disease
ESCS	electrical spinal cord	ESRF	end-stage renal failure
	stimulation	ESRS	Extrapyramidal Symptom
ESD	Emergency Services		Rating Scale
	Department	ESS	emotional, spiritual, and
	esophagus, stomach, and		social
	duodenum		endometrial stromal
ESE	exon splice enhancer		sarcoma
ESF	external skeletal fixation		endoscopic sinus surgery
ESFT	Ewing sarcoma family of		Epworth Sleepiness Scale
	tumors		essential
ESHAP	etoposide, methylpredniso-		euthyroid sick syndrome
	lone (Solu-Medrol),	EST	Eastern Standard Time
	high-dose cytarabine		endoscopic spincterotomy
	(ara-C), and cisplatin		electroshock therapy
	(Platinol AQ)		electrostimulation therapy
ESI	electrospray ionization		established patient
	epidural steroid injection		estimated
ESI-MS	electrospray ionization-		exercise stress test
	mass spectrometry		expressed sequence tag
ESIN	elastic stable	E-stim	electrical stimulation
	intramedullary nailing	ESTs	expressed sequence tags
ESKD	end-stage kidney disease	ESU	electrosurgical unit
ESL	English as a second	ESWL	extracorporeal shock
	language		wave lithotripsy

ESWT	extracorporeal shockwave therapy		eustachian tube dysfunction
ET	ejection time		eye-tracking dysfunction
	embryo transfer	ETDLA	esophageal-tracheal double lumen airway
	endometrial thickness		
	endothelin	ETE	end-to-end
	endotoxin	ETEC	enterotoxigenic *Escherichia coli*
	endotracheal		
	endotracheal tube	ETF	eustachian tubal function
	enterostomal therapy (therapist)		
		ETFN	empiric therapy in a febrile neutropenic (patient)
	epirubicin and paclitaxel (Taxol)		
	esotropia	ETG	Episodic Treatment Group
	essential thrombocythemia	ETGT	equal to or greater than
	essential tremor	ETH	elixir terpin hydrate
	eustachian tube		ethanol
	Ewing tumor		Ethrane
	exchange transfusion	ETHc̄C	elixir terpin hydrate with codeine
	exercise treadmill		
	exposure time	ETI	ejective time index
et	and		endotracheal intubation
ET′	esotropia at near	ETKTM	every test known to man
E(T)	intermittent esotropia at infinity		
		ETL	echo train length (radiology)
E(T′)	intermittent esotropia at near		
		ETLE	extratemporal lobe epilepsy
ET-1	endothelin-1		
ET @ 20′	esotropia at 6 meters (infinity)	ETLT	equal to or less than
		ETO	estimated time of ovulation
ETA	endotracheal airway		
	ethionamide (Trecator-SC)		ethylene oxide
ETAC	early treatment of the allergic child		etoposide (VePesid)
			eustachian tube obstruction
et al	and others		
ETBD	etiology to be determined	EtOH	alcohol (ethyl alcohol)
ETC	and so forth		alcoholic
	electrothermal capsulorrhaphy	ETOP	elective termination of pregnancy
	Emergency and Trauma Center	ETP	elective termination of pregnancy
	endoscopic tissue culture	ETS	elevated toilet seat
	epirubicin, paclitaxel (Taxol), and cyclophosphamide		endoscopic transthoracic sympathectomy
			endotracheal suction
	estimated time of conception		end-to-side
			environmental tobacco smoke
ETCH-C	Evaluation Tool of Children's Handwriting-Cursive		
			erythromycin topical solution
ETCO$_2$	end-tidal carbon dioxide	ETT	endotracheal tube
ETD	endoscopic transforma-tional diskectomy		endurance treadmill test
			esophageal transit time

E

138

	exercise tolerance test	eval	evaluate
	exercise treadmill test (time)	EVAR	endovascular aneurysm repair
	extrathyroidal thyroxine	EVC	Ellis-van Creveld (syndrome)
ETT-Tl	exercise treadmill test with thallium	EVG	endovascular grafting
ETU	emergency and trauma unit	EWB	emotional well-being
	emergency treatment unit	EWBH	extracorporeal whole body hyperthermia
ETX	edatrexate	EXC	excision
ETYA	eicosatetraynoic acid	EVD	external ventricular (ventriculostomy) drain
EU	Ehrlich units		
	endotoxin units		
	equivalent units	EVE	endoscopic vascular examination
	esophageal ulcer		
	etiology unknown		evening
	European Union	EVER	eversion
	excretory urography	EVG	endovascular grafting
EUA	examine under anesthesia	EVH	endoscopic (saphenous) vein harvesting
EUCD	emotionally unstable character disorder		
EUD	external urinary device	EVI	Exposure to Violence Interview
EUG	extrauterine gestation		
EUL	extra uterine life	EVL	endoscopic variceal ligation
EUM	external urethral meatus		
EUP	Experimental Use Permit	EVS	endoscopic variceal sclerosis
	extrauterine pregnancy	EW	expiratory wheeze
EUS	endoscopic ultrasonography		elsewhere
	esophageal ultrasound	EWB	estrogen withdrawal bleeding
	external urethral sphincter	EWCL	extended-wear contact lens
EUS-FNA	endoscopic ultrasonography with fine-needle aspiration	EWE	Eastern and Western encephalomyelitis vaccine
EUTH	euthanasia		
EV	epidermodysplasia verruciformis	EWHO	elbow-wrist-hand orthosis
	esophageal varices	EWL	estimated weight loss
	etoposide and vincristine		
	eversion	EWS	Early Warning Score
eV	electron volt (unit of radiation energy)		Ewing sarcoma
		EWSCLs	extended-wear soft contact lenses
EV71	enterovirus-71		
EVA	Entry and Validation Application	EWT	erupted wisdom teeth
		ex	examined
	ethylene vinyl acetate		example
	etoposide, vinblastine, and doxorubicin (Adriamycin)		excision
			exercise
		exam.	examination
EVAC	evacuation	EXE	exemestane (Aromasin)
EVAc	ethylene-vinyl acetate copolymer	EXEC 22	Executive 22 chemistry profile (see page 392)

E

EXECHO	exercise echocardiography
EXEF	exercise ejection fraction
EXGBUS	external genitalia, Bartholin (glands), urethral (glands), and Skene (glands)
EXH VT	exhaled tidal volume
EXIT	Ex-Utero Intrapartum Treatment
EXIT 25	Executive Interview (cognitive impairment test)
EXL	elixir
EXOPH	exophthalmos
EXP	experienced
	expired
	exploration
	expose
expect	expectorant
exp. lap.	exploratory laparotomy
EXT	extension
	extensor (tendon)
	external
	extract
	extraction
	extremities
	extremity
Ext mon	external monitor
extrav	extravasation
ext. rot.	external rotation
EXTUB	extubation
EX U	excretory urogram
EZ	Edmonston-Zagreb (vaccine)
EZ-HT	Edmonston-Zagreb high-titer (vaccine)

F

F	facial
	Fahrenheit
	fair
	false
	fasting
	father
	feces
	female
	finger
	firm
	flow
	fluoride
	French
	Friday
	fundi
	fundus
F/	full upper denture
/F	full lower denture
(F)	final
°F	degrees Fahrenheit
F=	firm and equal
F_1	offspring from the first generation
F_2	offspring from the second generation
F_3	Fluothane
14 F	14-hour fast required
F II-F XIII	factor 2 through 13
FA	Fanconi anemia
	fatty acid
	femoral artery
	fetus active
	fibroadenoma
	first aid
	fludarabine (Fludara)
	fluorescein angiogram
	fluorescent antibody
	folic acid
	forearm
	Friedreich ataxia
	functional activities
FAA	febrile antigen agglutination
	folic acid antagonist
FAAD	Fellow American Academy of Dermatology
FAAH	fatty acid amide hydrolase

E

FAAN	Food Allergy and Anaphylaxis Network	FACEP	Fellow of the American College of Emergency Physicians
FAAP	family assessment adjustment pass	FACES	pain scale for assessing pain intensity
FAA SOL	formalin, acetic, and alcohol solution	FACG	Fellow of the American College of Gastroenterology
FAAN	Fellow of the American Academy of Nursing	FACH	forceps to after-coming head
FAAP	Fellow of the American Academy of Pediatrics	FACIT-F	Functional Assessment of Chronic Illness Therapy Fatigue Subscale
FAB	digoxin immune Fab (Digibind)	FACLM	Fellow of the American College of Legal Medicine
	French-American-British Cooperative group	FACN	Fellow of the American College of Nutrition
	functional arm brace		
FABER	flexion, abduction, and external rotation	FACNP	Fellow of the American College of Neuropsychopharma-cology
FABF	femoral artery blood flow		
FAC	ferrite ammonium citrate		
	fluorouracil, doxorubicin (Adriamycin), and cyclophosphamide	FACO	Fellow of the American College of Otolaryngology
	fractional area change	FACOG	Fellow of the American College of Obstetricians & Gynecologists
	fractional area concentration		
	functional aerobic capacity	FACOS	Fellow of the American College of Orthopedic Surgeons
FACA	Fellow of the American College of Anaesthetists		
FACAG	Fellow of the American College of Angiology	FACP	Fellow of the American College of Physicians
FACAL	Fellow of the American College of Allergists	FACPRM	Fellow of the American College of Preventive Medicine
FACAN	Fellow of the American College of Anesthesiologists	FACR	Fellow of the American College of Radiology
FACAS	Fellow of the American College of Abdominal Surgeons	FACS	Fellow of the American College of Surgeons
			fluorescent-activated cell sorter
FACC	Fellow of the American College of Cardiology	FACSM	Fellow of the American College of Sports Medicine
FACCP	Fellow of the American College of Chest Physicians		
		FACT	focused appendix computed tomography
FACCPC	Fellow of the American College of Clinical Pharmacology & Chemotherapy	FACT-An	Functional Assessment of Cancer Therapy-Anemia
		FACT-B	....-Breast
FACD	Fellow of the American College of Dentists	FACT-F	....-Fatigue
		FACT-G	....-General
FACEM	Fellow of the American College of Emergency Medicine	FACT-L	....-Lung

F

FACT-O	....-Ovarian	
FACT-P	....-Prostate	
FAD	familial Alzheimer disease	
	Family Assessment Device	
	fetal abdominal diameter	
	fetal activity determination	
	flavin adenine dinucleotide	
FAE	fetal alcohol effect	
FAGA	full-term appropriate for gestational age	
FAH	fumarylacetoacetase hydrolase	
FAI	Functional Assessment Inventory	
FAK	focal adhesion kinase	
FAL	femoral arterial line	
FALL	fallopian	
FALS	familial amyotrophic lateral sclerosis	
FAM	family	
	fluorouracil, doxorubicin (Adriamycin), and mitomycin	
	full allosteric modulators	
FAMA	fluorescent antibody to membrane antigen	
FAME	fluorouracil, doxorubicin (Adriamycin), and semustin (methyl CCNU)	
FAMMM	familial atypical multiple mole melanoma	
FAM-S	fluorouracil, doxorubicin (Adriamycin), mitomycin, and streptozotocin	
FAMTX	fluorouracil, doxorubicin (Adriamycin), and methotrexate	
FANA	fluorescent antinuclear antibody	
FANG	fluorescent angiography	
FANSS&M	fundus anterior, normal size and shape and mobile	
FAO	fatty acid oxidation	
	Food and Agriculture Organization	
FAP	Facility Admission Profile	
	familial adenomatous polyposis	

	familial amyloid polyneuropathy
	femoral artery pressure
	fibrillating action potential
	functional ambulation profile
FAQ	frequently asked question(s)
FAR	frontal arousal rhythm
F-ara-A	fludarabine phosphate (Fludara)
FARS	Fatality Analysis Reporting System
FAS	fetal alcohol syndrome
FASAY	functional analysis of separated alleles in yeast
FASC	fluorescent-activated substrate conversion (assay)
	fasciculations
FASHP	Fellow of the American Society of Health-System Pharmacists
FASPS	familial advanced sleep-phase syndrome
FAST	fetal acoustic stimulation testing
	flow-assisted short-term
	fluorescent allergosorbent technique
	focused assessment with sonography for trauma
FAT	Fetal Activity Test
	fluorescent antibody test
	food awareness training
FAV	facio-auricular vertebral
FAZ	foveal avascular zone
FB	fasting blood (sugar)
	finger breadth
	flexible bronchoscope
	foreign body
F/B	followed by
	forward/backward
	forward bending
FBC	full (complete) blood count
FBCOD	foreign body, cornea, right eye
FBCOS	foreign body, cornea, left eye
FBD	familial British dementia
	fibrocystic breast disease
	functional bowel disease

F

142

FBF	forearm blood flow	FCA	Federal False Claims Act
FBG	fasting blood glucose	F. cath.	Foley catheter
	foreign-body-type granulomata	FCBD	fibrocystic breast disease
FBH	hydroxybutyric dehydrogenase	FCC	familial cerebral cavernoma
FBHH	familial benign hypocalciuric hypercalcemia		familial colonic cancer
			family centered care
			femoral cerebral catheter
FBI	flossing, brushing, and irrigation		follicular center cells
			fracture compound comminuted
	full bony impaction	FCCA	Final Comprehensive Consensus Assessment
FBL	fecal blood loss		
FBM	felbamate (Felbatol)	FCCC	fracture complete, compound, and comminuted
	fetal breathing motion		
	foreign body, metallic		
FBRCM	fingerbreadth below right costal margin	FCCL	follicular center cell lymphoma
		FCCU	family centered care unit
FBS	failed back syndrome	FCD	feces collection device
	fasting blood sugar		fibrocystic disease
	fetal bovine serum	FCDB	fibrocystic disease of the breast
	foreign body sensation (eye)		
FBSS	failed back surgery syndrome	FCE	fluorouracil, cisplatin, and etoposide
			functional capacity evaluation
FBU	fingers below umbilicus		
FBW	fasting blood work	FCFD	fluorescence capillary-fill device
FC	family conference		
	febrile convulsion	FCH	familial combined hyperlipidemia
	female child		
	fever, chills		fibrosing cholestatic hepatitis
	film coated (tablets)		
	financial class	FCHL	familial combined hyperlipemia
	finger clubbing		
	finger counting	FCI	flow cytometric immunophenotyping
	flexion contractor		
	flow compensation (radiology)	FCL	fibular collateral ligament
	flucytosine (Ancobon)	F-CL	fluorouracil and calcium leucovorin
	foam cuffed (tracheal or endotracheal tube)		
		FCM	facial choreic movements
	Foley catheter		flow cytometry
	follows commands	FCMC	family centered maternity care
	foster care		
	French Canadian	FCMD	Fukiyama congenital muscular dystrophy
	functional capacity		
	functional class	FCMN	family centered maternity nursing
F/C	film coated (tablet)		
F + C	flare and cells	FCNV	fever, cough, nausea, and vomiting
F & C	foam and condom		
5FC	flucytosine (this is a dangerous abbreviation as it can be seen as 5FU)	FCOU	finger count, both eyes

F

FCP	formocresol pulpotomu	FDGS	feedings
FCR	flexor carpi radialis	FDI	first dorsal interosseous
	fractional catabolic rate		food-drug interaction
FCRB	flexor carpi radialis brevis		Functional Disability Index
FCRT	fetal cardiac reactivity test	FDIU	fetal death in utero
	focal cranial radiation therapy	FDL	flexor digitorum longus
FCS	fever, chills, and sweating	FDLMP	first day of last menstrual period
FCSNVD	fever, chills, sweating, nausea, vomiting, and diarrhea	FDM	fetus of diabetic mother
			flexor digiti minimi
FCSRT	Free and Cued Selective Reminding Test	FDP	fibrin-degradation products
FCT	fever-clearance time		fixed-dose procedure
FCU	flexor carpi ulnaris (tendon)		flexor digitorum profundus
FCV	feline calicivirus	FDPCA	fixed-dose patient-controlled analgesia
FD	familial dysautonomia	FD-PET	fluorodopa-positron emission tomography
	fetal demise		
	fetal distress	FDQB	flexor digiti quinti brevis
	focal distance	FDR	first-dose reaction
	food diary	FDS	flexor digitorum superficialis
	forceps delivery		
	Forestier Disease		for duration of stay
	free drain	FDT	frequency-doubling technology (perimetry for visual field screening)
	full denture		
	fully dilated		
	functional deficits		fronto-dextra transversa (right frontotransverse)
F & D	fixed and dilated		
FDA	Food and Drug Administration		Functional Dexterity Test
		FE	field echo (radiology)
	fronto-dextra anterior		frequency encode (radiology)
FDB	first-degree burn		
	flexor digitorum brevis	Fe	female
FDBL	fecal daily blood loss		iron
FDC	fixed-dose combination (preparations)	F & E	full and equal
FDCA	Food, Drug, and Cosmetic Act	FEB	febrile
		FEC	fluorouracil, epirubicin, and cyclophosphamide
FDCs	follicular dendritic cells		fluorouracil, etoposide, and cisplatin
FDE	fixed-drug eruption		forced expiratory capacity
FDF	flexor digitorum profundus (tendon)	FECG	fetal electrocardiogram
FDG	feeding	FeCh	ferrochelatase
	fluorine-18-labeled deoxyglucose (^{18}fluorodeoxyglucose)	FECP	free erythrocyte coproporphyrin
		FECT	fibroelastic connective tissue
FDGB	fall down, go boom	FED	fish eye disease
FDG-PET	positron emission tomography with ^{18}fluorodeoxyglucose	FEE	Far-Eastern equine encephalitis

FEES	fiberoptic endoscopic evaluation (examination) of swallowing		forced expiratory spirogram
			functional electrical stimulation
FEF	forced expiratory flow rate	FeSO$_4$	ferrous sulfate
		FESS	functional endonasal sinus surgery
FEF$_{25\%-75\%}$	forced expiratory flow during the middle half of the forced vital capacity		functional endoscopic sinus surgery
		FET	familial essential tremor
FEF$_{x-y}$	forced expiratory flow between two designated volume points in the forced vital capacity		fixed erythrocyte turnover
		FETI	fluorescence (fluorescent) energy transfer immunoassay
FEHBP	Federal Employee Health Benefits Plan	FEUO	for external use only
		FEV	familial exudative vitreoretinopathy
FEL	familial erythrophagocytic lymphohistiocytosis	FEV$_1$	forced expiratory volume in one second
FeLV	feline leukemia virus		
FEM	femoral	FEVC	forced expiratory vital capacity
FEMA	Federal Emergency Management Agency	FEV$_{1\%VC}$	forced expiratory volume in one second as percent of forced vital capacity
FEM-FEM	femoral femoral (bypass)		
FEM-POP	femoral popliteal (bypass)		
FEM-TIB	femoral tibial (bypass)	FEVR	familial exudative vitreoretinopathy
FERGs	focal electroretinograms		
FEN	fluid, electrolytes, and nutrition	FF	fat free
			fecal frequency
FENa	fractional extraction of sodium		filtration fraction
			finger-to-finger
FENIB	familial encephalopathies with neuroserpin inclusion bodies		five-minute format
			flat feet
			force fluids
FEN-PHEN	fenfluramine and phentermine		formula fed
			forward flexion
FENS	field-electrical neural stimulation		foster father
			Fox-Fordyce (disease)
FEOM	full extraocular movements		fundus firm
			further flexion
FEP	free erythrocyte porphyrins	F/F	face-to-face
		F&F	filiform and follower
	free erythrocyte protoporphorin		fixes and follows
		F(ρ)F	finger to finger
	functional exercise program	FF1/U	fundus firm 1 cm above umbilicus
FER	flexion, extension, and rotation	FF2/U	fundus firm 2 cm above umbilicus
FERPA	Family Educational Rights and Privacy Act	FF@u	fundus firm at umbilicus
		FFA	free fatty acid
FERR	serum ferritin		fundus fluorescein angiogram
FES	fat embolism syndrome		fusiform face area
	floppy eyelid syndrome		

F

FFAT	Free Floating Anxiety Test	
FFB	flexible fiberoptic bronchoscopy	
FFD	fat-free diet	
	focal-film distance	
FFDM	freedom from distant metastases	
FFE	free-flow electrophoresis	
FFF	field-flow fractionation	
	freedom from (biochemical and/or clinical) failure	
FFI	fast food intake	
	fatal familial insomnia	
FFM	fat-free mass	
	Five-Factor Model (of personality)	
	five-finger movement	
	freedom from metastases	
FFP	free from progression	
	fresh frozen plasma	
FFPE	formalin-faxed, paraffin-embedded	
FFQ	food frequency questionnaire	
FFR	freedom from relapse	
FFROM	full, free range of motion	
FFS	failure-free survival	
	fee-for-service	
	Fight For Sight	
	flexible fiberoptic sigmoidoscopy	
FFT	fast-Fourier transforms	
	flicker fusion threshold	
FFTDWB	flat foot touchdown weight bearing	
FFTP	first full-term pregnancy	
FFU/1	fundus firm 1 cm below umbilicus	
FFU/2	fundus firm 2 cm below umbilicus	
FG	fibrin glue	
	fusiform gyrus	
FGAs	first-generation antihistamines	
	first-generation antipsychotics	
FGC	full gold crown	
FGF	fibroblast growth factor	
FGM	female genital mutilation	
FGP	fundic gland polyps	
FGR	fetal growth restriction	
FGS	fibrogastroscopy	

	focal glomerulosclerosis
FH	familial hypercholesterolemia
	family history
	favorable histology
	fetal head
	fetal heart
	fundal height
FH+	family history positive
FH−	family history negative
FHA	filamentous hemagglutinin
FHB	flexor hallucis brevis
FHC	familial hypertrophic cardiomyopathy
	family health center
FHCIC	Fuchs heterochromic iridocyclitis
FHD	family history of diabetes
FHF	fulminant hepatic failure
FHH	familial hypocalciuric hypercalcemia
	fetal heart heard
FHI	frontal horn index
	Fuchs heterochromic iridocyclitis
FHL	flexor hallucis longus
	functional hallux limitus
FHM	familial hemiplegic migraine
FHN	family history negative
FHNH	fetal heart not heard
FHO	family history of obesity
FHP	family history positive
FHR	fetal heart rate
FHRB	fetal heart rate baseline
FHRV	fetal heart rate variability
FHS	fetal heart sounds
	fetal hydantoin syndrome
FHT	fetal heart tone
FHVP	free hepatic vein pressure
FHX	fluorouracil, hydroxyurea, and radiotherapy
FHx	family history
FI	fecal incontinence
	fiscal intermediary
FIA	familial intracranial aneurysms
	Family Independence Agency (formerly Department of Social Services)
FIAC	fiacitabine

F

FIAU	fialuridine	FJROM	full joint range of motion
FIB	fibrillation		
	fibula	FJS	finger joint size
FICA	Federal Insurance Contributions Act (Social Security)	FJV	first jejunal vein
		FK506	tacrolimus (Prograf)
		FKA	failed to keep appointment
FiCO$_2$	fraction of inspired carbon dioxide		formally known as
		FKBP	FK-506 binding protein (tacrolimus; Prograf)
FICS	Fellow of the International College of Surgeons	FKD	Kinetic Family Drawing
		FKE	full-knee extension
FID	father in delivery	FKGL	Flesh-Kincaid Grade Level (score)
	free induction decay		
FIF	forced inspiratory flow	FL	fatty liver
FiF	Functional Intact Fibrinogen (test)		femur length
			fetal length
FIGE	field inversion gel electrophoresis		fluid
			fluorescein
FIGLU	formiminoglutamic acid		fluorouracil and leucovorin
FIGO	International Federation of Gynecology and Obstetrics		
			flutamide and leuprolide acetate
FIL	father-in-law		focal laser
	Filipino		focal length
FIM	functional independence measure		follicular lymphoma
			full liquids
FIN	flexible intramedullary nail		functional limitations
		fL	femtoliter (10^{-15} liter)
FIND	follow-up intervention for normal development	F/L	father-in-law
		FLA	free-living amebic (ameba)
FiO$_2$	fraction of inspired oxygen		low-friction arthroplasty
FIP	feline infectious peritonitis	FLAG	fludarabine, ara-C (cytarabine), and G-CSF (filgrastim)
	flatus in progress		
FIRI	fasting insulin resistance index	FLAIR	fluid-attenuated inversion recovery
FISH	fluorescent (fluorescence) in situ hybridization	FLAP	fluorouracil, leucovorin, doxorubicin (Adriamycin), and cisplatin (Platinol AQ)
FISP	fast imaging with steady state precision		
			5-lipoxygenase activating protein
FITC	fluorescein isothiocyanate conjugated		
		FLASH	fast low-angle shot
FIV	feline immunodeficiency virus	FLAVO	flavopiridol
		FLB	funny looking beat
	in vitro fertilization (French)	FLBS	funny looking baby syndrome (see note under FLK)
FIVC	forced inspiratory vital capacity		
		FLC	follicular large cell lymphoma
FIX	factor IX (nine)		
FJB	facet joint block		fuzzy logic control
FJN	familial juvenile nephrophthisis	FLD	fatty liver disease
			fluid
FJP	familial juvenile polyposis		

F

147

	flutamide and leuprolide acetate depot	F & M	firm and midline (uterus)
	full lower denture	F-MACHOP	fluorouracil, methotrexate, cytarabine (ara-C), cyclophosphamide, doxorubicin (hydroxydaunorubicin), vincristine (Oncovin), and prednisone
FL Dtr	full lower denture		
FLE	frontal lobe epilepsy		
FLe	fluorouracil and levamisole		
flexsig	flexible sigmoidoscopy		
FLF	funny looking facies (see note under FLK)	FMC	fetal movement count
FLGA	full-term, large for gestational age	FMD	family medical doctor fibromuscular dysplasia flow-mediated dilatation foot-and-mouth disease
FLIC	Functional Living Index–Cancer	FMDV	foot-and-mouth disease virus
FLIE	Functional Living Index–Emesis	FME	Frühsommer-meningoenzephalitis vaccine full-mouth extraction
FLK	funny looking kid (should never be used: unusual facial features, is a better expression)	FMEA	failure mode effects analysis
FLM	fetal lung maturity	FMEN-1	familial multiple endocrine neoplasia, type 1
fl. oz.	fluid ounce		
FLP	fasting lipid profile Functional Limitations Profile	FMF	familial Mediterranean fever fetal movement felt forced midexpiratory flow
FL REST	fluid restriction		
FLS	fibroblast-like synoviocytes flashing lights and/or scotoma flu-like symptoms	FMG	fine mesh gauze foreign medical graduate
FLT	fluorothymidine	FMH	family medical history fibromuscular hyperplasia
FLU	fluconazole (Diflucan) fludarabine (Fludara) flunisolide (Aero Bid) fluoxetine (Prozac) fluticasone propionate (Flonase) influenza	FmHx	family history
		FML(r)	fluorometholone
		FMLA	Family and Medical Leave Act of 1993
		FMN	first malignant neoplasm flavin mononucleotide
FLU A	influenza A virus	FMOA	full-mouth odontectomy and alveoloplasty
FLUO	Fluothane		
fluoro	fluoroscopy	FMOL	femtomole (10^{-15} mole)
FLUT	flutamide (Eulexin)	FMP	fasting metabolic panel first menstrual period functional maintenance program
FLV	Friend leukemia virus		
FLW	fasting laboratory work		
FLZ	flurazepam (Dalmane)		
FM	face mask fat mass fetal movements fibromyalgia (syndrome) fine motor floor manager fluorescent microscopy foster mother	FMPA	full-mouth periapicals
		FMR	fetal movement record focused medical review functional magnetic resonance (imaging) functional mitral regurgitation

FMR1	fragile X mental retardation 1	FNMTC	familial nonmedullary thyroid carcinoma
FMRD	full-mouth restorative dentistry	FNP	Family Nurse Practitioner
fMRI	functional magnetic resonance imaging	FNR	false-negative rate
		FNS	food and nutrition services
FMRP	fragile X mental retardation protein(s)		functional neuromuscular stimulation
FMS	fibromyalgia syndrome	F/NS	fever and night sweats
	fluorouracil, mitomycin, and streptozocin	FNT	finger-to-nose (test)
	full-mouth series	FNTC	fine-needle transhepatic cholangiography
F & MS	frontal and maxillary sinuses	FO	foot orthosis
FMT	fluorescein meniscus time (dry-eye test)		foramen ovale
			foreign object
	functional muscle test		fronto-occipital
FMTC	familial medullary thyroid carcinoma	FOB	father of baby
			fecal occult blood
FMU	first morning urine		feet out of bed
FMV	flow-mediated vasodilation		fiberoptic bronchoscope
	fluorouracil, semustine (methyl-CCNU), and vincristine		foot of bed
		FOBT	fecal occult blood test
		FOC	father of child
FMX	full-mouth x-ray		fluid of choice
FMZ	flumazenil (Romazicon)		fronto-occipital circumference
FN	facial nerve	FOCF	first observation carried forward
	false negative		
	febrile neutropenia	FOD	fixing right eye
	femoral neck		free of disease
	finger-to-nose (test)	FOEB	feet over edge of bed
	flight nurse	FOF	fell on floor
F/N	fluids and nutrition	FOG	Fluothane, oxygen and gas (nitrous oxide)
F to N	finger-to-nose		
FNA	femoral neck anteversion		full-on gain
	fine-needle aspiration	FOH	family ocular history
FNa	filtered sodium	FOI	flight of ideas
FNAB	fine-needle aspiration biopsy	FOIA	Freedom of Information Act
FNAC	fine-needle aspiratory cytology	FOID	fear of impending doom
		FOL	fiberoptic laryngoscopy
FNB	femoral nerve block	FOLFOX	leucovorin calcium (folinic acid), fluorouracil, and oxaliplatin
FNCJ	fine-needle catheter jejunostomy		
FND	fludarabine, mitoxantrone (Novantrone), and dexamethasone	FOM	floor of mouth
		FOMi	fluorouracil, Oncovin, (vincristine), and mitomycin
	focal neurological deficit		
FNF	femoral-neck fracture	FONSI	finding of no significant impact
	finger-nose-finger (test)		
FNH	focal nodular hyperplasia	FOO	family of origin
FNHL	follicular non-Hodgkin lymphoma		

F

FOOB	fell out of bed	FPHx	family psychiatric
FOOSH	fell on outstretched hand		history
FOP	fasting office profile	FPIA	fluorescence-polarization
	fibrodysplasia ossificans		immunoassay
	progressiva	FPIES	food protein-induced
FOPS	fiberoptic		enterocolitis syndrome
	proctosigmoidoscopy	FPL	flexor pollicis longus
FORMIL	foreign military		(tendon)
FOS	fiberoptic sigmoidoscopy		final printed labeling
	fixing left eye	FPLD	familial partial
	force of stream (urology)		lipodystrophy
	fosphenytoin (Cerebyx)	FPM	full passive movements
	fructooligosaccharides	FPNA	first-pass nuclear
	future order screen		angiocardiography
FOSC	freestanding outpatient	FPO	fetal pulse oximetry
	surgery center	FPOR	follicle puncture for
FOT	forced oscillation		oocyte retrieval
	technique	FPU	family participation unit
	form of thought	FPV	fosamprenavir (Lexiva)
	frontal outflow tract	FPZ	fluphenazine (Prolixin;
FOV	field of view		Permitil)
FOVI	field of vision intact	FPZ-D	fluphenazine decanoate
FOW	fenestration of oval		(Prolixin Decanoate)
	window	FQ	fluoroquinolones
FP	fall precautions	FR	fair
	false positive		father
	familial porencephaly		Father (priest)
	family planning		Federal Register
	family practice		first responder
	family practitioner		flow rate
	family presence		fluid restriction
	fibrous proliferation		fluid retention
	flat plate		fractional reabsorption
	fluorescence polarization		freestyle, no head or
	fluticasone propionate		lower-extremity fixation
	food poisoning		(aquatic therapy)
	frozen plasma		frequent relapses
F/P	fluid/plasma (ratio)		Friends
F-P	femoral popliteal		frothy
fpA	fibrinopeptide A		full range
FPAL	full term, premature,	Fr	French (catheter gauge)
	abortion, living	F/R	fire/rescue
FPB	femoral-popliteal	F & R	force and rhythm (pulse)
	bypass	FRA	fall risk assessment
	flexor pollicis brevis		fluorescent rabies antibody
FPC	familial polyposis coli	FRAC	fracture
	family practice center	FRACTS	fractional urines
FPD	feto-pelvic disproportion	FRAG	fragment
	fixed partial denture	FRAG-X	Fragile X Syndrome
FPDL	flashlamp-pumped pulsed	FRAP	family risk assessment
	dye laser		program
FPE	first-pass effect		fluorescence recovery
FPG	fasting plasma glucose		after photobleaching

F

FRC	frozen red cells	F & S	full and soft
	functional residual capacity	FSA	Family Services Association
FRCPC	Fellow of the Royal College of Physicians of Canada	FSAD	female sexual arousal disorder(s)
		FSALO	Fletcher suite after loading ovoids
FRCPE	Fellow of the Royal College of Physicians of Edinburgh	FSALT	Fletcher suite after loading tandem
FRCSC	Fellow of the Royal College of Surgeons of Canada	FSB	fetal scalp blood full spine board
		FSBG	fingerstick blood glucose
FRCSE	Fellow of the Royal College of Surgeons of Edinburgh	FSBM	full-strength breast milk
		FSBS	fingerstick blood sugar
		FSC	Fatigue Symptom Checklist
FRCSI	Fellow of the Royal College of Surgeons of Ireland		flexible sigmoidoscopy fracture, simple, and comminuted
FRE	flow-related enhancement		fracture, simple, and complete
FRET	fluoresence resonance energy transfer	FSCC	fracture, simple, complete, and comminuted
FRF	filtration replacement fluid	FSD	female sexual dysfunction focal-skin distance
FRG	Functional Related Groups		fracture, simple, and depressed
FRJM	full range of joint movement	FSE	fast spin-echo fetal scalp electrode
FRN	fetal rhabdomyomatous nephroblastoma	FSF	fibrin stabilizing factor
		FSG	fasting serum glucose focal and segmental glomerulosclerosis
FRNT	focus-reduction neutralization test		
FROA	full range of affect	FSGA	full-term, small for gestational age
FROM	full range of motion		
FROMAJE	functioning, reasoning, orientation, memory, arithmetic, judgment, and emotion (mental status evaluation)	FSGN	focal segmental glomerulonephritis
		FSGS	focal segmental glomerulosclerosis
		FSH	facioscapulohumeral follicle-stimulating hormone
FRP	follicle regulatory protein functional refractory period		
		FSHMD	facioscapulohumeral muscular dystrophy
FRSN	fluoroquinolone-resistant *Streptococcus pneumoniae*	FSIQ	Full-Scale Intelligence Quotient (part of Wechsler test)
FS	fetoscope fibromyalgia syndrome fingerstick	FSL	fasting serum level
		FSM	functional status measures
	flexible sigmoidoscopy foreskin	F-SM/C	fungus, smear and culture
	fractional shortenings frozen section full strength functional status	FSME	Frühsommer-meningoencephalitis

F

FSO	for screws only (prosthetic cups)		Federal Trade Commission
FSOP	French Society of Pediatric Oncology		frames to come
			full to confrontation
FSP	fibrin split products	FTD	failure to descend
FSR	fractionated stereotactic radiosurgery		frontotemporal degeneration
	fusiform skin revision		frontotemporal dementia
FSRS	fractionated stereotactic radiosurgery		full-term delivery
		FTE	failure to engraft
FSRT	fractionated stereotactic radiotherapy	FTEs	full-time equivalents
FSS	federal supply schedule (cost source)	FTF	finger-to-finger
			free thyroxine fraction
	fetal scalp sampling	FTFTN	finger-to-finger-to-nose
	Flinders Symptom Score	FTG	full-thickness graft
	French steel sound (dilated to #24FSS)	FTI	farnesyltransferase inhibitor
			force-time integral
	frequency-selective saturation		free thyroxine index
		F TIP	finger tip
	full-scale score	FTIUP	full-term intrauterine pregnancy
FSW	feet of sea water (pressure)	FTKA	failed to keep appointment
	field service worker	FTLB	full-term living birth
FT	family therapy	FTLD	frontotemporal lobar degeneration
	fast-twitch	FTLFC	full-term living female child
	feeding tube		
	filling time	FTLMC	full-term living male child
	finger tip		
	flexor tendon	FTM	fluid thioglycollate medium
	fluidotherapy		
	follow through	FTMH	full-thickness macular hole(s)
	foot (ft)		
	Fourier transform (radiology)	FTMS	Fourier transform mass spectrometer
	free testosterone	FTN	finger-to-nose
	full-term		full-term nursery
F_3T	trifluridine (Viroptic)	FTNB	full-term newborn
FT_3	free triiodothyronine	FTND	Fagerstrom Test for Nicotine Dependence
FT_4	free thyroxine		full-term normal delivery
FT_4I	free thyroxine index	FTNSD	full-term, normal, spontaneous delivery
FTA	fluorescent titer antibody		
	fluorescent treponemal antibody	FTO	full-time occlusion (eye patch)
FTA-ABS	fluorescent treponemal antibody absorption	FTOZ	frontotemporal orbitozygomatic
FTB	fingertip blood	FTOZ1	one-piece frontotemporal orbitozygomatic
FTBD	full-term born dead		
FTBI	fractionated total body irradiation	FTP	failure to progress
			full-term pregnancy
FTC	emtricitabine (Coviracil)	FTR	father
	fallopian tube carcinoma		

	failed to report	5FU/LV	fluorouracil and leucovorin
	failed to respond	FUN	follow-up note
	for the record	FUNASA	Fundão Naçional de Sade (Brazil's national health agency)
FTRAM	free transverse rectus abdominis myocutaneous (flap)		
FTSD	full-term spontaneous delivery	FUNG-C	fungus culture
		FUNG-S	fungus smear
FTSG	full-thickness skin graft	FUO	fever of undetermined origin
FTT	failure to thrive		
	fetal tissue transplant	FUOV	follow-up office visit
	Finger-Tapping Test	FU/LP	full upper denture, partial lower denture
Ftube	feeding tube		
FTUPLD	full-term uncomplicated pregnancy, labor, and delivery	FUP	follow-up
		FUS	fusion
		FUT	fibrinogen update test
FTV	Fortovase (saquinavir, soft gel cap)	FUV	follow-up visit
		FV	femoral vein
	functional trial visit	F & V	fruits and vegetables
FTW	failure to wean	FVC	false vocal cord(s)
FU	fraction unbound		forced vital capacity
	fluorouracil	FVD	fever, vomiting, and diarrhea
F & U	flanks and upper quadrants		
F/U	follow-up	FVFR	filled voiding flow rate
	fundus at umbilicus	FVH	focal vascular headache
F↑U	fingers above umbilicus	F VIII	factor VIII (factor eight; antihemophilic factor)
F↓U	fingers below umbilicus		
5-FU	fluorouracil	FVL	factor V-Leiden (mutation)
FUA	flat and upright (x-ray of the) abdomen		femoral vein ligation
			flow volume loop
FUB	function uterine bleeding		functional visual loss
FUCO	fractional uptake of carbon monoxide	FVP	foot venous pressure
		FVR	feline viral rhinotracheitis
FUD	fear, uncertainty, and doubt		forearm vascular resistance
	frequency, urgency, and dysuria	FW	fetal weight
	full upper denture	F/W	followed with
FUDR(r)	floxuridine	F waves	fibrillatory waves
FU Dtr	full upper denture		flutter waves
FUFA	fluorouracil and leucovorin (folinic acid)	FVWs	flow-velocity waveforms (umbilical artery Doppler)
FU/FL	full upper denture, full lower denture		
		FWB	full-weight bearing
FUFOL	fluorouracil and leucovorin calcium (folinic acid)		functional well-being
		FWCA	functional work capacity assessment
Fugl	Fugl-Meyer Assessment of Motor Recovery After Stroke	FWD	fairly well developed
		FWHM	full-width at half maximum (radiology)
FUL	federal upper limit (price list)	FWS	fetal warfarin syndrome
		FWW	front-wheel walker
FULG	fulguration	Fx	fractional urine

F

	fracture
Fx-BB	fracture both bones
Fx-dis	fracture-dislocation
F XI	Factor XI (eleven)
FXN	function
FXR	fracture
FXS	fragile X syndrome
FXTAS	fragile X associated tremor/ataxia syndrome
FY	fiscal year
FYC	facultative yeast carrier
FYI	for your information
FZ	flutamide and goserelin acetate (Zoladex)
FZRC	frozen red (blood) cells

G

G	gallop
	gastrostomy
	gauge
	gauss (a unit of magnetic flux density in radiology)
	gavage feeding
	gingiva
	good
	grade
	gram (g) (28.35 g = 1 ounce)
	gravida
	guaiac
	guanine
G +	gram-positive
	guaiac positive
G −	gram-negative
	guaiac negative
↑g	increasing
↓g	decreasing
G1-4	grade 1-4
G-11	hexachlorophene
GA	Gamblers Anonymous
	gastric analysis
	general anesthesia
	general appearance
	gestational age
	ginger ale
	glycyrrhetinic acid
	granuloma annulare
	glucose/acetone
Ga	gallium
^{67}Ga	gallium citrate Ga 67
GAA	alpha-glucosidase (gene)
	glacial acetic acid
GABA	gamma-aminobutyric acid
GABHS	group A beta hemolytic streptococci
GABS	group A beta (hemolytic) streptococci
GAD	generalized anxiety disorder
	glutamic acid decarboxylase
GAE	granulomatous amebic encephalitis

F

GAEB	good air entry bilaterally	Gas Anal F&T	gastric analysis, free and total
GAF	geographic adjustment factors	Ga scan	gallium scan
	Global Assessment of Functioning (scale)	Gastroc	gastrocnemius
		GAT	geriatric assessment team
GAG	glycosaminoglycan		Goldmann applanation tonometry
GAGS	global acne grading system		group adjustment therapy
GAHM	genioglossus advancement and hyoid myotomy	GATB	General Aptitude Test Battery
GAGPS	glycosaminoglycan polysulfate	GAU	geriatric assessment unit
		GAVE	gastric antral vascular ectasia
GAGS	global acne grading system	Gaw	airway conductance
GAHM	genioglossus advancement and hyoid myotomy	GB	gallbladder
			gingival bleeding
GAL	galanthamine hydrobromide (Reminyl)		*Ginkgo biloba*
			Guillain-Barré (syndrome)
	gallon	G & B	good and bad
G'ale	ginger ale	GBA	gingivobuccoaxial
GALI-PUT	galactose-1-phosphate uridye transferase enzyme		ganglionic-blocking agent
		GBBS	group B beta hemolytic streptococcus
GALT	galactose-1-phosphate uridyltransferase (gene)	GBD	global burden of disease
		GBE	*Ginkgo biloba* extract
	gut-associated lymphoid tissue	GBEF	gallbladder ejection fraction
GAM	Gamma Knife	GBG	gonadal-steroid binding globulin
	gene-activated matrices	GBH	gamma benzene hexachloride (lindane)
GAMT	guanidinoacetate methyltransferase	GBIA	Guthrie bacterial inhibition assay
GAN	giant axonal neuropathy	GBL	gamma butyrolactone
GAO	General Accounting Office	GBM	glioblastoma multiforme
GAP	GTPase activating protein		glomerular basement membrane
GAP-43	growth-associated protein-43	GBMI	guilty but mentally ill
GAR	gonnococcal antibody reaction	GBP	gabapentin (Neurontin)
			gastric bypass
GARFT	glycinamide ribonucleotide formyl transferase		gated blood pool (imaging)
		GBPS	gated blood pool scan
GAS	general adaption syndrome	GBR	gamma band response (audiology)
	ginseng-abuse syndrome		good blood return
	Glasgow Assessment Schedule		guided bone regeneration
	Global Assessment Scale	GBS	gallbladder series
	group A streptococcal (*Streptococcus pyogenes*) disease vaccine		gastric bypass surgery
			group B streptococcal (*Streptococcus agalactiae*) disease vaccine
	group *A* streptococci		

G

	group B streptococci	G-CSF	filgrastim (granulocyte
	Guillain-Barré syndrome		colony-stimulating
GBV-C	GB virus type C (also		factor)
	known as hepatitis G	GCST	Gibson-Cooke sweat test
	virus)	GCT	general care and treatment
GBW	generalized body		germ-cell tumor
	weakness		giant-cell tumor
GBX	gall bladder extraction		granulosa cell tumor
	(cholecystectomy)	GCU	gonococcal urethritis
GC	gas chromatography	GCV	ganciclovir (Cytovene)
	gastric cancer		great cardiac vein
	geriatric chair (Gerichair)	GCVF	great cardiac vein flow
	gingival curettage	GD	gastric distension
	gonococci (gonorrhea)		Gaucher disease
	good condition		generalized delays
	graham crackers		gestational diabetes
G−C	gram-negative cocci		good
G+C	gram-positive cocci		gravely disabled
GCA	ghost cell		Graves disease
	ameloblastoma	Gd	gadolinium
	giant cell arteritis	G & D	growth and development
GCBP	gated cardiac blood pool	GDA	gastroduodenal artery
GCC	glassy cell carcinoma	GDB	Guide Dogs for the Blind
	guanylyl cyclase C	Gd-	gadolinium
GCE	general conditioning	BOPTA	benzyloxypropionic
	exercise		tetra acetate
GCDFP	gross cystic disease fluid	GDC	Guglielmi detachable
	protein		coil
GCF	giant cell fibroblastoma	Gd-DTPA	gadopentetate (Magnevist)
	gingival crevicular fluid	Gd-DTPA-	gadodiamide (Omniscan)
GCI	General Cognitive Index	BMA	
GCIIS	glucose control insulin	GD FA	grandfather
	infusion system	GDH	glutamic dehydrogenase
GCL	generalized congenital	Gd-	gadoteridol
	lipodystrophy	HPD03A	
GCM	giant cell myocarditis	GDJ	gastroduodenal junction
	good central maintained	g/dl	grams per deciliter
GCMD	generalized cardiovascular	GDM	gestational diabetes
	metabolic disease		mellitus
GCMN	giant congenital	GDM A-1	gestational diabetes
	melanocytic nevus		mellitus, insulin
GC-MS	gas chromatography-mass		controlled, Type I
	spectroscopy	GDM A-2	gestational diabetes
GCP	gentamicin, clindamycin,		mellitus, diet
	and polymyxin topical		controlled, Type II
	preparation	GD MO	grandmother
	good clinical practice	Gd-MRI	gadolinium-enhanced
GCR	gastrocolonic response		magnetic resonance
	glucocerebrosidase		imaging
GCS	Glasgow Coma Scale	GDNF	glial (cell line) derived
	glucocorticosteroid(s)		neurotrophic factor
GCSE	generalized convulsive	GDP	gamma-detecting probe
	status epilepticus		gel diffusion precipitin

GDPs	general dental practitioners	GEU	geriatric evaluation unit
GDR	glucose disposal rate	GF	gastric fistula
GDS	Global Deterioration Scale		gluten free
GDx®	a scanning laser polarimeter		grandfather
		GFAAS	graphite furnace atomic absorption spectrometry
GE	gainfully employed	GFAP	glial fibrillary acidic protein
	gastric emptying		
	gastroenteritis	GF-BAO	gastric fluid, basal acid output
	gastroesophageal		
	group exercise	GFCL	Goldmann fundus contact lens
GEA	gastroepiploic artery		
GEC	galactose elimination capacity	GFD	gluten-free diet
		GFFF	gravitational field-flow fractionation
GED	General Educational Development (Test)	GFJ	grapefruit juice
GEE	gait energy expenditure	GFM	good fetal movement
	generalized estimating equations (statistics)	GFP	green fluorscent protein
		GFR	glomerular filtration rate
	Global Evaluation of Efficacy		grunting, flaring, and retractions
	glycine ethyl ester	GFS	glaucoma filtering surgery
	graft-enteric erosion	GG	gamma globulin
GEF	graft-enteric fistula		guaifenesin (glyceryl guaiacolate)
GEJ	gastroesophageal junction		
GEM	gemcitabine (Gemzar)	G=G	grips equal and good
	gemfibrozil (Lopid)	GGE	Gastrografin enema
	generalized erythema multiforme		generalized glandular enlargement
GEMOX	gemcitabine and oxaliplatin	GGF	great grandfather
		GGM	great grandmother
GEMU	geriatric evaluation and management unit	GGO	ground-glass opacity
		GGS	glands, goiter, and stiffness
GEN	genital		group G streptococci
GEN/ ENDO	general anesthesia with endotracheal intubation	GGT	gamma-glutamyl-transferase
GENT	gentamicin	GGTP	gamma-glutamyl-transpeptidase
GENTA/P	gentamicin-peak		
GENTA/T	gentamicin-trough	GH	general health
GEP	gastroenteropancreatic		genetic hemochromatosis
GEQ	generic equiavalent		gingival hyperplasia
GER	gastroesophageal reflux		glenohumeral
GERD	gastroesophageal reflux disease		good health
			growth hormone
GES	gastric emptying scintigraphy	GH₃	Gerovital
		GHAA	Group Health Association of America
GET	gastric emptying time		
	graded exercise test	GHB	gamma hydroxybutyrate (sodium oxybate; Xyrem)
GET 1/2	gastric emptying half-time		
GETA	general endotracheal anesthesia		
		GHb	glycosylated hemoglobin
GETV	gadolinium-enhancing tumor volume	GHD	growth hormone deficiency

G

GHDA	growth hormone deficiency (syndrome) in adults	GIPU	gastrointestinal procedure unit
GHI	growth hormone insufficiency	GIR	glucose infusion rate
		GIS	gas in stomach
GHJ	glenohumeral joint		gastrointestinal series
G-H jt	glenohumeral joint	GISA	glycopeptide intermediate-resistant *Staphylococcus aureus*
GHLC	glenohumeral ligament complex		
GHP(S)	gated heart pool (scan)	GIST	gastrointestinal stromal tumor
GHQ	General Health Questionnaire	GIT	gastrointestinal tract
		GITS	gastrointestinal therapeutic system
GHQ-30	General Health Questionnaire		gut-derived infectious toxic shock
GHRF	growth hormone releasing factor	GITSG	Gastrointestinal Tumor Study Group
GI	gastrointestinal	GITT	glucose insulin tolerance test
	glycemic index		
	granuloma inguinale	GIWU	gastrointestinal work-up
GIA	gastrointestinal anastomosis	giv	given
		GJ	gastrojejunostomy
GIB	gastric ileal bypass		grapefruit juice
	gastrointestinal bleeding	GJIC	gap junction intercellular communication
GIC	general immunocompetence		
		GJT	gastrojejunostomy tube
	Global Impression of Change	G1K	greater than one thousand
		GK	Gamma Knife
GID	gastrointestinal distress	GKRS	gamma-knife radiosurgery
	gender identity disorder	GKS	gamma-knife surgery
GIDA	Gastrointestinal Diagnostic Area	GL	gastric lavage
			glaucoma
GIFD #3	colonoscope		greatest length
GIFT	gamete intrafallopian (tube) transfer	GLA	gamolenic acid
			gingivolinguoaxial
GIH	gastrointestinal hemorrhage		glucose-lowering agents
		GLB	Graham-Leach-Bliley Act of 1999
GIK	glucose-insulin-potassium		
GIL	gastrointestinal (tract) lymphoma	GLC	gas-liquid chromatography
		GLD	Glanders (*Actinobacillus mallei*) vaccine
GING	gingiva		
	gingivectomy	GLF	ground-level fall
G1K	greater than one thousand	GLIO	glioblastoma
GIO	glucocorticoid-induced osteoporosis	GLM	general linear model
		GLN	glomerulonephritis
GIOP	glucocorticoid-induced osteoporosis	GLOC	gravity-induced loss of consciousness
GIP	gastric inhibitory peptide	GLP	Gambro Liendia Plate
			Good Laboratory Practice (Principles of)
	giant cell interstitial pneumonia		group-living program
	glucose-dependent insulinotropic polypeptide	GLP-1	glucagon-like peptide-1
		GLR	gravity lumbar reduction

G

GLU	glucose	
GLU 5	five-hour glucose tolerance test	
GLUC	glucose	
GLYCOS Hb	glycosylated hemoglobin	
GM	gastric mucosa	
	general medicine	
	genetically modified	
	geometric mean	
	gram (g)	
	grand mal	
	grandmother	
	gray matter	
G-M	Geiger-Müller (counter)	
GM +	gram-positive	
GM −	gram-negative	
gm %	grams per 100 milliliters	
GmbH	*Gesellschaft mit beschränkter Haftung* (a corporation with restricted liability or a private limited liability company)	
GMC	general medical clinic	
	geometric mean concentration	
GMCD	grand mal convulsive disorder	
GM-CSF	sargramostim (granulocyte-macrophage colony-stimulating factor; Leukine)	
GME	gaseous microemboli	
GMF	general medical floor	
GMFCS	Gross Motor Function Classification System	
GMFM	gross motor function measure	
GMH	germinal matrix hemorrhage	
GMLOS	geometric mean length of stay	
GMOs	genetically modified organisms	
GMP	general medical panel (see page 392)	
	Good Manufacturing Practices	
	guanosine monophosphate	
GMR	gallop, murmur or rub	
GMS	galvanic muscle stimulation	

	general medical services
	general medicine and surgery
	Gomori methenamine silver (stain)
GM&S	general medicine and surgery
GMSPS	Glasgow Meningococcal Septicemia Prognostic Score
GMTs	geometric mean antibody titers
GN	glomerulonephritis
	graduate nurse
	gram-negative
GNA	*Galanthus nivalis* agglutinin
GNB	ganglioneuroblastoma
	gram-negative bacilli
	gram-negative bacteremia
GNBM	gram-negative bacillary meningitis
GNC	gram-negative cocci
GND	gram-negative diplococci
GNID	gram-negative intracellular diplococci
GNP	Geriatric Nurse Practitioner
GNR	gram-negative rods
GnRH	gonadotropin-releasing hormone
GNS	gram-negative sepsis
GnSAF	gonadotropin surge attenuating factor
GNT	Graduate Nurse Technician
GO	Graves ophthalmopathy
	Greek Orthodox
GOAT	Galveston Orientation and Amnesia Test
GOBI	*g*rowth monitoring, *o*ral rehydration, *b*reast feeding, and *i*mmunization
GOCS	Global Obsessive-Compulsive Scale
GOD	glucose oxidase
GOG	Gynecologic Oncology Group
GOJ	gastro-oesophageal junction (UK and other countries)

G

GOK	God only knows	GPB	gram-positive bacilli
GOLD	Global Initiative for Chronic Obstructive Lung Disease (guidelines)	GPC	gel-permeation chromatography
			giant papillary conjunctivitis
GOMER	get out of my emergency room		glycerophosphorylcholine
			G-protein coupled
GON	gonococcal ophthalmia neonatorum		gram-positive cocci
		GPCL	gas-permeable contact lens
	greater occipital neuritis	GPCR	G protein-coupled receptors
GONA	glaucomatous optic nerve atrophy	GPC/TP	glycerylphosphorylcholine to total phosphate
GONIO	gonioscopy	G6PD	glucose-6-phosphate dehydrogenase
GOO	gastric outlet obstruction		
GOR	gastro-oesophageal reflux (United Kingdom)	GPGL	gamma probe guided lymphoscintigraphy
	general operating room	GPI	general paralysis of the insane
GORD	gastro-oesophageal reflux disease (United Kingdom)		glucose-6-phosphate isomerase
			glycoprotein IIb/IIIa receptor inhibitor(s)
GOS	galactose oxidase and Schiff reagent (test)	GPi	globus pallidus interna
	Glasgow Outcome Scale	G-PLT	giant platelets
GOT	glucose oxidase test	GPMAL	gravida, para, multiple births, abortions, and live births
	glutamic-oxaloacetic transaminase (aspartate aminotransferase)		
		GPN	graduate practical nurse
	goals of treatment	GPO	group purchasing organization
GOX	glucose oxidation		
GP	gabapentin (Neurontin)	GPP	Good Programming Practice
	general practitioner		
	globus pallidus	GPRD	General Practice Research Database (United Kingdom)
	glucose polymers		
	glycoprotein		
	gram-positive	GPS	Goodpasture syndrome
	grandparent	GPT	glutamic pyruvic transaminase
	gutta percha		
G/P	gravida/para	GPVP	good pharmacovigilance process
G4P3104	four pregnancies (gravid), 3 went to term, one premature, no abortion (or miscarriage), and 4 living children (p = para)		
		GPX	glutathione peroxidase
		GPx-1	glutathione peroxidase-1
		GR	gastric resection
			growth rate
GPA	gelatin particle agglutination	gr	grain (approximately 60 mg) (this is a dangerous abbreviation)
	global program on AIDS		
G#P#A#	gravida (number of pregnancies) para (number of live births) abortion (number of abortions)	G−R	gram-negative rods
		G+R	gram-positive rods
		GRA	granisetron (Kytril)
			glucocorticoid remediable aldosteronism

160

gravida 6, para 4- 0-2-3	6 pregnancies resulting in 4-full term deliveries with 0 premature births and 2 abortions or miscarriages and 3 living children		Gram stain
			grip strength
		G/S	5% dextrose (glucose) and 0.9% sodium chloride (saline) injection
		G & S	gait and stance
GRAS	generally recognized as safe	GSAP	greatest single allergen present
GRASE	Generally Recognized as Safe and Effective	G-SAS	Gambling Symptom Assessment Scale
GRASS	gradient recalled acquisition in a steady state	GS-Cbl	glutathionylcobalamin
		GSCU	geriatric skilled care unit
		GSD	gallstone disease
Grav.	gravid (pregnant)		glucogen storage disease
GRC	gastric remnant cancers	GSD-1	glycogen storage disease, type 1
GRD	gastroesophageal reflux disease	GSE	genital self-examination
GRD DTR	granddaughter		gluten sensitive enteropathy
GRD SON	grandson		grip strong and equal
GRE	glycopeptide-resistant enterococci	GSH	glutathione
		GSI	genuine stress incontinence
	graded resistive exercise	GSK	GlaxoSmithKline
	gradient-recalled echo	GSM	Global System of Mobile Communication
	gradient refocused echo		grey-scale median
GR-FR	grandfather	GSMD	gestational sack and maternal date
GRKP	gentamicin-resistant *Klebsiella pneumoniae*		
GR-MO	grandmother	GSP	generalized social phobia
GRN	granules		general survey panel
	green		Good Statistical Practice
GRO	growth-related oncogene	GSPN	greater superficial petrosal neurectomy
GRP	Good Regulatory Practice group		
		GSR	galvanic skin resistance (response)
$Gr_1P_0AB_1$	one pregnancy, no births, and one abortion		gastrosalivary reflex
GRP HM	group home	GSS	Gerstmann-Straüssler-Scheinker (syndrome)
GRT	gastric residence time		
	glandular replacement therapy	GST	glutathione S-transferase
			gold sodium thiomalate (Myochrysine)
	Graduate Respiratory Therapist	GSTM	gold sodium thiomalate (Myochrysine)
	grasp and release test		
	group-randomized trial	GSUI	genuine stress urinary incontinence
GRTT	Graduate Respiratory Therapist Technician		
		GSV	greater saphenous vein
GS	gallstone	GSW	gunshot wound
	generalized seizure	GSWA	gunshot wound to abdomen
	general surgery		
	Gleason score	GT	gait
	gliosarcoma		gait training
	glucosamine sulfate		gastrostomy
	gluteal sets		

G

	gastrotomy tube	GUM	Genitourinary Medicine (clinics)
	gene therapy		
	glucose tolerance	GUS	genitourinary sphincter
	great toe		genitourinary system
	greater trochanter	GUSTO	Global Utilization of
	green tea		Streptokinase and TPA
	group therapy		for Occluded Arteries
GTA	glutaraldehyde	GV	gentian violet
GTB	gastrointestinal tract bleeding		growth velocity
		GVF	Goldmann visual fields
GTC	generalized tonic-clonic (seizure)		good visual fields
		GVG	vigabatrin (gamma-vinyl GABA)
GTCS	generalized tonic-clonic seizure		
		GVH	generalized visceral hypersensitivity
GTD	gestational trophoblastic disease		
		GVHD	graft-versus-host disease
GTE	general therapeutic exercise	GVL	graft-versus leukemia
		GVM	Graft-versus malignancy
	Green tea extract	GVN	gentamicin, vancomycin, and nystatin
GTF	gastrostomy tube feedings		
	glucose tolerence factor	GVS	gastric vertical stapling
GTH	gonadotropic hormone	GVSDS	growth velocity standard deviation score
GTN	gestational trophoblastic neoplasms		
		GVT	graft-versus-tumor
	glomerulo-tubulo-nephritis	G/W	dextrose (glucose) in water
	glyceryl trinitrate (name for nitroglycerin in the United Kingdom)		
		G&W	glycerin and water (enema)
GTO	Golgi tendon organ(s)	GWA	gunshot wound of the abdomen
GTP	glutamyl transpeptidase		
	green tea polyphenols	GWBI	General Well-Being Index
	guanosine triphosphate	GWD	Guinea-worm disease
GTR	granulocyte turnover rate	GWMFT	Graded Wolf Motor Function Test
	gross total resection		
	guided tissue regeneration	GWS	Gulf-war syndrome
GTS	Gilles de la Tourette syndrome	GWT	gunshot wound of the throat
gtt.	drops	GWX	guide-wire exchange
GTT	gestational trophoblastic tumor	GXP	graded exercise program
		GXT	graded exercise test
	glucose tolerance test	Gy	gray (radiation unit)
GTT agar	gelatin-tellurite-taurocholate agar	GYN	gynecology
		GZTS	Guilford-Zimmerman Temperament Survey
GTT3H	glucose tolerence test, 3 hours (oral)		
gtts.	drops		
G-tube	gastrostomy tube		
GU	gastric upset		
	genitourinary		
	gonococcal urethritis		
GUAR	guarantor		
GUD	genital ulcer disease		
GUI	genitourinary infection		

G

H

H	*Haemophilis*
	head
	heart
	height
	Helicobacter
	heroin
	Hispanic
	hour
	husband
	hydrogen
	hyperopia
	hypermetropia
	hyperphoria
	hypodermic
	isoniazid [part of tuberculosis regimen, see RHZ(E/S)/HR]
	objective angle
	trastuzumab (Herceptin)
H′	hip
H	hypodermic injection
H²	hiatal hernia
H₂	hydrogen
3H	high, hot, and a helluva lot
H24	24 hour
HA	headache
	hearing aid
	heart attack
	hemadsorption
	hemagglutination
	hemolytic anemia
	Hispanic American
	hospital admission
	hyaluronan
	hyaluronic acid
	hyperalimentation
	hypermetropic astigmatism
	hypothalmic amenorrhea
H/A	head-to-abdomen (ratio)
	holding area
HA-1A®	nebacumab
HAA	hepatitis-associated antigen
HAAB	hepatitis A antibody
HAART	highly active antiretroviral treatment

HABF	hepatic artery blood flow
HAc	acetic acid
HACA	human antichimeric antibodies
HACCP	Hazard Analysis Critical Control Point(s)
HACE	hepatic artery chemoembolization
	high-altitude cerebral edema
HACEK group	*Haemophilus parainfluenzae, H. aphrophilus,* and *H. paraphrophilus, Actinobacillus actinomycetemcomitans, Cardiobacterium hominis, Eikenella corrodens,* and *Kingella kingae*
HACS	hyperactive child syndrome
HAD	HIV (human immunodeficiency virus)-associated dementia
	human adjuvant disease
	hypertonic acetate dextran
HADH	the reduced form of nicotinamide-adenine dinucleotide (hydride donors in biochemical redox reactions)
HADS	Hospital Anxiety and Depression Scale
HAE	hearing aid evaluation
	hepatic artery embolization
	herb-related adverse event
	hereditary angioedema
HAEC	Hirschprung associated enterocolitis
HAF	hyperalimentation fluid
HAFM	hospital-acquired *Plasmodium falciparum* malaria
HAGG	hyperimmune antivariola gamma globulin
HAGHL	humeral avulsion of the glenohumeral ligament
HAGL	humeral avulsion of the glenohumeral ligament
HAH	high-altitude headache

H

HAI	hemagglutination inhibition assay	HAPS	hepatic arterial perfusion scintigraphy
	hepatic arterial infusion	HAPTO	haptoglobin
HAIC	hepatic arterial infusional chemotherapy	HAQ	Headache Assessment Questionnaire
HAK	hyperalimentation kit		Health Assessment Questionnaire
HAL	hemorrhoidal artery ligation	HAR	high-altitude retinopathy
	hip axis length		hyperacute rejection
	hyperalimentation	HARDI	high-angular resolution diffusion-weighted imaging
HALE	health-adjusted life expectancy		
HALN	hand-assisted laparoscopic (radical) nephrectomy	HARH	high-altitude retinal hemorrhage
HALO	halothane (Fluothane)	HARP	hypoprebetalipoproteinemia, acanthocytosis, retinitis pigmentosa, and pallidale degeneration (syndrome)
	hours after light onset		
HALRI	hospital-acquired lower respiratory infections		
HALRN	hand-assisted laparoscopic radical nephrectomy		
		HARS	Hamilton Anxiety Rating Scale
HAM	Haldol, Ativan, and morphine		HIV-associated adipose redistribution syndrome
	high-dose cytarabine (ara-C) and mitoxantrone	HAS	Hamilton Anxiety (Rating) Scale
	HTLV-1-associated myelopathy		headache associated with sexual activity
	human albumin microspheres		Holmes-Adie syndrome home assessment service
HAMA	human antimurine antibody		hyperalimentation solution
HAM-A	Hamilton Anxiety (scale)	HASCI	head and spinal cord injury
HAM D	Hamilton Depression (scale)	HASCVD	hypertensive arteriosclerotic cardiovascular disease
HAMS	hamstrings	HASHD	hypertensive arteriosclerotic heart disease
HAN	heroin-associated nephropathy		
HANE	hereditary angioneurotic edema	HAT	head, arms, and trunk
HAO	hearing aid orientation		heterophile antibody titer
HAP	hearing aid problem		histone acetyltransferase
	heredopathia atactica polyneuritiformis		hormone ablative therapy
			hospital arrival time
	hospital-acquired pneumonia		human African trypanosomiasis (sleeping sickness)
	hydroxyapatite		
HAPC	hospital-acquired penetration contact	HAV	hallux abducto valgus
			hepatitis A vaccine
HAPD	home-automated peritoneal dialysis		hepatitis A virus
		HAV-HBV	hepatitis A virus, and hepatitis B virus vaccine
HAPE	high-altitude pulmonary edema		

H

HAZWO PER	Hazardous Waste Operations and Emergency Response	HBGM	home blood glucose monitoring
HB	heart-beating (donor)	HBH	Health Belief Model
	heart block	HBHC	hospital based home care
	heel-to-buttock	HBI	Harvey-Bradshaw Index
	hemoglobin (Hb)		hemibody irradiation
	hepatitis B	HBID	hereditary benign intraepithelial dyskeratosis
	high calorie		
	hold breakfast		
	housebound	HBIG	hepatitis B immune globulin
	hydrocodone bitartrate		
1^0HB	first degree heart block	Hb Kansas	mutant hemoglobin with a low affinity for oxygen
HB1°	first degree heart block		
HB2°	second degree heart block	HBLs	hemangioblastomas
		HBLV	B-lymphotropic virus human
HB3°	third degree heart block		
HBAB	hepatitis B antibody	HBM	human bone marrow
Hb A_{1c}	glycosylated hemoglobin	HBNK	heparin-binding neurotrophic factor
HBAC	hyperdynamic beta-adrenergic circulatory		
		hBNP	human B-type natriuretic peptide (nesiritide [Natrecor])
HbAS	sickle cell trait		
HBBW	hold breakfast for blood work		
		HBO	hyperbaric oxygen (HBO_2 preferred)
HBC	health and beauty care		
	hereditary breast cancer	HBO_2	hyperbaric oxygen
	hit by car	HbO_2	hemoglobin, oxygenated
HBcAb	hepatitis B core antibody (antigen)		hyperbaric oxygen (HBO_2 preferred)
HBc AB	hepatitis B core antibody	HBOC	hemoglobin-based oxygen carrier
HBc Ag	hepatitis B core antigen		
HbCO	carboxyhemoglobin		hereditary breast and ovarian cancer
HB core	hepatitis B core antigen		
HbCV	*Haemophilus* b conjugate vaccine	HBOT	hyperbaric oxygen treatment/therapy (HBO_2T preferred)
HBD	has been drinking		
	hydroxybutyrate dehydrogenase	HBO_2T	hyperbaric oxygen treatment
HBDH	hydroxybutyrate dehydrogenase	HBP	high blood pressure
		HBPM	home blood pressure monitoring
HBE	hepatitis B epsilon		
	human bronchial epithelial (cells)	HBr	hydrobromide
		HBS	Health Behavior Scale
	hypopharyngoscopy, bronchoscopy, and esophagoscopy	HbS	sickle cell hemoglobin
		HBsAg	hepatitis B surface antigen
HBeAb	hepatitis Be antibody (antigen)	HbSC	sickle cell hemoglobin C
		HBSS	Hank balanced salt solution
HBED	hydroxybenzylethylene-diamine diacetic acid	HbSS	sickle cell anemia
HbF	fetal hemoglobin	HBT	hydrogen breath test
HBF	hepatic blood flow	HBV	hepatitis B vaccine
HBGA	had it before, got it again		hepatitis B virus
			honey-bee venom

H

HBVig	hepatitis B virus immune globulin	HCI	home care instructions
		HCL	hairy cell leukemia
HBVP	high biological value protein	HCl	hydrochloric acid (when it appears separately [not as part of a drug name])
HBW	high birth weight		hydrochloride (when part of a drug name, as in thiamine HCl [thiamine hydrochloride])
H/BW	heart-to-body weight (ratio)		
HC	hair count		
	hairy cell		
	handicapped		
	head circumference		
	healthy controls	HCLF	high carbohydrate, low fiber (diet)
	heart catheterization		
	heel cords	HCLs	hard contact lenses
	Hickman catheter	HCLV	hairy cell leukemia variant
	home care		
	hot compress	HCM	health care maintenance
	housecall		heterogeneous cation-exchange membrane
	Huntington chorea		
	hydrocephalus		hypercalcemia of malignancy
	hydrocortisone		
4-HC	4-hydroperoxycyclo-phosphamide		hypertrophic cardiomyopathy
H & C	hot and cold	HCMV	human cytomegalovirus
HCA	health care aide	HCO₃	bicarbonate
	heterocyclic antidepressant	HCP	handicapped
			healthcare provider
	hypercalcemia		hearing conservation programs
	hypothermic circulatory arrest		hereditary coporphyria
HCAO	hepatitis C-associated osteosclerosis		hexachlorophene
			home chemotherapy program
H-CAP	altretamine (hexamethyl-melamine), cyclophosphamide, doxorubicin (Adriamycin), and cisplatin (Platinol AQ)		hospital chemistry profile
			hydrocephalus
		HCPCS	HCFA (Health Care Financing Administration) Common Procedural Coding System
HCB	hexachlorobenzene		
HCBR	human carbonyl reductase	HCQ	hydroxychloroquine (Plaquenil)
HCC	hepatocellular carcinoma		
		HCR	health care review
HCD	herniate cervical disk	HCS	heel-cord stretches
	hydrocolloid dressing		human chorionic somatomammotropin
HCFA	Health Care Financing Administration		
			hypercoagulable states
HCFC	hydrochlorofluorocarbon	17-HCS	17-hydroxycorticosteroids
HCFU	1-hexylcarbamoyl-5-fluorouracil (Camofur)	HCSE	horse chestnut seed extract
hCG	human chorionic gonadotropin	HCSS	hypersensitive carotid sinus syndrome
HCH	hexachlorocyclohexane	HCT	head computerized (axial) tomography
	hygroscopic condenser humidifier		

H

	hematopoietic cell transplantation
	hematocrit
	histamine challenge test
	human chorionic thyrotropin
	hydrochlorothiazide (this is a dangerous abbreviation)
	hydrocortisone
HCTU	home cervical traction unit
HCTZ	hydrochlorothiazide (this is a dangerous abbreviation)
HCV	hepatitis C vaccine
	hepatitis C virus
HCVD	hypertensive cardiovascular disease
HCWs	healthcare workers
HCY	homocysteine
HCYS	homocysteine
HD	haloperidol decanoate
	Hansen disease
	hearing distance
	heart disease
	Heller-Dor (procedure)
	heloma durum
	hemodialysis
	herniated disk
	high dose
	hip disarticulation
	Hodgkin disease
	hospital day
	hospital discharge
	house dust
	Huntington disease
HDA	heteroduplex analysis
	high-dose arm
HDAC	histone deacetylase
HD-AC	high-dose cytarabine
HDAC2	histone deacetylase 2
HD-ara-C	high-dose cytarabine (ara-C)
HDBQ	Hilton Drinking Behavior Questionnaire
HDC	habilitative day care
	high-dose chemotherapy
	histamine dihydrochloride
HDC-ASCS	high-dose chemotherapy with autologous stem cell support
HDCC	high-dose combination chemotherapy

HD-CPA	high-dose cyclophosphamide
HDCPT	high-dose cyclophosphamide therapy
HDC-SCR	high-dose chemotherapy with stem-cell rescue
HDCT	high-dose chemotherapy
HDCV	rabies virus vaccine, human diploid (human diploid cell vaccine)
HDE	Humanitarian Device Exemption (FDA)
HDF	hemodiafiltration
HDG	hydrogel (dressing)
HDH	high-density humidity
HDI	high-definition image
HDIs	histone deacetylase inhibitors
HDL	high-density lipoprotein
HDL-C	high-density lipoprotein cholesterol
HDLW	hearing distance for watch to be heard in left ear
HDM	home-delivered meals
	house dust mite
HDMEC	human dermal microvascular endothelial cells
HDMP	high-dose methylprednisolone
HD-MTX	high-dose methotrexate
HD-MTX-CF	high-dose methotrexate and leucovorin (citrovorum factor)
HD-MTX/LV	high-dose methotrexate and leucovorin
HDN	hemolytic disease of the newborn
	heparin dosing nomogram
	high-density nebulizer
HDNS	Hodgkin disease, nodular sclerosis
HDP	high-density polyethylene
	hydroxymethyline diphosphonate
HDPA	high-dose pulse administration
HDPAA	heparin-dependent platelet-associated antibody
HDPC	hand piece
HDPE	high-density polyethylene

H

HDR	heparin dose response	HeLa	Helen Lake (tumor cells)
	husband to delivery room	HELLP	hemolysis, elevated liver
HDRA	histoculture drug response	Syn-	enzymes, and low
	assay	drome	platelet count
HDRB	high-dose rate	HEM	hypertensive emergency
	brachytherapy	HEMA	hydroxyethylmethacrylate
HDRS	Hamilton Depression	HEMI	hemiplegia
	Rating Scale	HEMOSID	hemosiderin
HDRW	hearing distance for watch	HEMPAS	hereditary erythrocytic
	to be heard in right ear		multinuclearity with
HDS	Hamilton Depression		positive acidified serum
	(Rating) Scale		test
	herniated disk syndrome	HEMS	helicopter emergency
HDSCR	health deviation self-care		medical services
	requisite	HEN	hemorrhages, exudates,
HDT	habilitative day treatment		and nicking
	hearing distraction test		home enteral nutrition
HDU	hemodialysis unit	He-Ne	helium-neon
	high-dependency unit (an	HEP	hemoglobin
	intensive care unit)		electrophoresis
HDV	hepatitis D virus		hemorrhage, exudates, and
HDW	hearing distance (with)		papilledemaa
	watch		heparin
HDYF	how do you feel		hepatic
HE	hard events		hepatoerythropoietic
	hard exudate		porphyria
	health educator		hepatoma
	hepatic encephalopathy		histamine equivalent prick
H&E	hematoxylin and eosin		home exercise program
	hemorrhage and exudate	HEPA	hamster egg penetration
	heredity and environment		assay
HEA	health		high-efficiency particulate
HEAR	hospital emergency		air (filter)
	ambulance radio	hep cap	heparin cap
HEAT	human erythrocyte	HER2	human epidermal growth
	agglutination test		factor 2
HEB	hydrophilic emollient base	HERP	human exposure (dose)/
HEC	Health Education Center		rodent potency (dose)
HeCOG	Hellenic Cooperative	HES	hetastarch (hydroxyethyl
	Oncology Group		starch; Hespan)
HEDIS	Health Employer Data		hypereosinophilic
	and Information Set		syndrome
HEENT	head, eyes, ears, nose,	HEs	hypertensive emergencies
	and throat	hES	human embryonic stem
HeFH	heterozygous familial	20-HETE	20-hydroxyeico-
	hypercholesterolemia		satetraenoic acid
HEICS	Hospital Emergency	HETF	home enteral tube feeding
	Incident Command	HEV	hepatitis E vaccine
	System		hepatitis E virus
HEK	human embryonic kidney		high-endothelial venule
HEL	*Helicobacter pylori*	Hex	altretamine
	vaccine		(hexamethylmelamine;
	human embryonic lung		Hexalen)

Hexa-CAF	altretamine (hexamethylmelamine), cyclophosphamide, methotrexate (amethopterin), and fluorouracil		Hoffa fat pad
		HFPPV	high-frequency positive pressure ventilation
		HFR	hemorrhagic fever with renal syndrome vaccine
HF	Hageman factor		
	hard feces	HFRS	hemorrhagic fever with renal syndrome
	hay fever		
	head of fetus	HFRT	hyperfractionated radiotherapy
	heart failure		
	high frequency	HFS	hand-foot skin (reaction)
	Hispanic female		hand-foot syndrome
	hot flashes	HFSH	human follicle-stimulating hormone
	house formula		
HFA	health facility administrator	HFST	hearing-for-speech test
		HFUPR	hourly fetal urine production rate
	high-functioning autism		
	hydrofluoroalkane-134a	HFV	high-frequency ventilation
HFAS	hereditary flat adenoma syndrome		high-fruit/vegetable (diet)
		HFX RT	hyperfractionated radiation therapy
HFB	high-frequency band		
HFC	hydrofluorocarbon	HG	handgrasp
HFCB	horizontal flow clean bench		handgrip
			hemoglobin
HFCC	high-frequency chest compression		hyperemesis gravidarum
		Hg	mercury
HFD	high-fiber diet	HGA	high-grade astrocytomas
	high-forceps delivery	Hgb	hemoglobin
	high-frequency discharges	Hgb ELECT	hemoglobin electrophoresis
hFH	heterozygous familial hypercholesterolemia	Hgb F	fetal hemoglobin
		Hgb S	sickle cell hemoglobin
HFHL	high-frequence hearing loss	HGD	high grade dysplasia
		HGE	human granulocytic ehrlichiosis
HFI	hereditary fructose intolerance		
		HGES	handgrasp equal and strong
HFIP	hexafluoro-isopropranolol		
HFJV	high-frequency jet ventilation	HGF	hepatocyte growth factor
			hereditary gingival fibromatosis
H flu	*Haemophilus influenzae*		
HFM	hand-foot-and-mouth (disease) (often caused by coxsackievirus A16)	HGG	human gamma globulin
		HGH	human growth hormone
		HGI	Human Genome Initiative
	hemifacial microsomia	HGM	home glucose monitoring
HFMD	hand-foot-and-mouth disease (often caused by coxsackievirus A16)	HGN	hypogastric nerve
		HGNT	high-grade neuroendocrine tumors
		HGO	hepatic glucose output
HFO	high-frequency oscillation		hip guidance orthosis
HFOV	high-frequency oscillatory ventilation	HGP	Human Genome Project
		HGPIN	high-grade prostatic intraepithelial neoplasia
HFP	hepatic function panel (see page 392)		

H

HGPRT	hypoxanthine-guanine phosphoribosyl-transferase
HGS	hand-grip strength
	human genome sequence
HGSIL	high-grade squamous intraepithelial lesion
HGV	hepatitis G vaccine
	hepatitis G virus
HH	hard of hearing
	head hood
	hiatal hernia
	home health
	homonymous hemiopia
	household
	hyperhomocystinemia
	hypogonadotropic hypogonadism
	hypoeninemic hypoaldosteronism
H/H	hemoglobin/hematocrit
H&H	hematocrit and hemoglobin
HHA	health hazard appraisal
	hereditary hemolytic anemia
	home health agency
	home health aid
HH Assist	hand-held assist
HHC	home health care
HHCA	home health care agency
	hypothermic hypokalemic cardioplegic arrest
HHcy	hyperhomocystinemia
HHD	Doctor of Holistic Health
	hand-held dynamometer
	home hemodialysis
	household distance (physical therapy goal of mobility)
	hypertensive heart disease
HHFM	high-humidity face mask
HHH	hypermethionemia, hyperammonemia, and homocitrolinemia (syndrome)
HHHQ	Health Habits and History Questionnaire (Block-National Cancer Institute)
HHM	high-humidity mask
	humoral hypercalcemia of malignancy

HHN	hand-held nebulizer
HHNC	hyperosmolar hyperglycemic nonketotic coma
HHNK	hyperglycemic hyperosmolar nonketotic (coma)
HHNS	hyperosmolar-hyperglycemic nonketotic syndrome
HHRG	Home Health Resource Group (reimbursement categories for home health)
HHS	Health and Human Service (US Department of)
HHT	hereditary hemorrhagic telangiectasis
HHTC	high-humidity trach collar
HHTM	high-humidity trach mask
HHTS	high-humidity tracheostomy shield
HHV-8	human herpesvirus 8
HI	*Haemophilus influenzae*
	head injury
	health insurance
	hearing impaired
	hemagglutination inhibition
	homicidal ideation
	hospital insurance
	human insulin
HIA	hemagglutination inhibition antibody
HIAA	hydroxyindoleacetic acid
5-HIAA	5-hydroxyindoleacetic acid
HIAP	human intracisternal A-type particle
HIB	*Haemophilus influenzae* type b (vaccine)
HIB$_{cn}$	*haemophilus influenzae* type b conjugate vaccine
HIB$_{HbOC}$	*haemophilus influenzae* type b vaccine, HbOC conjugate vaccine
HIB$_{PRP-D}$	*haemophilus influenzae* type b vaccine, PRP-D conjugate vaccine
HIB$_{PRP-OMP}$	*haemophilus influenzae* type b vaccine, PRP-OMP conjugate vaccine

HIB$_{PRP-T}$	*haemophilus influenzae* type b vaccine, PRP-T conjugate vaccine	HINN	Hospital-issued Notice of Noncoverage
HIB$_{ps}$	*haemophilus influenzae* type b polysaccharide vaccine	HIO	health insuring organization
			hepatic iron overload
HIC	Human Investigation Committee	HIP	health insurance plan
		HIPA	heparin-induced platelet aggregation
	Humphriss immediate contrast (astigmatism test)	HIPAA	Health Insurance Portability and Accountability Act of 1996
hi-cal	high caloric		
HID	headache, insomnia, and depression		
	herniated intervertebral disk	HIPC	hormone-independent prostate cancer
HIDA	hepato-iminodiacetic acid (lidofenin)	HIPPS	Health Insurance Prospective Payment System
HiDAC	high-dose cytarabine (ara-C)	hi-pro	high-protein
		HIR	head injury routine
HIDS	hyperimmunoglobulinemia D syndrome	HIS	Hanover Intensive Score
			Health Intention Scale
HIE	hyperimmunoglobulinemia E		high-intermittent suction
			histidine
	hypoxic-ischemic encephalopathy		Home Incapacity Scale
			hospital (healthcare) information system
HIF	*Haemophilus influenzae*		
	higher integrative functions	HISMS	How I See Myself Scale
		HISTO	histoplasmin skin test
HIFU	high-intensity focused ultrasonography		histoplasmosis
		HIT	heparin-induced thrombocytopenia
HIHA	high impulsiveness, high anxiety		histamine-inhalation test
			home infusion therapy
HIHARS	hyperventilation-induced high-amplitude rhythmic slowing	HITS	high-intensity transient signals
HII	hepatic-iron index	HITTS	heparin-induced thrombotic thrombocytopenia syndrome
HIIC	heated intraoperative intraperitoneal chemotherapy		
HIL	hypoxic-ischemic lesion	HIU	head injury unit
HILA	high impulsiveness, low anxiety	HIV	human immunodeficiency virus
HILP	hyperthermic isolated limb perfusion		human immunodeficiency virus vaccine
HIM	health information management	HIV-1	human immunodeficiency virus type 1
	hexyl-insulin monoconjugate	HIV-2	human immunodeficiency virus type 2
HIN	*haemophilus influenzae* nontypable strain(s) vaccine	HIVAN	human immunodeficiency virus-associated nephropathy
HINI	hypoxic-ischemic neuronal injury	HIVAT	home intravenous antibiotic therapy

H

171

HIVD	herniated intervertebral disk		human luteinizing hormone
HIV-D	human immunodeficiency virus-related dementia	HLHS	hypoplastic left-heart syndrome
hi-vit	high-vitamin	HLI	head lice infestation
HIVMP	high-dose intravenous methylprednisolone	HLK	heart, liver, and kidneys
		HLM	hemosiderin-laden macrophages
HIVN	human immunodeficiency virus nephropathy	HLOS	hypertensive lower oesophageal sphincter (United Kingdom and other countries)
HJB	Howell-Jolly bodies		
HJR	hepatojugular reflux		
HK	hand-to-knee		
	heel-to-knee	HLP	hyperlipoproteinemia
	hexokinase	hLS	human lung surfactant
hK6	human kallikrein 6	HLT	heart-lung transplantation (transplant)
HKAFO	hip-knee-ankle-foot orthosis		
		HLV	herpes-like virus
HKAO	hip-knee-ankle orthosis		hypoplastic left ventricle
HKMN	Hickman (catheter)		
HKO	hip-knee orthosis	HM	hand motion
HKS	heel-knee-shin (test)		head movement
HKT	heterotopic kidney transplant		heart murmur
			heavily muscled
HL	hairline		heloma molle
	half-life		Hispanic male
	hallux limitus		Holter monitor
	haloperidol		home
	harelip		human milk
	hearing level		human semisynthetic insulin
	hearing loss		
	heavy lifting		humidity mask
	hemilaryngectomy	HMA	hemorrhages and microaneurysms
	heparin lock		
	hepatic lipase		heteroduplex mobility assay
	Hickman line		
H&L	heart and lung	HMB	beta-hydroxy-beta methylbutyrate (a leucine metabolite)
HLA	human leukocyte antigen		
	human lymphocyte antigen		
HLA negative	heart, lungs, and abdomen negative		homatropine methylbromide
			hypersensitivity to mosquito bites
HLB	head, limbs, and body		
HLD	haloperidol decanoate (Haldol)	HMBA	hexamethylene bisacetamide
	herniated lumbar disk	HMD	hyaline membrane disease
	high-lipid disorder	HMDP	hydroxymethyline diphosphonate
HLDP	hypoglossia-limb deficiency phenotype		
		HME	heat and moisture exchanger
HLES	hypertensive lower esophageal sphincter		
			heat, massage, and exercise
HLGR	high-level gentamicin resistance		
			hereditary multiple exostoses
HLH	hemophagocytic lymphohistiocytosis		

	home medical equipment	HMX	heat massage exercise
	human monocytic ehrlichiosis	HN	head and neck
			head nurse
HMEF	heat moisture exchanging filter		high nitrogen
			home nursing
HMETSC	heavy metal screen	H&N	head and neck
HMF	human milk fortifier	HN2	mechlorethamine HCl (Mustargen)
HMG	human menopausal gonadotropin		
		HNC	head and neck cancer
HMG CoA	hydroxymethyl glutaryl coenzyme A		human neutrophil collagenase
HMI	healed myocardial infarction		hyperosmolar nonketotic coma
	history of medical illness	HNCa	head and neck cancer
HMIS	hospital medical information system	HNCCG	Head and Neck Cancer Cooperative Group
HMK	homemaking	HNE	human neutrophil elastase
HM & LP	hand motion and light perception	HNI	hospitalization not indicated
HMM	altretamine (hexamethyl-melamine; Hexalen)	HNKDC	hyperosomolar nonketotic diabetic coma
HMO	Health Maintenance Organization	HNKDS	hyperosmolar nonketotic diabetic state
	hypothetical mean organism	HNLN	hospitalization no longer necessary
HMP	health maintenance plan	¹H-NMR	proton nuclear magnetic resonance (spectroscopy)
	hexose monophosphate		
	hot moist packs		
HMPAO	hexylmethylpropylene amineoxine	HNN	hybrid neural network
		HNP	herniated nucleus pulposus
HMR	histocytic medullary reticulosis	HNPCC	heredity nonpolyposis colorectal cancer
	Hoechst Marion Roussel	HNPP	hereditary neuropathy with liability to pressure palsies
¹H-MRS	proton magnetic resonance spectroscopy		
HMS	hyper-reactive malarial splenomegaly	HNRNA	heterogeneous nuclear ribonucleic acid
	hypodermic morphine sulfate (this is a dangerous abbreviation)	HNS	0.45% sodium chloride injection (half-normal saline)
HMS®	medrysone		head and neck surgery
hMSCs	human mesenchymal stem cells		head, neck, and shaft
		HNSCC	squamous cell carcinoma of the head and neck
HMSN I	hereditary motor and sensory neuropathy type I		
		HNSN	home, no services needed
		HNT	hantaan (hantavirus) vaccine
HMSR	high medical-social risk		
HMSS	hyperactive malarial splenomegaly syndrome	HNV	has not voided
		HNWG	has not worn glasses
HMV	home mechanical ventilation	HO	hand orthosis
			heme oxygenase
HMWK	high-molecular weight kininogen		Hemotology-Oncology
			heterotropic ossification

	hip orthosis	HOVT	letter symbols used in pediatric visual acuity testing
	house officer		
H/O	history of		
H₂O	water	Ho:YAG	holmium: yttrium-aluminum-garnet
H₂O₂	hydrogen peroxide		
HOA	hip osteoarthritis	HP	hard palate
	hypertropic osteoarthropathy		Harvard pump
			Helicobacter pylori
HOB	head of bed		hemipelvectomy
HOB UPSOB	head of bed up for shortness of breath		hemiplegia
			herbal products
HOC	Health Officer Certificate		high-protein (supplement)
HOCM	high-osmolality contrast media		hot packs
			house physician
	hypertrophic obstructive cardiomyopathy		hydrogen peroxide
			hydrophilic petrolatum
HOD	heroin overdose	Hp	*Helicobacter pylori*
HOG	halothane, oxygen, and gas (nitrous oxide)	H&P	history and physical
		HPA	hybridization protection assay
HOH	hand-over-hand (rehabilitation term)		hypothalamic-pituitary-adrenal (axis)
	hard of hearing		
HOI	hospital onset of infection	HPAE-PAD	high-pH anion exchange chromatography coupled with pulsed amperometric detection
HOM	high-osmolar contrast media		
HOMA	homeostatic assessment model algorithm (index)		
		HPAI	highly pathogenic avian influenza A virus
	homeostatic model assessment	HPAT	home parenteral antibiotic therapy
HOME	Home Observation for Measurement of the Environment		
		HPB	Health Protection Branch (the Canadian equivalent of the U.S. Food and Drug Administration)
HONC	Hooked on Nicotine Checklist		
	hyperosmolar, nonketotic coma		
		HPC	hemangiopericytoma
HONK	hyperosmolar nonketotic (coma)		hereditary prostate cancer
HOP	hourly output		history of present condition (complaint)
HOPI	history of present illness		
Hopkins-25	Hopkins Symptom Checklist-25	HPCE	high-performance capillary electrophoresis
HOR	higher-order repeat	HPD	high-protein diet
HORF	high-output renal failure		home peritoneal dialysis
HORS	Hemiballism/Hemichorea Outcome Rating Score		hours post dose
		HpD	hematoporphyrin derivative
HOS	Health Outcomes Survey	HP&D	hemoprofile and differential
HOSP	hospital		
	hospitalization	HPE	hemorrhage, papilledema, exudate
HOT	home oxygen therapy		
HOTV	letter symbols used in pediatric visual acuity testing		history and physical examination
			holoprosencephaly

HPET	*Helicobacter pylori* eradication therapy	HPTD	highly permeable transparent dressing
HPF	high-power field	hPTH	human parathyroid hormone I_{34} (teriparatide)
HPFH	hereditary persistence of fetal hemoglobin		
HPG	human pituitary gonadotropin	HPTM	home prothrombin time monitoring
HPI	history of present illness	HPTX	hemopneumothorax
HPIP	history, physical, impression, and plan	HPV	human papilloma virus human papilloma virus vaccine human parvovirus
HPK	hyperkeratosis		
HPL	human placenta lactogen hyperlipidemia hyperplexia	*H pylori*	*Helicobacter pylori*
		HPZ	high-pressure zone
HPLC	high-performance (pressure) liquid chromatography	HQC	hydroquinone cream
		HQL	health-related quality of life
HPM	hemiplegic migraine	HR	hallux rigidus Harrington rod hazard ratio health related heart rate hemorrhagic retinopathy histamine release hospital record hour
HPMC	high-performance membrane chromatography hydroxypropyl methylcellulose		
HPN	home parenteral nutrition		
HPNI	hemodialysis prognostic nutrition index	Hr 0	zero hour (when treatment starts)
HPNS	high-pressure nervous syndrome	Hr -2	minus two hours (two hours prior to treatment)
HPO	hydrophilic ointment hypertrophic pulmonary osteoarthropathy	H & R	hysterectomy and radiation
HPOA	hypertrophic pulmonary osteoarthropathy	HRA	high-right atrium histamine-releasing activity
2HPP	2-hour postprandial (blood sugar)	H2RA	histamine$_2$-receptor antagonist
2HPPBS	2-hour postprandial blood sugar		
HPPM	hyperplastic persistent pupillary membrane	HRC	Human Rights Committee
		HRCT	high-resolution computed tomography
hPRL	prolactin, human	HRD	human retroviral disease hypertension renal disease hypoparathyroidism, retardation, and dysmorphism (syndrome)
HPS	hantavirus pulmonary syndrome hepatopulmonary syndrome hypertrophic pyloric stenosis		
HpSA	*Helicobacter pylori* stool antigen	HRE	high-resolution electrocardiography
HPT	heparin protamine titration histamine provocation test home pregnancy test hyperparathyroidism	HRECG	high-resolution electrocardiography
		HRF	Harris return flow health-related facility

H

175

	histamine-releasing factor		high-risk transfer
	hypertensive renal failure		hormone replacement
	hypoxic respiratory failure		therapy
HRI	HMG-CoA (3-hydroxy-3-methylglutaryl-coenzyme A) reductase inhibitors	HRV	hyperfractioned radiotherapy
			heart rate variability
			heterogeneous resistance to vancomycin
HRIF	histamine inhibitory releasing factor	HS	bedtime
			half-strength
HRIG	human rabies immune globulin		hamstrings
			hamstring sets
HRL	head rotated left		Harmonic scalpel
HRLA	human reovirus-like agent		Hartman solution (lactated Ringers)
HRLM	high-resolution light microscopy		
			heart size
hRLX-2	synthetic human relaxin		heart sounds
HRMPC	hormone-refractory metastatic prostate cancer		heavy smoker
			heel spur
			heel stick
HRMS	high-resolution mass spectrometry		hereditary spherocytosis
			herpes simplex
HRNB	Halstead-Reitan Neuropsychological Battery		hidradenitis suppurativa
			high school
			hippocampal sclerosis
HRP	high-risk pregnancy		Hurler syndrome
	horseradish peroxidase	H → S	heel-to-shin
HRP-2	histidine-rich protein-2	H&S	hearing and speech
HRPC	hormone-refractory prostate cancer		hemorrhage and shock
			hysterectomy and sterilization
HRQL	health-related quality of life	HSA	Health Services Administration (Administrator)
HRQOL	health-related quality of life		
			Health Systems Agency
HRR	head rotated right		human serum albumin
HRRC	Human Research Review Committee		hypersomnia-sleep apnea
		HSAN	hereditary sensory and autonomic neuropathy (types I-IV)
HRS	Haw River syndrome		
	hepatorenal syndrome		
	Hodgkin-Reed-Sternberg (cells)	HSB	husband
HRSD	Hamilton Rating Scale for Depression	HSBS	evening blood sugar
		HSBG	heel-stick blood gas
HRSEM	high-resolution scanning electron microscopy	HSC	hematopoietic stem cell
		HSCL	Hopkins Symptom-Check List
HRST	heat, reddening, swelling, or tenderness		
		hs-CRP	high-sensitivity C-reactive protein
	heavy-resistance strength training		
		HSCSS	hypersensitive carotid sinus syndrome
HRT	heart rate		
	heart rate turbulence	HSCT	hematopoietic stem cell transplant
	Heidelberg retina tomograph		
	heparin-response test		

HSD	Honestly Significant Difference (test) (Turkey)	HSS	half-strength saline (0.45% Sodium Chloride)
	hypoactive sexual desire (disorder)	HSSE	high soap-suds enema
HSDD	hypoactive sexual desire disorder	HS-tk	herpes simplex thymidine kinase
HSE	herpes simplex encephalitis	HSV	herpes simplex virus highly selective vagotomy
	human skin equivalent	HSV-1	herpes simplex virus type 1
	hypertonic saline-epinephrine		herpes simplex virus type 1 vaccine
HSEES	Hazardous Substances Emergency Events Surveillance	HSV_2	herpes simplex virus type 2 vaccine
HSES	hemorrhagic shock and encephalopathy	HSV_{12}	herpes simplex virus types 1, 2 vaccine
HSG	herpes simplex genitalis	HSV-2	herpes simplex virus type 2
	hysterosalpingogram	HSVE	herpes simplex virus encephalitis
HSGYV	heat, steam, gum, yawn, and Valsalva maneuver (for otitis media)	HT	hammertoe
			head trauma
			healing time
H-SIL	high-grade squamous intraepithelial lesions		hearing test
			heart
HSJ	hepatic schistosomiasis japonica		heart transplant
			height
HSK	herpes simplex keratitis		heparin trap (hep-trap; heparin lock; a venous access device)
HSL	herpes simplex labialis		
	hormone-sensitive lipase		high temperature
HSM	hepatosplenomegaly		hormonotherapy
	holosystolic murmur		Hubbard tank
HSN	Hansen-Street nail		hypermetropia
	heart sounds normal		hyperopia
	hereditary sensory neuropathy		hypertension
			hyperthermia
HSOs	health services organizations		hyperthyroid
		H/T	heel and toe (walking)
HSP	heat shock protein	H&T	hospitalization and treatment
	Henoch-Schönlein purpura		
	hereditary spastic paraplegia	H(T)	intermittent hypertropia
		HT-1	hereditary tyrosinemia type 1
	hysterosalpingography		
HSPC	hydrogenated soy phosphatidyl choline	$5\text{-}HT_1$	serotonin (5-hydroxytryptamine)
HSPE	high-strength pancreatic enzymes	HTA	Health Technology Assessment (Program)
HSQ	Health Status Questionnaire		hypertension (French)
		ht. aer.	heated aerosol
HSR	heated serum reagin	HTAT	human tetanus antitoxin
	hypersensitivity reaction	HTB	hot tub bath
	hypofractionated stereotactic radiotherapy	HTC	heated-tracheostomy collar
			hypertensive crisis

H

HTDS	high-throughput drug screening	HUH	Humana Hospital
		HUI	Health Utilities Index
HTE	highly-treatment experienced (patients)	HUI2	Health Utilities Index Mark 2
hTERT	human telomerase reverse transcriptase	HUIFM	human leukocyte interferon meloy
HTF	house tube feeding	HUK	human urinary kallikrein
HTGL	hepatic triglyceride lipase	HUM	heat, ultrasound, and massage
HTK	heel-to-knee (test)		
HTL	hearing threshold level	HUM 70/30	human insulin, regular 30 units/mL with human insulin isophane suspension 70 units/mL (Humulin® 70/30 insulin)
	honey-thick liquid (diet consistency)		
	human T-cell leukemia		
	human thymic leukemia		
HTLV III	human T-cell lymphotrophic virus type III	HUMARA	human androgen receptor assay
HTM	*Haemophilus* test medium	HUM L	human insulin zinc suspension (Humulin® L Insulin)
	high threshold mechanoceptors		
HTML	hypertext markup language	HUM N	human insulin isophane suspension (Humulin® N Insulin)
HTN	hypertension		
HTO	high tibial osteotomy		
HTP	House-Tree-Person-test	HUM R	human insulin, regular (Humulin® R Insulin)
5-HTP	serotonin (5-hydroxytryptophan)		
		HUR	hydroxyurea
HTR	hard tissue replacement	HUS	head ultrasound
hTRT	human telomerase reverse transcriptase		hemolytic uremic syndrome
HTS	head traumatic syndrome		husband
	heel-to-shin (test)	husb	husband
	Hematest(r) stools	HUT	head-upright tilt (test)
	high-throughput screening		hyperplasia of usual type
HTSCA	human tumor stem cell assay	HUVEC	human umbilical vein endothelial cells
HtSDS	height standard deviation score	HV	hallux valgus
H-TSH	human thyroid-stimulating hormone		Hantavirus
			has voided
HTT	hand thrust test		Hemovac®
HTV	herpes-type virus		hepatic vein
HTVD	hypertensive vascular disease		herpesvirus
			home visit
HTX	hemothorax	H&V	hemigastrecotomy and vagotomy
HTx	heart transplant		
HU	head unit	HVII	hypervariable segment II
	hydroxyurea	HVA	homovanillic acid
	hypertensive urgencies	HVD	hypertensive vascular disease
Hu	Hounsfield units		
HUAEC	human umbilical endothelial cells	HVDO	hypovitaminosis D osteopathy
HUCB	human umbilical cord blood	HVE	high-voltage electrophoresis

HVES	high-voltage electrical stimulation	Hypo K	hypokalemia
HVF	Humphrey visual field	hypopit	hypopituitarism
HVGS	high-voltage galvanic stimulation	HYs	healthy years of life
		Hyst	hysterectomy
HVI	hollow viscus injury	Hz	Hertz
HVL	half-value layer	HZ	herpes zoster
	hippocampal volume loss	HZD	herpes zoster dermatitis
HVOD	hepatic veno-occlusive disease	HZO	herpes zoster ophthalmicus
HVOO	hepatic venous outflow obstruction	HZV	herpes zoster virus

HVPC   high-voltage pulsed current

HVPG   hepatic venous pressure gradient

HYPT   hyperventilation provocation test

HVR   hypoxic ventilatory response

HVS   hyperventilation syndrome

HVS-TK   herpes simplex virus thymidine kinase

HW   heparin well
homework
housewife

HWB   hot water bottle

HWFE   housewife

HWG   has worn glasses

HWH   halfway house

HWP   hot wet pack

HWPG   has worn prescription glasses

Hx   history
hospitalization

HXM   altretamine (hexamethylmelamine; Hexalen)

Hx & Px   history and physical (examination)

Hy   hypermetropia

HYDRO   hydronephrosis
hydrotherapy

HYG   hygiene

HYPER   above
higher than

Hyper Al   hyperalimentation

Hyper K   hyperkalemia

HYPER T & A   hypertrophic tonsils and adenoids

HYPO   below
hypodermic injection
lower than

H

I

I	impression
	incisal
	incontinent
	independent
	initial
	inspiration
	intact (bag of waters)
	intermediate
	iris
	one
I_2	iodine
I^{131}	radioactive iodine
I-3+7	idarubicin and cytarabine
IA	ideational apraxia
	idiopathic anaphylaxis
	incidental appendectomy
	incurred accidentally
	indigenous Australian(s)
	intra-amniotic
	intra-arterial
	invasive aspergillosis
I & A	irrigation and aspiration
IAA	ileoanal anastomosis
	insulin autoantibodies
	interrupted aortic arch
	intra-abdominal abscess
IAAA	inflammatory abdominal aortic aneurysms
IAAT	intra-abdominal adipose tissue
IAB	incomplete abortion
	induced abortion
	intermittent androgen blockade
IABC	intra-aortic balloon counterpulsation
IABCP	intra-aortic balloon counterpulsation
IABP	intra-aortic balloon pump
	intra-arterial blood pressure
IAC	internal auditory canal
	intra-arterial chemotherapy
	isolated adrenal cell
IAC-CPR	interposed abdominal compressions—cardiopulmonary resuscitation

IACG	intermittent angle-closure glaucoma
IACNS	isolated angiitis of central nervous system
IACP	intra-aortic counterpulsation
IAD	implantable atrial defibrillator
	intermittent androgen deprivation
	intractable atopic dermatitis
	intraoperative autologous (blood) donation
IADHS	inappropriate antidiuretic hormone syndrome
IADL	Instrumental Activities of Daily Living
IA DSA	intra-arterial digital subtraction arteriography
IAEA	International Atomic Energy Agency
IAET	International Association for Enterostomal Therapy (Standards of Care Dermal Wounds: Pressure Ulcers)—see WOCN
IAF	intra-abdominal fat
IAG	indolyl-3-acryloylglycine
IAGT	indirect antiglobulin test
IAHA	immune adherence hemagglutination
IAHC	intra-arterial hepatic chemotherapy
IAHD	idiopathic acquired hemolytic disease
IAI	intra-abdominal infection
	intra-abdominal injury
	intra-amniotic infection
IALD	instrumental activities of daily living
IAM	internal auditory meatus
IAN	indinavir (Crixivan) associated nephrolithiasis
	inferior alveolar nerve
	intern's admission note
IAO	immediately after onset
IAP	independent adjudicating panel

	intermittent acute porphyria	IBG	iliac bone graft
	intra-abdominal pressure	IBI	intermittent bladder irrigation
	intracarotid amobarbital procedure	*ibid*	at the same place
IAPP	islet amyloid polypeptide	IBILI	indirect bilirubin
IAQ	indoor air quality	IBM	ideal body mass
IARC	International Agency for Research on Cancer		inclusion body myositis
IART	intra-atrial reentrant tachycardia	IBMI	initial body mass index
IAS	idiopathic ankylosing spondylitis	IBMTR	International Bone Marrow Transplant Registry
	intermittent androgen suppression	IBNR	incurred but not reported
	internal anal sphincter	IBOW	intact bag of waters
	Interpersonal Adjective Scales	IBP	ibuprofen
IASD	interatrial septal defect		intrableb pigmentation
IAT	immunoaugmentive therapy	IBPB	interscalene brachial plexus block
	indirect antiglobulin test	IBPS	Insall-Burstein posterior stabilizer
	intracarotid amobarbital test	IBR	immediate breast reconstruction
	intraoperative autologous transfusion		infectious bovine rhinotracheitis
IATT	intra-arterial thrombolytic therapy	IBRS	Inpatient Behavior Rating Scale
IAV	intermittent assist ventilation	IBS	irritable bowel syndrome
IAVC	intrinsic atrioventricular conduction	IBS-D	Irritable Bowel Syndrome–Diarrhea Type
IB	ileal bypass	IBT	ink blot test (Rorschach test)
	insulin-receptor binding test		interblinking time
	isolation bed		immune-based therapy
	investigator's brochure	IBTR	intrabreast-tumor recurrence
IB1A	interferon beta-1a (Avonex)		ipsilateral breast tumor recurrence
IBAM	idiopathic bile acid malabsorption	IBU	ibuprofen
IBBB	intra-blood-brain barrier	IBW	ideal body weight
IBBBB	incomplete bilateral bundle branch block	IC	between meals
IBC	Institutional Biosafety Committee		iliac crest
	invasive bladder cancer		immune complex
	iron binding capacity		immunocompromised
IBD	infectious bursal disease		incipient cataract (grade 1+ to 4+)
	inflammatory bowel disease		incomplete
	isosulfan blue dye		indirect calorimetry
IBDQ	Inflammatory Bowel Disease Questionnaire		indirect Coombs (test)
IBE	individual bioequivalence		individual counseling
			informed consent
			inspiratory capacity
			intensive care
			intercostal
			intercourse
			intermediate care

I

	intermittent catheterization		intermediate coronary care unit
	intermittent claudication		
	interstitial changes	ICD	implantable cardioverter defibrillator
	interstitial cystitis		
	intracerebral		indigocarmine dye
	intracranial		informed consent document
	intraincisional		
	ion chromatography		instantaneous cardiac death
	irritable colon		
I/C	imipenem-cilastatin (Primaxin)		isocitrate dehydrogenase
ICA	ileocolic anastomosis		irritant contact dermatitis
	intermediate care area	ICDA	International Classification of Disease, Adapted
	internal carotid artery		
	intracranial abscess		
	intracranial aneurysm	ICDB	incomplete database
	islet-cell antibody	ICDC	implantable cardioverter defibrillator catheter
ICa	calcium, ionized		
ICAAC	Interscience Conference on Antimicrobial Agents and Chemotherapy	ICD 9 CM	International Statistical Classification of Diseases, 9th Revision, Clinical Modification
ICAM	intracellular adhesion molecule	ICD-10	International Classification of Diseases and Related Health Problems, 10th revision
ICAM-1	intercellular adhesion molecule-1		
ICAO	internal carotid artery occlusion	ICD-10-PCS	International Statistical Classification of Diseases, 10th Revision, Procedure Coding Classification System
ICAS	intermediate coronary artery syndrome		
ICAT	infant cardiac arrest tray		
ICB	intracranial bleeding		
ICBG	iliac crest bone graft	ICDO	International Classification of Diseases for Oncology
ICBT	intercostobronchial trunk		
ICC	idiopathic chronic cough	ICE	ice, compression, and elevation
	immunocytochemistry		
	Indian childhood cirrhosis		ifosfamide, carboplatin, and etoposide
	Infection Control Committee		
	intracluster correlation coefficient		individual career exploration
	intraclass correlation coefficient		interleukin-1 alpha converting enzyme
	invasive cervical carcinoma		interleukin-1 beta converting enzyme
	islet cell carcinoma		intracardiac echocardiography
ICCD	intensified charge-coupled device	+ ice	add ice
		ICECI	International Classification of External Causes of Injuries
ICCE	intracapsular cataract extraction		
ICCU	intensive coronary care unit	ICER	incremental cost-effectiveness ratio

ICES	ice, compression, elevation, and support	ICPP	intubated continuous positive pressure
ICF	intermediate care facility	ICR	intercaudate nucleus ratio
	intracellular fluid		intercostal retractions
ICFDH	International Classification of Functioning, Disability, and Health		intrastromal corneal ring
		ICRC	International Committee of the Red Cross
		ICRF-159	razoxane
ICG	indocyanine green	ICRP	International Commission on Radiological Protection
ICGA	indocyanine green angiography		
ICH	immunocompromised host	ICRS	intrastromal corneal ring segments
	International Conference on Harmonization (of Technical Requirements for Registration of Pharmaceuticals for Human Use)	ICS	ileocecal sphincter
			inhaled corticosteroid(s)
			intercostal space
		ICSC	idiopathic central serous choroidopathy
	intracerebral hemorrhage	ICSH	interstitial cell-stimulating hormone
	intracranial hemorrhage		
ICHI	International Classification of Health Interventions	ICSI	intracytoplasmic sperm injection
ICI	intracranial injury	ICSR	Individual Case Safety Reports
ICIT	intensified conventional insulin therapy		intercostal space retractions
ICL	intracorneal lens	ICT	icterus
	isocitrate lyase		indirect Coombs test
ICLE	intracapsular lens extraction		inflammation of connective tissue
ICM	intercostal margin		intensive conventional therapy
	intercostal muscle		intermittent cervical traction
	ischemic cardiomyopathy		
ICN	infection control nurse		intracranial tumor
	intensive care nursery		intracutaneous test
ICN2	neonatal intensive care unit level II		islet cell transplant
		ICTX	intermittent cervical traction
ICP	inductively coupled plasma		
	intercostal position (for chest lead)	ICU	intensive care unit
			intermediate care unit
	intracranial pressure	ICV	intracerebroventricular
	intrahepatic cholestasis of pregnancy	ICVH	ischemic cerebrovascular headache
ICPC	International Classification of Primary Care	ICW	in connection with
			intact canal wall
ICPC-2	International Classification of Primary Care, 2nd revision		intercellular water
		ID	identification
			identify
ICP-MS	inductively-coupled plasma—mass spectrometer		idiotype
			ifosfamide, mesna uroprotection, and doxorubicin
ICP-OES	inductively-coupled plasma—optical emission spectrometry		

I

		immunodiffusion		intrathecal drug infusion
		induction delivery	IDK	internal derangement of knee
		infectious disease (physician or department)	IDL	intermediate-density lipoprotein
		initial diagnosis		ischemic digital loss
		initial dose	IDLH	immediately dangerous to life or health
		intellectual disability	IDM	infant of a diabetic mother
		internal derangement	IDMC	immature dead male child
		intradermal		Independent Data Monitoring Committee
id		the same		
I & D		incision and debridement	IDNA	iron-deficient, not anemic
		incision and drainage	IDP	initiate discharge planning
		irrigation and debridement		inosine diphosphate
IDA		idarubicin (Idamycin)	IDPN	intradialytic parenteral nutrition
		iron deficiency anemia	IDR	idarubicin (Zavedos)
IDAM		infant of drug abusing mother		idiosyncratic drug reaction
				intradermal reaction
IDB		incomplete database	IDS	infectious disease service
IDC		idiopathic dilated cardiomyopathy		integrated delivery system
		invasive ductal cancer		intradermal smears
IDCF		immunodiffusion complement fixation	IDSA	Infectious Disease Society of America (guidelines)
IDCM		idiopathic dilated cardiomyopathy	IDT	intensive diabetes treatment
				interdisciplinary team
IDD		insulin-dependent diabetes		intradermal test
		intervertebral disk disease	IDTP	immunodiffusion tube precipitin
		iodine-deficiency disorders	IDU	idoxuridine
I/DD		intellectual and developmental disabilities		infectious disease unit
				injecting drug user
IDDD		Interview for Deterioration in Daily Life in Dementia	IDV	indinavir (Crixivan)
				intermittent demand ventilation
IDDM		insulin-dependent diabetes mellitus	IDVC	indwelling venous catheter
IDDS		implantable drug delivery system	IE	ifosfamide, and etoposide with mesna
IDE		Investigational Device Exemption		immunoelectrophoresis
				induced emesis
IDEA		Individuals with Disabilities Education Act		infective endocarditis
				inner ear
				internal/external (rotation)
				international unit (European abbreviation)
IDET		intradiskal electrothermal therapy	I & E	ingress and egress (tubes)
IDFC		immature dead female child	*i.e.*	internal and external
				that is
IDH		isocitric dehydrogenase	IEC	independent ethics committee
IDI		Interpersonal Dependency Inventory		inpatient exercise center

I

	intradiskal electrothermal	IFM	internal fetal monitoring
	coagulation	IFN	interferon
IEF	isoelectric focusing	IFN α-1	interferon alfa-1
IEI	idiopathic environmental	IFNB	interferon beta-1 b
	intolerance		(Betaseron)
IEL	internal elastic lamina	IFO	ifosfamide (Ifex)
	intestinal-intraepithelial		in front of
	lymphocyte	IFOS	ifosfamide (Ifex)
IEM	immune electron	IFP	inflammatory fibroid
	microscopy		polyps
	inborn errors of	IFPMA	International Federation of
	metabolism		Pharmaceutical
iEMG	integrated		Manufacturers
	electromyography		Associations
IEMR	integrated electronic	IFSAC	Inventory of Functional
	medical records		Status After Childbirth
IEN	intraepithelial neoplasia	IFSE	internal fetal scalp
IEP	immunoelectrophoresis		electrode
	Individualized Education	IFSP	individualized family
	Plan		service plan
IEPA	immunoelectrophoresis	IgA	immunoglobulin A
	analysis	IGCS	inpatient geriatric
I:E ratio	inspiratory to expiratory		consultation services
	time ratio	IgD	immunoglobulin D
IES	Impact of Event Scale	IGDE	idiopathic gait disorders
IET	infantile estropia		of the elderly
IF	idiopathic flushing	IGDM	infant of gestational
	ifosfamide (Ifex)		diabetic mother
	immunofluorescence	IgE	immunoglobulin E
	index finger	IGF-I	insulin-like growth
	injury factor		factor I
	interferon	IGFA	indocyanine-green fundus
	interfrontal		angiography
	intermaxillary fixation	IGFBP-3	insulin-like growth factor-
	internal fixation		binding protein 3
	intrinsic factor	IgG	immunoglobulin G
	involved field	IGHL	inferior glenohumeral
	(radiotherapy)		ligament
IFA	immunofluorescent assay	IGIM	immune globulin
	imported fire ants		intramuscular
	indirect fluorescent	IGIV	immune globulin
	antibody		intravenous
IFAT	immunofluorescence	IgM	immunoglobulin M
	antibody test (technique)	IGP	interstitial glycoprotein
IFC	interferential current	IGR	intrauterine growth
IFE	immunofixation		retardation
	electrophoresis	IGT	impaired glucose
	in-flight emergency		tolerance
IFG	impaired fasting glucose	IGTN	impaired glucose
IFL	indolent follicular		tolerance and
	lymphoma		neuropathy
	irinotecan, fluorouracil,		ingrown toenail
	and leucovorin	IH	indirect hemagglutination

	infectious hepatitis	IHW	inner-heel wedge
	inguinal hernia	II	internal iliac (artery)
	in-house	IIA	internal iliac artery
IHA	immune hemolytic anemia	IICP	increased intracranial
	indirect hemagglutination		pressure
	infusion hepatic	IICU	infant intensive care unit
	arteriography	IID	infectious intestinal
	intrahepatic arterial		disease
IHC	idiopathic hypercalciuria	IIEF	International Index of
	immobilization		Erectile Function
	hypercalcemia	IIF	indirect
	immunohistochemistry		immunofluorescence
	inner hair cell	IIH	idiopathic infantile
	(in cochlea)		hypercalcemia
IHD	intermittent hemodialysis		iodine-induced
	intraheptic duct (ule)		hyperthyroidism
	ischemic heart disease	IIHT	iodide-induced
IHDN	integrated health delivery		hyperthyroidism
	network	IIM	idiopathic inflammatory
IHES	idiopathic		myopathies
	hypereosinophilic		intracortical interaction
	syndrome		mapping
IHH	idiopathic	IINB	iliohypogastric
	hypogonadotrophic		ilioinguinal nerve block
	hypogonadism	IIP	idiopathic interstitial
IHHE	infantile hepatic		pneumonitis
	hemangioendothelioma	IIPF	idiopathic interstitial
IHO	idiopathic hypertrophic		pulmonary fibrosis
	osteoarthropathy	IJ	ileojejunal
IHP	idiopathic		internal jugular
	hypoparathyroidism	I&J	insight and judgment
	inferior hypogastric plexus	IJC	internal jugular catheter
	isolated hepatic perfusion	IJD	inflammatory joint disease
IHPH	intrahepatic portal	IJO	idiopathic juvenile
	hypertension		osteoporosis
IHPS	infantile hypertrophic	IJP	internal jugular pressure
	pyloric stenosis	IJR	idiojunctional rhythm
IHR	inguinal hernia repair	IJT	idiojunctional tachycardia
	intrinsic heart rate	IJV	internal jugular vein
IHS	Indian Health Service	IK	immobilized knee
	integrated healthcare		interstitial keratitis
	system	IKDC	International Knee
	International Headache		Documentation
	Society (criteria)		Committee (evaluation;
	Idiopathic Headache		score; form)
	Score	IL	immature lungs
IHs	iris hamartomas		interleukin (1, 2, etc.)
IHSA	iodinated human serum		intralesional
	albumin		Intralipid®
IHSS	idiopathic hypertrophic	IL-2	aldesleukin (Proleukin;
	subaortic stenosis		interleukin-2)
IHT	insulin hypoglycemia test	IL-11	oprelvekin (Neumega;
IHU	inpatient hospice unit		interleukin-11)

I

ILA	inferior lateral angle		intramedullary
	insulin-like activity		intramuscular
ILB	incidental Lewy body	IMA	inferior mesenteric artery
ILBBB	incomplete left bundle		internal mammary artery
	branch block	IMAC	ifosfamide, mesna
ILBW	infant, low birth weight		uroprotection,
	(less than 2,500 g)		doxorubicin
ILC	interstitial laser		(Adriamycin), and
	coagulation		cisplatin
	invasive lobular cancer		immobilized metal
ILD	immature lung disease		affinity chromatography
	indentation load deflection	IMAE	internal maxillary artery
	interlaminar distance in		embolization
	flexion	IMAG	internal mammary artery
	intermediate density		graft
	lipoproteins	IMARD	immunomodulating
	interstitial lung disease		antirheumatic drugs
	ischemic leg disease	IMAT	intensity-modulated arc
ILE	infantile lobar emphysema		therapy
	involutional lateral	IMB	intermenstrual bleeding
	entropion	IMBP	immobilized mismatch
ILF	indicated low forceps		binding protein
ILFC	immature living female	IMC	intermittent catheterization
	child		intramedullary catheter
ILHP	ipsilateral	IMCI	Integrated Management of
	hemidiaphragmatic		Childhood Illness
	paresis	IMCU	intermediate care unit
ILI	influenza-like illness	IME	important medical event
ILM	internal limiting		independent medical
	membrane		examination
ILMC	immature living male		(evaluation)
	child		isometric exercise
ILMI	inferolateral myocardial	IMF	idiopathic myelofibrosis
	infarct		ifosfamide, mesna
ILP	interstitial laser		uroprotection,
	photocoagulation		methotrexate, and
	isolated limb perfusion		fluorouracil
ILQTS	idiopathic long QT		immobilization
	(interval) syndrome		mandibular fracture
ILR	implantable loop recorder		inframammary fold
ILS	intralabyrinthine		intermaxillary fixation
	schwannomas	IMG	internal medicine group
ILT	interstitial laser therapy	IMGU	insulin-mediated glucose
ILVEN	inflammatory linear		uptake
	verrucal epidermal nevus	IMH	idiopathic myocardial
IM	ice massage		hypertrophy
	imatinib mesylate		intramural hematoma
	(Gleevec) (This is a	IMH	indirect
	very dangerous		microhemagglutination
	abbreviation)		(test)
	infectious mononucleosis	IMI	imipramine
	intermetatarsal		impending myocardial
	internal medicine		infarction

	inferior myocardial infarction	In	indium
		in.	inch
	intramuscular injection	INAD	in no apparent distress
^{131}I-MIBG	iodine^{131}-metaiodobenzyl-guanidine (iobenguane ^{131}I)		Investigational New Animal Drug
		INB	intercostal nerve blockade
IMIG	intramuscular immunoglobulin	INC	incisal
			incision
IMLC	incomplete mitral leaflet closure		incomplete
			incontinent
IMM	immunizations		increase
IMN	idiopathic membranous nephropathy		inside-the-needle catheter
		INCC	Institut National du Cancer du Canada
	immune modulating nutrition (immunonutrition)	Inc Spir	incentive spirometer
	internal mammary (lymph) node	IND	indinavir (Crixivan)
			induced
IMP	impacted		Investigational New Drug (application)
	important		
	impression	INDA	Investigational New Drug Application
	improved		
	inosine monophoshate	INDIGO	interstitial laser ablation of the prostate
IMPX	impaction		
IMR	infant mortality rate	INDM	infant of nondiabetic mother
IMRA	immunoradiometric assay		
IMRS	intensity-modulated radiosurgery	INDO	indomethacin
		^{111}In-DTPA	indium pentetate
IMRT	intensity-modulated radiation therapy	INE	infantile necrotizing encephalomyelopathy
IMS	immunosuppressants		
	incurred in military service	INEX	inexperienced
		INF	infant
	involuntary movements		infarction
	ion mobility spectrometry		infected
IMT	inspiratory muscle training		infection
	intimal medial thickness		inferior
IMU	intermediate medicine unit		influenza virus vaccine, not otherwise specified
IMV	inferior mesenteric vein		
	intermittent mandatory ventilation		information
			infused
	intermittent mechanical ventilation		infusion
IMVP-16	ifosfamide, mesna uroprotection, methotrexate, and etoposide		intravenous nutritional fluid
		INF$_a$	influenza virus, attenuated live vaccine
		INFas	influenza virus attenuated live vaccine, intranasal
IN	insulin	INFC	infected
	intranasal (this is a dangerous abbreviation as it can be read as IV [intravenous] or IM [intramuscular]; use nasally or intranasal)		infection
		INFi	influenza virus inactivated vaccine
		INFs	influenza virus vaccine, split viron

I

INFs-AB3	influenza virus inactivated vaccine, split virion, types A and B, trivalent		intraocular pressure intra-Ommaya intraoperative intraosseous
INF$_w$	influenza virus vaccine, whole viron	I&O	intake and output
ING	inguinal	IOA	intact on admission
√ing	checking	IOC	intern on call
INH	isoniazid (isonicotinic acid hydrazide)		intraoperative cholangiogram
INI	intranuclear inclusion	IOCG	intraoperative cholangiogram
inj	injection injury	IOD	implant-supported overdenture
INK	injury not known		interorbital distance
INN	International Nonproprietary Name	IODM	infant of diabetic mother
INO	inhaled nitrous oxide internuclear ophthalmoplegia	IOF IOFB IOFNA	intraocular fluid intraocular foreign body intraoperative fine needle
INOP	internodal ophthalmoplegia	IOH	aspiration idiopathic orthostatic
iNOS	inducible nitric oxide synthase	IO-HDRBT	hypotension intraoperative high-dose-
inpt	inpatient		rate brachytherapy
INQ	inferior nasal quadrant	IOI	idiopathic orbital
INR	international normalized ratio (for anticoagulant monitoring)		inflammation intraosseous infusion
INS	idiopathic nephrotic syndrome	IOL	induction of labor intraocular lens
	inspection insurance	IOLI	intraocular lens implantation
INSS	International Neuroblastoma Staging System	IOLM	intraoperative lymphatic mapping
INST	instrumental delivery	IOM	Institute of Medicine
INT	intermittent needle therapy	ION IONIS	ischemic optic neuropathy indirect optic nerve injury
	internal	IONTO	syndrome iontophoresis
Int mon	internal monitor	IOOA	inferior oblique
INTERP	interpretation		overaction
Int Med	internal medicine	IOP	intraocular pressure
intol	intolerance		intraosseous puncture
int-rot	internal rotation	IOR	ideas of reference
int trx	intermittent traction		immature oocyte retrieval
intub	intubation		inferior oblique
INV	Invirase (saquinavir, hard gel cap)	IO-RB	recession intraocular retinoblastoma
inver	inversion	IORT	intraoperative radiation
INVOS	in vivo optical spectroscopy	IOS	therapy intraoperative sonography
IO	inferior oblique	IOSH	Institute for Occupational
	initial opening		Safety and Health
	intestinal obstruction	IOT	intraocular tension

I

IOTEE	intraoperative transesophageal echocardiography		interpupillary distance
			invasive pneumococcal disease
IOTT	intensification-of-treatment trigger (criteria)	IPEX	immune dysregulation, polyendocrinopathy, enteropathy, X-linked (syndrome)
IOUS	intraocular ultrasound		
IOV	initial office visit		
IP	ice pack	IPF	idiopathic pulmonary fibrosis
	incubation period		
	individualized plan		interstitial pulmonary fibrosis
	Infrapatellar		
	inpatient	IPFD	intrapartum fetal distress
	in plaster	IPG	immobilized pH gradient
	interphalangeal		impedance plethysmography
	interstitial pneumonia		
	intestinal permeability		individually polymerized grass
	intraperitoneal		
	invasive procedures	IPH	idiopathic pulmonary hemosiderosis
	inverted (inverting) papilloma		
			interphalangeal
I/P	iris/pupil		intraparenchymal hemorrhage
IP3	inositol triphosphate		
IPA	independent practice association		intraperitoneal hemorrhage
	interpleural analgesia	IPHC	intraperitoneal hyperthermic chemotherapy
	invasive pulmonary aspergillosis		
	isopropyl alcohol	IPHEP	independent progressive home exercise program
IPAA	ileo-pouch anal anastamosis		
IPAP	inspiratory positive airway pressure	IPHP	intraperitoneal hyperthermic chemotherapy
IPB	infrapopliteal bypass		
IPC	indirect pulp cavity	IPI	International Prognostic Index
	intermittent pneumatic compression (boots)	IPJ	interphalangeal joint
	intraperitoneal chemotherapy	IPK	intractable plantar keratosis
IPCD	idiopathic paroxysmal cerebral dysrhythmia	IPL	intense pulsed light
		IPM	intranodal-palisaded myofibroblastoma
	infantile polycystic disease		
IPCK	infantile polycystic kidney (disease)		intrauterine pressure monitor
IPCT	intraperitoneal chemotherapy		interventional pain management
IPD	idiopathic Parkinson disease	IPMI	inferoposterior myocardial infarct
	immediate pigment darkening	IPMN	intraductal papillary mucinous neoplasm
	inflammatory pelvic disease	IPN	infantile periarteritis nodosa
	intermittent peritoneal dialysis		intern's progress note
			interstitial pneumonia

IPOF	immediate postoperative fitting	IPW	interphalangeal width
		IQ	intelligence quotient
IPOM	intraperitoneal onlay mesh	IQR	interquartile range
IPOP	immediate postoperative prosthesis	IQWiG	Leiter des Institus für Qualität and Wirtschaftlichkeit im Gesundheitswesen (Institute for Quality and Economy in Healthcare)
IPP	inflatable penile prosthesis		
	intrapleual pressure		
	intravesical protrusion of the prostate		
	isolated pelvic perfusion		
IPPA	inspection, palpation, percussion, and auscultation	IR	immediate-release (tablets)
			immunoreactive
IPPB	intermittent positive-pressure breathing		inferior rectus
			infrared
IP-PDT	intraperitoneal photodynamic therapy		insulin resistance
			internal reduction
IPPF	immediate postoperative prosthetic fitting		internal resistance
			internal rotation
IPPI	interruption of pregnancy for psychiatric indication	I&R	insertion and removal
		IRA	infarct-related artery
		IRAAF	intraoperative radiofrequency ablation for chronic atrial fibrillation
IPPV	intermittent positive pressure ventilation		
IPS	idiopathic pneumonia syndrome	IRA-EEA	ileorectal anastomoses with end-to-end anastomosis
	infundibular pulmonic stenosis		
	initial prognostic score	IRAP	interleukin-1 receptor antagonist protein
	intermittent photic stimulation	IRB	Institutional Review Board
IPSCs	islet-producing stem cells		
		IRBBB	incomplete right bundle branch block
IPSF	immediate postsurgical fitting		
		IRBC	immature red blood cell
IPSID	immunoproliferative small intestinal disease		irradiated red blood cells
IPSP	inhibitory postsynaptic potential	IRBP	implantable rotary blood pump
IPSS	inferior petrosal sinus sampling		interphotoreceptor retinoid-binding protein
I-PSS	International Prostate Symptom Score	IRC	indirect radionuclide cystography
I PSY	intermediate psychiatry		infrared coagulation
IPT	intermittent pelvic traction		Institutional Review Committee (Board)
iPTH	parathyroid hormone by radioimmunoassay	IRCU	intensive respiratory care unit
IPTX	intermittent pelvic traction	IRD	immune renal disease(s)
IPV	inactivated poliovirus vaccine	IRDA	intermittent rhythmic delta activity
	intimate partner violence	IRDM	insulin-resistant diabetes mellitus
IPVC	interpolated premature ventricular contraction		

I

191

IR-DRGs	International Refined Diagnosis Related Groups	IRT	immunoreactive trypsin
			incident response team
IRDS	idiopathic respiratory distress syndrome	IRV	inspiratory reserve volume
			inverse ratio ventilation
	infant respiratory distress syndrome	IS	incentive spirometer
			induced sputum
IRE	internal rotation in extension		Information Services (Department)
IRED	infrared-emission detection		*in situ*
			intercostal space
IRF	inpatient rehabilitation facilities		inventory of systems
			ipecac syrup
	internal rotation in flexion	I-S	Ionescu-Shiley (prosthetic heart valve)
IRH	intraretinal hemorrhage		
IRI	immunoreactive insulin	I & S	intact and symmetrical
IRIV	immunopotentiating reconstituted influenza virosomes	I/S	instruct/supervise
		ISA	ileosigmoid anastomosis
			Incest Survivors Anonymous
IRM	magnetic resonance imaging (French)		intrinsic sympathomimetic activity
IRMA	immediate response mobile analysis (blood analysis system)	ISAAC	International Study of Asthma and Allergies in Childhood (questionnaire; protocol)
	immunoradiometric assay		
	intraretinal microvascular abnormalities	ISADH	inappropriate secretion of antidiuretic hormone
IRMS	isotope-ratio mass spectrometry	ISB	incentive spirometry breathing
IRN	iterated rippled noise		
IRNS	intercostal repetitive nerve stimulation	ISBN	International Standard Book Number
IROS	ipsilateral routing of signals	ISBP	interscalen brachial plexus
		ISC	carcinoma *in situ* (also CIS)
IROX	irinotecan and oxaliplatin		
IRP	intellectual property rights		indwelling subclavian catheter
IRR	infrared radiation		infant servo-control
	intrarenal reflux		infant skin control
	irregular rate and rhythm		intermittent self-catheterization
IRRC	Institutional Research Review Committee		
			intermittent straight catheterization
irreg	irregular		
IRR HYDRO	irreversible hydrocolloid		isolette servo-control
IRRs	incidence rate ratios	ISCM	intramedullary spinal cord metastases
IRS	Information and Referral Society		
		I/SCN	urinary iodine/thiocyanate ratio
	insulin-resistance syndrome	ISCOM	immunostimulating complex
IRSB	intravenous regional sympathetic block	ISCP	infection surveillance and control program
IRSG	Intergroup Rhabdomyo-sarcoma Study Group		

ISCs	irreversible sickle cells	ISRCTN	International Standard Randomized Controlled Trial Number
ISCU	infant special care unit		
ISD	inhibited sexual desire		
	initial sleep disturbance	ISS	idiopathic short stature
	intrinsic (urethral) sphincter deficiency		Individual Self-Rating Scale
	isosorbide dinitrate (Isordol)		Injury Severity Score
			irritable stomach syndrome
ISDN	isosorbide dinitrate (Isordol)		Integrated Summary of Safety
ISE	ion-sensitive electrode		
ISEL	*in situ* end labeling	IS10S	10% invert sugar in 0.9% sodium chloride (saline) injection
ISF	interstitial fluid		
ISFET	ion-selective field effect transistor		
		ISSP	Infant Support Services Program
ISG	immune serum globulin (immune globulin)	IST	immunosuppressive therapy
ISH	isolated systolic hypertension		injection sclerotherapy
			insulin sensitivity test
ISHH	*in situ* hybridization histochemistry		insulin shock therapy
		ISU	intermediate surgical unit
ISHLT	International Society for Heart and Lung Transplantation		
		ISW	interstitial water
		IS10W	10% invert sugar injection (in water)
ISHT	isolated systolic hypertension		
		ISWI	incisional surgical wound infection
ISI	International Sensitivity Index		
		IT	incentive therapy
ISK	isokinetic		individual therapy
ISMA	infantile spinal muscular atrophy		inferior-temporal
			inferior turbinate
ISMN	isosorbide mononitrate		information technology
ISMO®	isosorbide mononitrate		Information Technology (Department)
ISMP	Institute for Safe Medication Practices		
			Inhalation Therapist
ISNA	iron-sufficient, not anemic		inhalation therapy
ISO	isodose		inspiratory time
	isolette		intensive therapy
	isoproterenol		intermittent traction
ISOE	isoetharine		interpreted
ISOF	isoflurane (Florane)		intertrochanteric
ISOK	isokinetic		intertuberous
ISOM	isometric		intrathecal (dangerous abbreviation)
ISOs	isoenzymes		
ISP	inferior spermatic plexus		intratracheal (dangerous, could be interupted as intrathecal)
	interspace		
ISPP	individualized sleep promotion plan		intratumoral
		ITA	individual treatment assessment
ISQ	as before; continue on (*in status quo*)		
			inferior temporal artery
ISR	injection site reaction		itasetron
	integrated secretory response		

ITAG	internal thoracic artery graft	ITT	identical twins (raised) together
ITAL	intrathoracic artificial lung		incremental treadmill test
ITB	iliotibial band		insulin tolerance test
	intrathecal baclofen		intention-to-treat
ITBC	intraluminal typical bronchial carcinoid		(analysis)
		ITU	infant-toddler unit
ITBS	iliotibial band syndrome		intensive therapy unit
	Iowa Tests of Basic Skills		intensive treatment unit
ITC	Incontinence Treatment Center	ITVAD	indwelling transcutaneous vascular access device
	in-the-canal (hearing aid)	ITX	immunotoxin(s)
	isothermal titration calorimetry	ITZ	itraconazole (Sporanox)
		IU	international unit (this is a dangerous abbreviation as it is read as intravenous; use "units")
ITCP	idiopathic thrombocytopenic purpura		
ITCU	intensive thoracic cardiovascular unit	IUC	intrauterine catheter
		IUCD	intrauterine contraceptive device
ITE	insufficient therapeutic effect	IUD	intrauterine death
	in-the-ear (hearing aid)		intrauterine device
ITF	inpatient treatment facility	IUDE	intravenous drug exposure
ITFF	intertrochanteric femoral fracture	IUDR	idoxuridine (Herplex)
		IUFB	intrauterine foreign body
ITGV	intrathoracic gas volume	IUFD	intrauterine fetal death (demise)
ITM	Institute of Tropical Medicine, (Antwerp, Belgium)		intrauterine fetal distress
		IUFT	intrauterine fetal transfusion
ITMTX	intrathecal methotrexate		
ITN	irinotecan (Camptosar)	IUGR	intrauterine growth retardation (restriction)
ITNs	insecticide treated nets	IUI	intrauterine insemination
ITOC	intratracheal oxygen catheter	IULN	institutional upper limit of normal
ITOP	intentional termination of pregnancy	IUMR	intrauterine myelomeningocele repair
ITOU	intensive therapy observation unit	IUP	intrauterine pregnancy
ITP	idiopathic thrombocytopenic purpura	IUPC	intrauterine pressure catheter
	interim treatment plan	IUPD	intrauterine pregnancy delivered
ITPA	Illinois Test of Psycholinguistic Ability	IUP,TBCS	intrauterine pregnancy, term birth, cesarean section
ITQ	inferior temporal quadrant		
ITR	isotretinoin (Accutane)	IUP,TBLC	intrauterine pregnancy, term birth, living child
ITRA	itraconazole (Sporanox)		
ITS	internal transcribed spacer	IUR	intrauterine retardation
	isometric trunk stabilization	IUS	intrauterine system
		IUT	intrauterine transfusion
ITSCU	infant-toddler special care unit	IUTD	immunizations up to date

IV	four	IVGTT	intravenous glucose tolerance test
	interview		
	intravenous (i.v.)	IVH	intravenous hyperalimentation
	intravertebral		
	invasive		intraventricular hemorrhage
	inversion		
	symbol for class 4 controlled substances	IVID	intravenous iron dextran (INFeD; DexFerrum)
IVA	Intervir-A	IVIG	intravenous immunoglobulin
IVAD	implantable venous access device	IVJC	intervertebral joint complex
	implantable vascular access device	IVL	intravascular lymphomatosis
IVBAT	intravascular bronchoalveolar tumor		intravenous lock
IVC	inferior vena cava	IVLBW	infant of very low birth weight (less than 1,500 g)
	inspiratory vital capacity		
	intravenous chemotherapy		
	intravenous cholangiogram	IVMP	intravenously administered methylprednisolone
	intraventricular catheter		
	intraventricular conduction	IVNC	isolated ventricular noncompaction
IVCD	intraventricular conduction defect (delay)	IVO	intraoral vertical osteotomy
		IVOX	intravascular oxygenator (oxygenation)
IVCF	inferior vena cava filter		
IVCI	intravenous continuous infusion	IVP	intravenous push (this is a dangerous meaning as it is read as intravenous pyelogram)
IVCP	inferior vena cava pressure		
IVCV	inferior venacavography		intravenous pyelogram
IVD	intervertebral disk	IVPB	intravenous piggyback
	intravenous drip	IVPF	isovolume pressure flow
	in vitro diagnostic	IVPU	intravenous push
IVDA	intravenous drug abuse	IVR	idioventricular rhythm
IVDSA	intravenous digital subtraction angiography		interactive voice-response (system)
			intravaginal ring
IVDU	intravenous drug user		intravenous retrograde
IVET	in vivo expression technology		intravenous rider (this is a dangerous abbreviation as it has been read as IVP-intravenous push)
IVF	intervertebral foramina		
	intravenous fluid(s)		
	in vitro fertilization		isovolumic relaxation (time)
IVFA	intravenous fluorescein angiography		
IVFE	intravenous fat emulsion	IVRA	intravenous regional anesthesia
IVF-ET	in vitro fertilization-embryo transfer	IVRAP	intravenous retrograde access port
IVFT	intravenous fetal transfusion	IVRG	intravenous retrograde
IVGG	intravenous gamma globulin	IV-RNV	intravenous radionuclide venography

I

195

IVRO	intraoral vertical ramus osteotomy	
IVRS	interactive voice response system	
IVRT	isovolumic relation time	
IVS	intraventricular septum irritable voiding syndrome	
IVSD	intraventricular septal defect	
IVSE	interventricular septal excursion	
IVSO	intraoral vertical segmental osteotomy	
IVSS	intravenous Soluset®	
IVST	interventricular septum thickness	
IVT	intravenous transfusion intraventricular	
IVTTT	intravenous tolbutamide tolerance test	
IVU	intravenous urography (urogram)	
IVUC	intravenous ultrasound catheter	
IVUS	intravascular ultrasound	
IW	inspiratory wheeze	
IWD	individual with a disability	
IWI	inferior wall infarction	
IWL	insensible water loss involuntary weight loss	
IWMI	inferior wall myocardial infarct	
IWML	idiopathic white matter lesion	
IWT	ice-water test impacted wisdom teeth	

J

J	Jaeger measure of near vision with 20/20 about equal to J1
	jejunostomy
	Jewish
	joint
	joule
	juice
J 1-16	Jaeger near acuity notation (1 to 16 scale)
JA	joint aspiration
Jack	jackknife position
JAFAR	Juvenile Arthritis Functional Assessment Report
JAMA	*Journal of the American Medical Association*
JAMG	juvenile autoimmune myasthenia gravis
JAN	Japanese Accepted Name
JAR	junior assistant resident
JARAN	junior assistant resident admission note
JBE	Japanese B encephalitis
JBS	Johanson Blizzard syndrome
JC	junior clinicians (medical students)
JCA	juvenile chronic arthritis
JCAHO	Joint Commission on Accreditation of Healthcare Organizations
JCC	Jackson cross cylinder (astigmatism test)
JCOG	Japanese Clinical Oncology Group
JCQ	Job Content Questionnaire
JD	Doctor of Jurisprudence (a law degree)
	jaundice
JDG	jugulodigastric
JDM	juvenile diabetes mellitus
JDMS	juvenile dermatomyositis
JE	Japanese encephalitis
JEB	junctional escape beat
JEJ	jejunum

JEN	Japanese encephalitis vaccine		respiratory papillomatosis
JER	junctional escape rhythm	JP	Jackson-Pratt (drain)
			Jobst pump
JET	jejunal extension tube		joint protection
	junctional ectopic tachycardia	JPB	junctional premature beats
JEV	Japanese encephalitis virus	JP BS	Jackson-Pratt to bulb suction
JF	joint fluid	JPC	junctional premature contraction
JFS	Jewish Family Service		
JGCT	juvenile granulosa cell tumor	JPS	joint position sense
		JR	junctional rhythm
JHR	Jarisch-Herxheimer reaction	JRA	juvenile rheumatoid arthritis
JI	jejunoileal	JRAN	junior resident admission note
JIA	juvenile idiopathic arthritis	Jr BF	junior baby food
JIB	jejunoileal bypass	JRC	joint replacement center
JIS	juvenile idiopathic scoliosis	JSF	Japanese spotted fever
		JSRV	jaagziekte sheep retrovirus
JJ	jaw jerk	JT	jejunostomy tube
J & J	Johnson & Johnson Health Care Systems, Inc.		joint
			junctional tachycardia
		JTF	jejunostomy tube feeding
JLO	Judgment of Line Orientation (test)	JTJ	jaw-to-jaw (position)
		JTP	joint projection
JLP	juvenile laryngeal papillomatosis	JTPS	juvenile tropical pancreatitis syndrome
JM-9	iproplatin	J-Tube	jejunostomy tube
JME	juvenile myoclonic epilepsy	JUV	juvenile
		JV	jugular vein
JMS	junior medical student	JVC	jugular venous catheter
JNA	juvenile nasopharyngeal angiofibroma	JVD	jugular venous distention
		JVI	jugular-valve incompetencce
JNB	jaundice of newborn		
JNCL	juvenile-onset neuronal ceroid lipofuscinosis	JVP	jugular venous pressure
			jugular venous pulsation
JND	just noticeable difference		jugular venous pulse
JNT	joint	JVPT	jugular venous pulse tracing
JNVD	jugular neck vein distention		
		JW	Jehovah's Witness
JODM	juvenile-onset diabetes mellitus	Jx	joint
		JXG	juvenile xanthogranuloma
JOF	juvenile ossifying fibroma		
JOMAC	judgment, orientation, memory, abstraction, and calculation		
JOMACI	judgment, orientation, memory, abstraction, and calculation intact		
JOR	jaw-opening reflex		
JORRP	juvenile-onset recurrent		

J

K

K	cornea
	kelvin
	ketamine (Ketalar, Vitamin K, Special K, and Super K)
	kilodalton
	Kosher
	potassium
	thousand
	vitamin K
K′	knee
K$^+$	potassium
K$_1$	phytonadione (AquaMETHYTON)
K$_2$	menatetrenone
K$_3$	menadione
K$_4$	menadiol sodium diphosphate
17K	17-ketosteroids
510(k)	Medical Device Premarket Notification
KA	kainic acid
	kala-azar
	keratoacanthoma
	ketoacidosis
Ka	first order absorption constant in hr.$^{-1}$
KAB	knowledge, attitude, and behavior
K-ABC	Kaufman Assessment Battery for Children
KABINS	knowledge, attitude, behavior, and improvement in nutritional status
KACT	kaolin-activated clotting time
KAFO	knee-ankle-foot orthosis
KAO	knee-ankle orthosis
KAS	Katz Adjustment Scale
KASH	knowledge, abilities, skills, and habits
kat	katal
K-A units	King-Armstrong units
KB	ketone bodies
	kilobase
	knee-bearing
KBD	Kashin-Beck disease

KC	kangaroo care
	keratoconjunctivitis
	keratoconus
	knees-to-chest
	Korean conflict
kcal	kilocalorie
KCCT	kaolin cephalin clotting time
KChIPs	potassium channel-interacting proteins
kCi	kilocurie
KCl	potassium chloride
KCS	keratoconjunctivitis sicca
KCZ	ketoconazole (Nizoral)
KD	Kawasaki disease
	Keto Diastix®
	ketogenic diet
	kidney donors
	knee disarticulation
	knowledge deficit
kd	kilodalton
KDA	known drug allergies
KDC®	brand name of infant warmer
KDQ	Kidney Disease Questionnaire
KDU	Kidney Dialysis Unit
KE	first order elimination rate constant in hr.$^{-1}$
KED	Kendrick extrication device
k$_{el}$	elimination rate constant
KET	ketamine (Ketalar)
	ketoconazole (Nizoral)
	ketones
KETO	ketoconazole (Nizoral)
17 Keto	17 ketosteroids
keV	kilo-electron volts
KEVD	Krupin eye valve with disk
KF	kidney function
KFA	kinetic fibrinogen assay
KFAB	kidney-fixing antibodies
KFAO	knee-foot-ankle orthosis
KFD	Kyasanur Forrest disease
KFE	knee flexion and extension
KFR	Kayser-Fleischer ring
KFS	Klippel-Feil syndrome
kg	kilogram (1 Kg = 2.2 pounds)
K-G	Kimray-Greenfield (filter)
KGF	keratinocyte growth factor
KGC	Keflin, gentamicin, and carbenicillin

17-KGS	17-ketogenic steroids	kPa	kilopascal
KGy	kiloGray	KPE	Kelman phacoemulsification
KHF	Korean hemorrhagic fever		
K24H	potassium, urine 24-hour	KPM	kilopounds per minute
kHz	kilohertz	KPS	Karnofsky performance
KI	karyopyknotic index		status (scores)
	knee immobilizer		(scale)
	potassium iodide	KQI	key quality indicators
KID	keratitis, ichthyosis, and	Kr	krypton
	deafness (syndrome)	K-rod	Küntscher rod
	kidney	KS	Kawasaki syndrome
kilo	kilogram		Kaposi sarcoma
	thousand		kidney stone
KIN	kinetic		Klinefelter syndrome
KISS	saturated solution of	17-KS	17-ketogenic steroids
	potassium iodide		17-ketosteroids
KIT	Kahn Intelligence Test	KSA	knowledge, skills, and
KIU	kallikrein inhibitor units		abilities
KJ	kilojoule	K-SADS	Kiddie Schedule for
	knee jerk		Affective Disorders and
KJR	knee-jerk reflex		Schizophrenia
KK	knee kick	KSE	knee sling exercises
	knock-knee	KSHV	Kaposi sarcoma-
KKS	kallikrein-kinin system		associated herpesvirus
K & L	Kellgren and Lawrence	KS/OI	Kaposi sarcoma and
	(scale for osteoarthritis		opportunistic infections
	assessment)	KSP	Karolinska Scales of
KLB	klebsiella vaccine		Personality
KL-BET	Kleihauer-Betke	KSR	potassium chloride
Kleb	*Klebsiella*		sustained release
KLH	keyhole limpet hemocyanin		(tablets)
K-Lor®	potassium chloride tablets	KSS	Kearns-Sayre syndrome
KLS	kidneys, liver, and spleen	KSW	knife stab wound
	Kleine-Levin syndrome	KT	kidney transplant
KM	kanamycin		kinesiotherapy
KMC	kangaroo-mother care		known to
KMnO₄	potassium permanganate	KTC	knee-to-chest
KMO	Kaiser-Meyer-Olkin	KTP	potassium-titanyl-
	(measure of statistical		phosphate (laser)
	sampling adequacy)	KTS	Klippel-Trenaunay
KMV	killed measles vaccine		syndrome
KN	knee	KTU	kidney transplant unit
KNO	keep needle open		known to us
KNSA	Kron Nutritive Sucking	KTx	kidney transplantation
	Apparatus	KTZ	ketoconazole (Nizoral)
KO	keep open	KUB	kidney(s), ureter(s), and
	knee orthosis		bladder
	knocked out		kidney ultrasound biopsy
KOH	potassium hydroxide	KUS	kidney(s), ureter(s),
KOR	keep open rate		and spleen
KP	hot pack	KV	kilovolt
	keratoprecipitate	KVO	keep vein open
	kinetic perimetry	KVP	kilovolt peak

K

KW	Keith-Wagener (ophthalmoscopic finding, graded I-IV)
	Kimmelstiel-Wilson
KWB	Keith, Wagener, Barker
KWIC	keywork in context
K-wire	Kirschner wire

L	fifty
	Laribacter
	left (this is a dangerous abbreviation; spell out "left" to avoid surgical errors)
	lente insulin (this is a dangerous abbreviation, since there is also a Lantus insulin available)
	levorotatory
	lingual
	Listeria
	liter (1 L = 1,000 mL = 1 quart plus about 2 ounces)
	liver
	lumbar
	lung
l	levorotatory
L′	lumbar
Ⓛ	left (this is a dangerous abbreviation; spell out "left" to avoid surgical errors)
$L_1...L_5$	lumbar nerve 1 through 5
	lumbar vertebra 1 through 5
L1-2	lumbar spine, between first and second vertebrae (the disk space)
LA	language age
	latex agglutination
	Latin American
	left arm
	left atrial
	left atrium
	leukoaraiosis (a radiologic finding)
	light adaptation
	linguoaxial
	linoleic acid
	local anesthesia
	long acting
	lupus anticoagulant
L + A	light and accommodation
	living and active

K

200

LAA	large artery atherosclerosis	LADD	left anterior descending diagonal
	left atrium and its appendage	LAD-MIN	left axis deviation minimal
LAAM	levomethadyl acetate (L-alpha acetylmeth-adol, Orlaam)	LADPG	laparoscopically assisted distal partial gastrectomy
LAAs	leukemia-associated antigens	LAE	left atrial enlargement long above elbow
LAB	laboratory left abdomen (LAb)	LAEC	locally advanced esophageal cancer
LABA	laser-assisted balloon angioplasty long-acting beta-2 agonist	LAF	laminar air flow Latin-American female low animal fat
LABBB	left anterior bundle branch block		lymphocyte-activating factor
LABC	locally advanced breast cancer	LAFB	left anterior fascicular block
LABD	linear immunoglobulin A bullous dermatosis	LAFF	lateral arm free flap
		LAFM	locally acquired *Plasmodium falciparum* malaria
LABR	laparoscopic-assisted bowel resection		
LAC	laceration	LAFR	laminar airflow room
	lactobacillus acidophilus vaccine	LAG	lymphangiogram
		LAGB	laparoscopic-adjustable gastric banding
	laparoscopic-assisted colectomy	LAH	left anterior hemiblock left atrial hypertrophy
	left antecubital		
	left atrial catheter	LAHB	left anterior hemiblock
	locally advanced cancer	LAI	left atrial isomerism
	long arm cast	LAIT	latex agglutination inhibition test
	lupus anticoagulant		
LAc	Licensed Acupuncturist	LAIV	live, attenuated influenza vaccine
LACC	locally advanced cervical carcinoma		
		LAK	lymphokine-activated killer
LACI	lacunar circulation infarct		
	lipoprotein-associated coagulation inhibitor	LAL	left axillary line *limulus* amebocyte lysate
LACS	laser-assisted capsular shrinkage		
		LALLS	low-angle laser light scattering
LACT-ART	lactate arterial		
		LALT	larynx-associated lymphoid tissue low-air loss therapy (mattress)
LAD	laser anesthesia device		
	left anterior descending		
	left atrial dimension		
	left axis deviation	LAM	lactational anovulatory method (birth control)
	leukocyte adhesion deficiency		laminectomy
	ligament augmentation device		laminogram laparoscopic-assisted myomectomy
LADA	left anterior descending (coronary) artery		Latin-American male lymphangioleiomyomatosis
LADCA	left anterior descending coronary artery	lam✓	laminectomy check

L

LAMA	laser-assisted microanastomosis		lymphangioscintigraphy
			lysine acetylsalicylate
LAMB	mucocutaneous lentigines, atrial myxoma, and blue nevus (syndrome)	LASA	Linear Analogue Self-Assessment (scales)
			lipid-associated sialic acid
L-AMB	liposomal amphotericin B	LASCC	locally advanced squamous cell carcinoma
LAMMA	laser microprobe mass analysis	LASEC	left atrial spontaneous echo contrast
LAN	lymphadenopathy		
LANC	long arm navicular cast	LASER	light amplification by stimulated emission of radiation
LA-NSCLC	locally-advanced nonsmall-cell lung cancer		
		LASGB	laparoscopic-adjustable silicone gastric banding
LAO	left anterior oblique		
LAP	laparoscopy	LASIK	laser in situ keratomileusis
	laparotomy	L-ASP	asparaginase (Elspar)
	left abdominal pain	LAST	left anterior small thoracotomy
	left atrial pressure		
	leucine amino peptidase	LASW	Licensed Advanced Social Worker
	leukocyte alkaline phosphatase		
		LAT	lateral
	lower abdominal pain		latex agglutination test
LAPA	locally-advanced pancreatic adenocarcinoma		left anterior thigh
		LATCH	literature attached to chart
lap-appy	laparoscopic appendectomy	lat.men.	lateral meniscectomy
LAPC	locally-advanced prostate cancer	LATS	long-acting thyroid stimulator
		LAUP	laser-assisted uvula-palatoplasty
lap chole	laparoscopic cholecystectomy		
		LAV	left atrial volume
LAPMS	long arm posterior molded splint		live attenuated flavivirus
			lymphadenopathy associated virus
LAPW	left atrial posterior wall		
LAQ	long arc quad	LAVA	laser-assisted vasal anastomosis
LAR	left arm, reclining		
	long-acting release	LAVH	laparoscopically assisted vaginal hysterectomy
	low anterior resection		
LARC	Locally-advanced rectal cancer	LAVM	laparoscopic-assisted vaginal myomectomy
		LAW	left atrial wall
LARM	left arm		
LARS	laparoscopic antireflux surgery	LAWER	life-terminating acts without the explicit request
LARSI	lumbar anterior-root stimulator implants		
		LAX	laxative
LAS	lactic acidosis syndrome	LB	large bowel
	laxative abuse syndrome		lateral bend
	left arm, sitting		left breast
	leucine acetylsalicylate		left buttock
	long arm splint		live births
	low-amplitude signal		low back
	lymphadenopathy syndrome		lung biopsy
			lymphoid body

L

lb	pound (1 lb = 0.454 Kg)		low birth weight (less than 2,500 g)
L&B	left and below		
LB3	colonoscope	LBWI	low birth weight infant
LBA	laser balloon angioplasty	LC	Laënnec cirrhosis
	lower-body adiposity		laparoscopic cholecystectomy
	lymphocyte blastogenesis assay		lethal concentration
LBB	left breast biopsy		left circumflex
	long-back board		leisure counseling
LBBB	left bundle branch block		level of consciousness
			levocarnitine (Carnitor)
LBBx	left breast biopsy		living children
LBCD	left border of cardiac dullness		low calorie
			lung cancer
L/B/Cr	electrolytes, blood urea nitrogen, and serum creatinine (see page 392)	L & C	lids and conjunctivae
		3LC	triple-lumen catheter
		LC50	median lethal concentration
LBD	large bile duct	LCA	Leber congenital amaurosis
	left border dullness		left circumflex artery
	Lewy body dementia		left coronary artery
	low back disability		leukocyte common antigen
LBE	long below elbow		
LBG	Landry-Guillain-Barré (syndrome)		life cycle assessment
			light contact assist
LBH	length, breadth, and height		
LBI	Lewy body-like inclusions	LCAD	long-chain acyl-coenzyme A dehydrogenase
	low back injury		
LBM	last bowel movement	LCAH	life-care at home
	lean body mass	LCAL	large-cell anaplastic lymphoma
	loose bowel movement		
LBMI	last body mass index	LCAT	lecithin cholesterol acyltransferase
LBNA	lysis bladder neck adhesions		
		LCB	left costal border
LBNP	lower-body negative pressure	LCCA	left circumflex coronary artery
LBO	large bowel obstruction		left common carotid artery
LBOTC	laryngeal and base-of-tongue carcinomas		leukocytoclastic angiitis
LBP	low back pain	LCCS	low cervical cesarean section
	low blood pressure		
LBQC	large base quad cane	LCD	coal tar solution (*liquor carbonis detergens*)
LBRF	louse-borne relapsing fever		localized collagen dystrophy
LBS	low back syndrome		low-calcium diet
	pounds		
LBT	low back tenderness	LCDC	Laboratory Centre for Disease Control (Canada)
	low back trouble		
LBV	left brachial vein	LCDCP	low-contact dynamic compression plate
	low biological value		
LBVO	left brachial vein occlusion	LCDE	laparoscopic common duct exploration
LBW	lean body weight		

L

LCE	laparoscopic cholecystectomy	LCSG	left cardiac sympathetic ganglionectomy
	left carotid endarterectomy		lost child support group
LCF	left circumflex	LCSS	Lung Cancer Symptom Score
LCFA	long-chain fatty acid	LCSW	Licensed Clinical Social Worker
LCFM	left circumflex marginal		
LCGU	local cerebral glucose utilization		low continuous wall suction
LCH	Langerhans cell histiocytosis	LCT	long-chain triglyceride
			low cervical transverse
	local city hospital		lymphocytotoxicity
LCIS	lobular cancer *in situ*	LCTA	lungs clear to auscultation
LCL	lateral collateral ligament	LCTCS	low cervical transverse cesarean section
	localized cutaneous leishmaniasis	LCTD	low-calcium test diet
LCLC	large-cell lung carcinoma	LCV	leucovorin
LCM	laser-capture microdissection		leukocytoclastic vasculitis
			low cervical vertical
	left costal margin	LCX	left circumflex coronary artery
	lower costal margin		
	lymphocytic choriomeningitis	LD	lactic dehydrogenase (formerly LDH)
LCMI	left ventricular mass index		laser Doppler
LC-MS-MS	liquid chromatography coupled to tandem mass spectrometry		last dose
			latissimus dorsi
			learning disability
LCN	lidocaine		learning disorder
LCNB	large-core needle biopsy		left deltoid
LCNEC	large-cell neuroendocrine carcinoma		Legionnaires disease
			lethal dose
LCO	low cardiac output		levodopa
LCP	long, closed, posterior (cervix)		Licensed Dietician
			liver disease
LCPD	Legg-Calvé-Perthes disease		living donor
			loading dose
LCPUFAs	long-chain polyunsaturated fatty acids		long dwell
			low density
			low dosage
LCR	cerebrospinal fluid (French)		Lyme disease
		L&D	labor and deliver
	late cortical response	L/D	labor and delivery
	late cutaneous reaction		light to dark (ratio)
	ligase chain reaction	LD-1	lactic dehydrogenase 1
	locus control region	LD-5	lactic dehydrogenase 5
LCRS	Living Conditions Rating Scale	LD$_{50}$	median lethal dose
		LDA	laser-Doppler anemometry
LCS	Leydig cell stimulation		low density areas
	lids, conjunctiva, and sclera		low-dose arm
		LDB	Legionnaires disease bacterium
	low constant suction		
	low continuous suction	LDCOC	low-dose combination oral contraceptive
	Lung Cancer Subscale		

L

204

LDD	laser disk decompression	left ear
	Lee and Desu D (test)	left eye
	light-dark discrimination	lens extraction
LDDS	local dentist	leptin
LDEA	left deviation of electrical axis	live embryo
		local excision
LDF	laser-Doppler flowmetry	lower extremities
LDH	lactic dehydrogenase	lupus erythematosus
LDIH	left direct inguinal hernia	LEA	lower extremity amputation
LDIR	low-dose of ionizing radiation		lumbar epidural anesthesia
LDI-TOF-MS	laser desorption/ionization time-of-flight-mass spectrometer	LEAD	lower extremity arterial disease
		LEAP	Lower Extremity Amputation Prevention (program)
LDL	limitation of daily life low-density lipoprotein	LEB	lumbar epidural block
		LEC	lens epithelial cell
LDL-C	low-density lipoprotein cholesterol	LECBD	laparoscopic exploration of the common bile duct
LDLT	living donor liver transplantation	LE-CEMRA	lower extremity contrast-enhanced magnetic resonance angiography
LDM	lorazepam, dexamethasone, and metoclopramide	LED	liposomal encapsulated doxorubicin (Doxil)
LDMRT	low-dose mediastinal radiation therapy		lowest effective dose
			lupus erythematosus disseminatus
LDN	living-donor nephrectomy	LEEP	loop electrosurgical excision procedure
LDNF	lung-derived neurotrophic factor		
LDO	Licensed Dispensing Optician	LEF	lower extremity fracture
		LEH	liposome-encapsulated hemoglobin
l-dopa	levodopa		
LDP	laparoscopic distal pancreatectomy	LEHPZ	lower esophageal high pressure zone
LD-PCR	limiting dilution polymerase chain reaction	LEJ	ligation of the esophagogastric junction
LDPM	laser Doppler perfusion monitoring	LEL	low-energy laser
		LEM	lateral eye movements
LDR	labor, delivery, and recovery		light electron microscope
	length-to-diameter ratio	LEMS	Lambert-Eaton myasthenic syndrome
	long-duration response		
LDR/P	labor, delivery, recovery, and postpartum	LENT-SOMA	Late Effect of Normal Tissue—Subjective Objective Management Analytic (toxicity table)
LDT	left dorsotransverse		
LD-T	lactic dehydrogenase total		
LDUB	long double upright brace		
		LEP	leptospirosis
LDUH	low-dose unfractionated heparin		limited English proficiency
			liposome-encapsulated paclitaxel
LDV	laser-Doppler velocimetry		
LE	labor epidural		lower esophageal pressure

L

LEP 2	leptospirosis 2
LE prep	lupus erythematosus preparation
L-ERX	leukoerythroblastic reaction
LES	local excitatory state
	lower esophageal sphincter
	lumbar epidural steroids
	lupus erythematosus systemic
LESEP	lower extremity somatosensory evoked potential
LESG	Late Effects Study Group
LESI	lumbar epidural steroid injection
LESP	lower esophageal sphincter pressure
LET	left esotropia
	leukocyte esterase test
	lidocaine, epinephrine and tetracaine gel
	linear energy transfer
LEU	leucine
LEV	levamisole (Ergamisol)
	levator muscle
LEVA	levamisole (Ergamisol)
LeY	Lewis Y (antigen)
LF	laparoscopic fundoplications
	Lassa fever
	left foot
	left frontal
	living female
	low fat
	low forceps
	low frequency
	lymphatic filariasis
LFA	left femoral artery
	left forearm
	left fronto-anterior
	leukocyte function-associated antigen
	low-friction arthroplasty
	lymphocyte function-associated antigen
LFA-1	leukocyte function-associated antigen-1
LFB	low-frequency band
LFC	living female child
	low-fat and cholesterol
LFCS	low-flap cesarean section

LFD	lactose-free diet
	low-fat diet
	low-fiber diet
	low-forceps delivery
	lunate fossa depression
LFGNR	lactose fermenting gram-negative rod
LFI	local-field irradiation
LFL	left frontolateral
LFM	lateral force microscopy
LFP	left frontoposterior
LFS	leukemia-free survival
	Li-Fraumeni syndrome
	liver function series
LFT	latex flocculation test
	left fronto-transverse
	liver function tests
	low-flap transverse
LFU	limit flocculation unit
	lost to follow-up
LG	large
	laryngectomy
	left gluteal
	linguogingival
	lymphography
L-G	Lich-Gregoire (ureteroneocystostomy)
LGA	large for gestational age
	left gastric artery
	localized granuloma annulare
LGBP/LC	laparoscopic gastric bypass with simultaneous cholecystectomy
LGBT	lesbian, gay, bisexual, and transsexual
LGG	low-grade gliomas
L-GG	*Lactobacillus rhamnosus* strain GG
LGI	lower gastrointestinal (series)
LGIOS	low-grade intraosseous-type osteosarcoma
LGL	large granular lymphocyte
	low-grade lymphoma(s)
	Lown-Ganong-Levine (syndrome)
LGLS	Lown-Ganong-Levine syndrome
LGM	left gluteus medius (maximus)
LGN	lateral geniculate leaflet

L

	lobular glomerulonephritis	LIC	left iliac crest
LG-NHL	low-grade non-Hodgkin lymphoma		left internal carotid
			leisure interest class
LGS	Lennox-Gastaut syndrome	LICA	left internal carotid artery
	low-Gomco suction	LICD	lower intestinal Crohn disease
LGSIL	low-grade squamous intraepithelial lesion	LICM	left intercostal margin
LGV	lymphogranuloma venerum	Li_2CO_3	lithium carbonate
		LICS	left intercostal space
LH	learning handicap	LID	levodopa-induced dyskinesia
	left hand		
	left hemisphere	Lido	lidocaine
	left hyperphoria	LIF	laser-induced fluorescence
	luteinizing hormone		left iliac fossa
	lymphoid hyperplasia		left index finger
LHA	left hepatic artery		leukemia-inhibiting factor
LHC	left heart catheterization		liver (migration) inhibitory factor
LHD	left-hand dominant		
LHF	left heart failure	LIFE	laser-induced fluorescence emission
LHG	left hand grip		
LHH	left homonymous hemianopsia		lung imaging fluorescence endoscopy
LHI	Labor Health Institute	LIG	ligament
LHL	left hemisphere lesions		lymphocyte immune globulin
	left hepatic lobe		
LHON	Leber hereditary optic neuropathy	LIGHTS	phototherapy lights
		LIH	laparoscopic inguinal herniorrhaphy
LHP	left hemiparesis		
LHR	legal health record		left inguinal hernia
	leukocyte histamine release	LIHA	low impulsiveness, high anxiety
LHRH	luteinizing hormone-releasing hormone	LIJ	left internal jugular
		LILA	low impulsiveness, low anxiety
LHRH-A	luteinizing hormone-releasing hormone analogue		
		LILT	low-intensity laser therapy
LHRT	leukocyte histamine release test	LIM	limited toxicology screening
LHS	left hand side	LIMA	left internal mammary artery (graft)
	long-handled sponge		
LHSH	long-handled shoe horn	LIMS	laboratory information management system(s)
LHT	left hypertropia		
LI	lactose intolerance	LINAC	linear accelerator
	lamellar ichthyosis	LINCL	late-infantile neuronal ceroid lipofuscinosis
	large intestine		
	laser iridotomy	LINDI	lithium-induced nephrogenic diabetes insipidus
	learning impaired		
	linguoincisal		
	liver involvement	LING	lingual
Li	lithium	LIO	laser-indirect ophthalmoscope
LIA	laser interference acuity		
	left iliac artery		left inferior oblique (muscle)
LIB	left in bottle		

L

LIOU	laparoscopic intraoperative ultrasound	LKM-3	liver-kidney microsomal antibodies type 3
LIP	lithium-induced polydipsia	LKS	Landau-Kleffner syndrome
			liver, kidneys, spleen
	lymphocytic interstitial pneumonia	LKSB	liver, kidneys, spleen, and bladder
LIPV	left inferior pulmonary vein	LKSNP	liver, kidneys, and spleen not palpable
LIQ	liquid	LL	large lymphocyte
	liquor		left lateral
	lower inner quadrant		left leg
LIR	left iliac region		left lower
	left inferior rectus		left lung
LIR-1	leucocyte immunoglobulin-like receptor-1		lepromatous leprosy
			lid lag
			long leg (brace or cast)
LIS	late-onset idiopathic scoliosis		lower lid
			lower lip
	left intercostal space		lower lobe
	locked-in syndrome		lumbar laminectomy
	low intermittent suction		lumbar length
			lymphocytic leukemia
	lung injury score		lymphoblastic lymphoma
LISS	low ionic strength saline	L&L	lids and lashes
		LL2	limb lead two
LISW	Licensed Independent Social Worker	LLA	lids, lashes, and adnexa
			limulus lysate assay
LIT	literature	LLAs	lipid-lowering agents
	liver injury test	LLAT	left lateral
LITA	left internal thoracic artery	LLB	last living breath
			left lateral bending
LITH	lithotomy		left lateral border
LITHO	lithotripsy		long leg brace
LITT	laser-induced thermotherapy	LLC	laparoscopic laser cholecystectomy
LIV	left innominate vein		Lewis lung carcinoma
L-IVP	limited intravenous pyelogram		limited liability corporation
LIVB	live birth		long leg cast
LIVC	left inferior vena cava	LLBCD	left lower border of cardiac dullness
LIVPRO	liver profile (see page 392)	LLD	late-life depressions
			left lateral decubitus
LIWS	low intermittent wall suction		left length discrepancy
			leg length differential
LJ	left jugular	LLE	left lower extremity
	lockable joints		little league elbow
LJL	lateral joint line	LLETZ	large-loop excision of the transformation zone
LJM	limited joint mobility		
LK	lamellar keratoplasty	LLFG	long leg fiberglas (cast)
	left kidney	LLG	left lateral gaze
LKA	Lazare-Klerman-Armour (Personality Inventory)	LL-GXT	low-level graded exercise test

LLI	leg-length inequality		low molecular weight dextran
LLL	left lower lid		
	left lower lobe (lung)	LME	left mediolateral episiotomy
LLLE	lower lid, left eye		
LLLNR	left lower lobe, no rales	LMEE	left middle ear exploration
LLLT	low-level laser therapy	LMF	left middle finger
LLN	lower limit of normal		melphalan (L-PAM), methotrexate, and fluorouracil
LLO	Legionella-like organism		
LLOD	lower lid, right eye		
	lower limit of detection	LMFT	Licensed Marriage and Family Therapist
LLOS	lower lid, left eye		
LLP	Limited Liability Partnership	LMHC	Licensed Mental Health Counselor
	long leg plaster	LMI	large multivalent immunogen
LLPDD	late luteal phase dysphoric disorder		
		L/min	liters per minute
LLPS	low-load prolonged stress	LML	left medial lateral
			left middle lobe
LLQ	left lower quadrant (abdomen)	LMLE	left mediolateral episiotomy
LLR	left lateral rectus	LMM	lentigo maligna melanoma
LLRE	lower lid, right eye	LMN	letter of medical necessity
LLS	lazy leukocyte syndrome		lower motor neuron
LLSB	left lower sternal border	LMNL	lower motor neuron lesion
LLSD	laser light scattering detector	LMP	last menstrual period
			left mentoposterior
LLT	left lateral thigh		low malignant potential
	lowest level term	LMP1	latent membrane protein 1
LLWC	long leg walking cast	LMR	left medial rectus
LLX	left lower extremity	LMRM	left modified radical mastectomy
LM	landmarks		
	left main	LMRP	Local Medical Review Policy
	light microscopy		
	linguomesial	LMS	lateral medullary syndrome
	living male		
	lung metastases		leiomyosarcomas
L/M	liters per minute	LMT	left main trunk
LMA	laryngeal mask airway		left mentotransverse
	left mentoanterior		Licensed Massage Therapist
	liver membrane autoantibody		
			light moving touch
LMAM	left message on answering machine	LMW	low molecular weight
		LMWD	low molecular weight dextran
LMB	Laurence-Moon-Biedl syndrome		
		LMWH	low molecular weight heparins
	left main bronchus		
LMC	living male child	LN	latent nystagmus
LMCA	left main coronary artery		left nostril (nare)
	left middle cerebral artery		lymph nodes
LMCAT	left middle cerebral artery thrombosis	LN₂	liquid nitrogen
		LNA	alpha-linolenic acid
LMCL	left midclavicular line	LNB	lymph node biopsy
LMD	local medical doctor	LNCs	lymph node cells

LND	light-near dissociation	LOE	left otitis externa
	lonidamine	LOEL	lowest-observed-effect level
	lymph node dissection		
LNE	lymph node enlargement	LOF	leaking of fluids
	lymph node excision		leave on floor
LNF	laparoscopic Nissen fundoplication	LOFD	low-outlet forceps delivery
		LOG	Logmar chart
LNG	levonorgestrel	LOH	loss of heterozygosity
LNM	lymph node metastases	LOHF	late-onset hepatic failure
LNMC	lymph node mononuclear cells	LOHP	oxaliplatin (Eloxatin)
		LOIH	left oblique inguinal hernia
LNMP	last normal menstrual period		
		LOI	level of injury
LNNB	Luria-Nebraska Neuropsychological Battery		Leyton Obsessional Inventory
			loss of imprinting
LNS	lymph node sampling	LOINC	Logical Observation Identifier Names and Codes
LNT	late neurological toxicity		
LO	lateral oblique (x-ray view)		
		LOL	laughing out loud
	linguo-occlusal		left occipitolateral
	lumbar orthosis		little old lady
5-LO	5-lipoxygenase	LOLINAD	little old lady in no apparent distress
LOA	late-onset agammaglobulinemia		
		LOM	left otitis media
	leave of absence		limitation of motion
	left occiput anterior		little old man
	long-acting opioid		loss of motion
	looseness of associations		low-osmolar (contrast) media
	lysis of adhesions		
LOAD	late-onset Alzheimer disease	LOMSA	left otitis media, suppurative, acute
LOAEL	lowest observed adverse effect level	LOMSC	left otitis media, suppurative, chronic
LOB	loss of balance	LoNa	low sodium
LOC	laxative of choice	LOO	length of operation
	level of care	LOP	laparoscopic orchiopexy
	level of comfort		leave on pass
	level of concern		left occiput posterior
	level of consciousness		level of pain
	local	LOQ	limit(s) of quantitation
	loss of consciousness		lower outer quadrant
LOCF	last observation carried forward (used for inputting data missing due to dropouts in longitudinal clinical trials)	LOR	loss of resistance
		LORS-I	Level of Rehabilitation Scale-I
		LOS	length of stay
			loss of sight
			low-output syndrome
LOCM	low-osmolality contrast media	LOT	left occiput transverse
			Licensed Occupational Therapist
LOD	limit of detection		
	line of duty	LOV	loss of vision
	log of odds	LOVA	loss of visual acuity

L

LOX	lipid oxidation	LPIH	left-posterior-inferior hemiblock
LOZ	lozenge		
LP	Licensed Psychologist	LPL	laparoscopic pelvic lymphadenectomy
	light perception		
	linguopulpal		left posterolateral
	lipid panel (see page 392)		lipoprotein lipase
	lipoprotein	LPLC	low-pressure liquid chromatography
	low protein		
	lumbar puncture	LPLND	laparoscopic pelvic lymph node dissection
L/P	lactate-pyruvate ratio		
LP5	Life-Pak 5	LPM	latent primary malignancy
LPA	left pulmonary artery		
Lp(a)	lipoprotein (a)		liters per minute
LPA%	left pulmonary artery oxygen saturation	LPME	liquid-phase microextraction
L-PAM	melphalan (Alkeran)	LPN	Licensed Practical Nurse
LPC	laser photocoagulation	LPO	left posterior oblique
	Licensed Professional Counselor		light perception only
		LPPC	leukocyte-poor packed cells
LPCC	Licensed Professional Certified Counselor	LPPH	late postpartum hemorrhage
LPC-L	lymphoplasmacytoid lymphoma		
		LPR	laryngopharyngeal reflux
LPcP	light perception with projection		leprosy (Hansen disease) vaccine
LPD	leiomyomatosis peritonealis disseminata	LPS	last Pap smear
			lipopolysaccharide
	low-potassium dextran	LPSDT	laryngopharyngeal sensory discrimination testing
	low-protein diet		
	luteal phase defect	LP SHUNT	lumboperitoneal shunt
	luteal phase deficiency		
	lymphoproliferative disease	LPsP	light perception without projection
LPDA	left posterior descending artery	LPT	leptospirosis (Leptospira-Leptospires sp.) vaccine
LPEP	left pre-ejection period		
LPF	liver plasma flow		Licensed Physical Therapist
	low-power field	LPTN	Licensed Psychiatric Technical Nurse
	lymphocytosis-promoting factor		
		LPV	left portal vein
LPFB	left posterior fascicular block		left pulmonary vein
			lopinavir (Kaletra)
LPH	left posterior hemiblock	LQTS	long QT (interval) syndrome
	lumbar puncture headache		
LPHB	left posterior hemiblock	LR	labor room
LPI	laser peripheral iridectomy		lactated Ringer (injection)
			laser resection
	last patient in		lateral rectus
	leukotriene pathway inhibitor		left-right
			light reflex
LPICA	left posterior internal carotid artery		likelihood ratios
		L&R	left and right

L

L → R	left to right	LRTI	ligament reconstruction with tendon interposition
LR1A	labor room 1A		lower respiratory tract infection
LRA	left radial artery		
	left renal artery	LRV	left renal vein
LRC	locoregional control		log reduction value
	lower rib cage	LRW	LAL (*Limulus* amebocyte lysate) reagent water
LRCP	Licentiate of the Royal College of Physicians	LRZ	lorazepam (Ativan)
LRCS	Licentiate of the Royal College of Surgeons	LS	left side
			legally separated
LRD	limb reduction defects		Leigh syndrome
	living-related donor		liver scan
	living renal donor		liver-spleen
LRDT	living-related donor transplant		low salt
			lumbosacral
LRE	localization-related epilepsy		lung sounds
LREH	low-renin essential hypertension	L/S	lecithin-sphingomyelin ratio
LRF	left rectus femoris	L&S	ligation and stripping
	left ring finger		liver and spleen
	local-regional failure	L5-S1	lumbar fifth vertebra to sacral first vertebra (where the lumbar and sacral spines join)
L&R gtt	Levophed and Regitine drip (infusion)		
LRHT	living-related hepatic transplantation		
LRI	lower respiratory infection	LSA	left sacrum anterior
			lipid-bound sialic acid
LRLT	living-related liver transplantation		lymphosarcoma
LRM	left radical mastectomy	LSAs	low-sedating antihistamines
	local regional metastases	LSB	left scapular border
LRMP	last regular menstrual period		left sternal border
			local standby
LRND	left radical neck dissection		lumbar spinal block
			lumbar sympathetic block
LRO	long-range objective		
Lrot	left rotation	LS BPS	laparoscopic bilateral partial salpingectomy
LRP	laparoscopic radical prostatectomy	LSC	laser-scanning cytometry
	lung-resistance protein		last sexual contact
LRQ	lower right quadrant		late systolic click
LROU	lateral rectus, both eyes		least significant change
LRR	light reflection rheography		left subclavian (artery) (vein)
	locoregional recurrences		lichen simplex chronicus
LRRT	locoregional radiotherapy		liquid scintillation counting
LRS	lactated Ringer solution		
LRT	living renal transplant	LSCA	left scapuloanterior
	local radiation therapy	LSCC	laryngeal squamous cell carcinoma
	lower respiratory tract		
LRTD	living relative transplant donor	LSCCB	limited-state small-cell cancer of the bladder

LSCM	laser-scanning confocal microscopy		lumbar spinal stenosis
		LSSS	Liverpool Seizure Severity Scale
LSCP	left scapuloposterior		
LSCS	lower segment cesarean section	LST	left sacrum transverse
		LSTAT	life support for trauma and transport
LSD	least significant difference		
	low-salt diet	LSTC	laparoscopic tubal coagulation
	lumbosacral derangement		
	lysergide	LSTL	laparoscopic tubal ligation
LSE	local side effects	LSTM	lean soft tissue mass
LSed	level of sedation	L's & T's	lines and tubes
LSF	low-saturated fat	LSU	life support unit
LSFA	low-saturated fatty acid (diet)	LSV	left subclavian vein
			lesser saphenous vein
LSH	laparoscopic supracervical hysterectomy	LSVC	left superior vena cava
		LSW	left-side weakness
	leishmaniasis vaccine		Licensed Social Worker
LSI	levonorgestrel subdermal implant	LT	laboratory technician
			left
L-SIL	low-grade squamous intraepithelial lesions		left thigh
			left triceps
LSK	liver, spleen, and kidneys		leukotrienes
			Levin tube
LSKM	liver-spleen-kidney-megalgia		light
			light touch
LSL	left sacrolateral		low transverse
	left short leg (brace)		lumbar traction
LSLF	low sodium, low fat (diet)		lung transplantation
LSM	laser scanning microscope		lunotriquetral
	late systolic murmur		lymphotoxin
	least squares mean	L&T	lettuce and tomato
	limited sampling model	LT3	liothyronine sodium (Cytomel)
	liver, spleen masses		
LSMFT	liposclerosing myxofibrous tumor	LT4	levothyroxine
		LTA	laryngotracheal applicator
LSMT	life-sustaining medical treatment		laryngeal tracheal anesthesia
LSO	left salpingo-oophorectomy		lateral thoracic arteries
			local tracheal anesthesia
	left superior oblique	LTAC	long-term acute care
	lumbosacral orthosis	LTAS	left transatrial septal
LSP	left sacrum posterior	LTB	laparoscopic tubal banding
	liver-specific (membrane) lipoprotein		laryngotracheobronchitis
		LTB$_4$	leukotriene B$_4$
L–Spar	Elspar (asparaginase)	LTBI	latent tuberculosis infection
L-spine	lumbar spine	LTC	left to count
LSQ	Life Situation Questionnaire		long-term care
			long thick closed
LSR	left superior rectus	LTC$_4$	leukotriene C$_4$
L/S ratio	lecithin/sphingomyelin ratio	LTC-101	long-term care form-101
		LTCBDE	laparoscopic transcystic common bile duct exploration
LSS	limb-sparing surgery		
	liver-spleen scan		

L

LTCCS	low-transverse cervical cesarean section		lymphocyte transformation test
LTCF	long-term care facility	LTUI	low transverse uterine incision
LTCH	long-term care hospital		
LTC-IC	long-term culture-initiating cells	LTV	long-term variability long-term ventilation Luche tumor virus
LTCR	long-term complete remission(s)	LTV+	long-term variability–average to moderate
LTCS	low-transverse cesarean section	LTV 0	long-term variability–absent
LTD	largest tumor dimension	LTVC	long-term venous catheter
	leg transfer device	LTWN	long-term low-level white noise
	lipid tear deficiency long-term depression	LTx	lung transplantation
	long-term disability	LTZ	letrozole (Femara)
LTD$_4$	leukotriene D$_4$	LU	left upper
LTE	less than effective		left ureteral
LTE$_4$	leukotriene E$_4$		living unit
LTED	long-term estrogen deprivation		Lutheran
LTF	lost to follow-up	L & U	lower and upper
LTFU	long-term follow-up	LUA	left upper arm
LTG	lamotrigine (Lamictal)	LUD	left uterine displacement
	long-term goal	LUE	left upper extremity
	low-tension glaucoma	Lues I	primary syphilis
LTGA	left transposition of great artery	Lues II	secondary syphilis
		Lues III	tertiary syphilis
LTH	left total hip (arthroplasty) luteotropic hormone	LUFF	lateral upper arm free flap (reconstruction of pharyngeal defect)
LTK	laser thermal keratoplasty		
	left total knee (arthroplasty)	LUL	left upper lid left upper lobe (lung)
LTL	laparoscopic tubal ligation	LUM	laparoscopic-ultraminilaparotomic myomectomy
	left temporal lobectomy		
LTM	long-term memory long-term monitoring	LUNA	laparoscopic uterosacral nerve ablation
LTNPs	long-term nonprogressors (AIDS patients)	LUOB	left upper outer buttock
		LUOQ	left upper outer quadrant
LTOT	long-term oxygen therapy	LUQ	left upper quadrant
LTP	laser trabeculoplasty	LURD	living-unrelated donor
	long-term plan long-term potentiation	LUS	laparoscopic ultrasonography
LTPA	leisure-time physical activity		lower uterine segment
		LUSB	left upper scapular border
LTR	long terminal repeats		left upper sternal border
	lower trunk rotation	LUST	lower uterine segment transverse
LTRA	leukotriene receptor antagonist		
		LUT	lower urinary tract
LTS	laparoscopic tubal sterilization	LUTD	lower urinary tract dysfunction
	long-term survivors	LUTS	lower urinary tract symptoms
LTT	lactose tolerance test		

L

LUTT	lower urinary tract tumor	LVET	left ventricular ejection time
LUW	lungworm vaccine		
LUX	left upper extremity	LVF	left ventricular failure
LV	leave		left visual field
	left ventricle	LVFP	left ventricular filling pressure
	leucovorin		
	live virus	LVFU	leucovorin and fluorouracil
LVA	left ventricular aneurysm		
LVC	laser vision correction	LVFWR	left ventricular free wall rupture
	low-viscosity cement		
	low-vision clinic	LVG	left ventrogluteal
LVAD	left ventricular assist device	LVH	left ventricular hypertrophy
LV Angio	left ventricular angiogram	LVHR	laparoscopic ventral hernia repair
L-VAM	leuprolide acetate, vinblastine, doxorubicin (Adriamycin), and mitomycin		
		LVID	left ventricular internal diameter
		LVIDd	left ventricle internal diameter at end-diastole
LVAS	left ventricular assist system		
		LVIDs	left ventricle internal dimension systole
LVAT	left ventricular activation time		
		LVL	large volume leukapheresis
LVBP	left ventricle bypass pump		
LVD	left ventricular dimension		left vastus lateralis
	left ventricular dysfunction	LVM	left ventricular mass
		LVMI	left ventricular mass index
LVDd	left ventricular end-diastolic diameter	LVMM	left ventricular muscle mass
LVDP	left ventricular diastolic pressure	LVN	Licensed Visiting Nurse
			Licensed Vocational Nurse
LVDs	left ventricular systolic diameter	LVO	left ventricular overactivity
LVDT	linear variable differential transformer	LVOT	left ventricular outflow tract
LVDV	left ventricular diastolic volume	LVOTO	left ventricular outflow tract obstruction
LVE	left ventricular enlargement	LVP	large volume parenteral
LVEDD	left ventricular end-diastolic diameter		left ventricular pressure
		LVPW	left ventricular posterior wall
LVEDP	left ventricular end diastolic pressure		
		LVR	leucovorin
LVEDV	left ventricular end-diastolic volume	LVRS	lung-volume reduction surgery
LVEF	left ventricular ejection fraction	LVRT	liver-volume replaced by tumor
LVEP	left ventricular end pressure	LVS	laryngeal videostroboscopy
LVESD	left ventricular end-systolic dimension		left ventricular strain
		LVS EMI	left ventricular subendocardial myocardial ischemia
LVESV	left-ventricular end-systolic volumes		
LVESVI	left ventricular end-systolic volume index	LVSF	left ventricular systolic function

L

		M
LVSI	lymph-vascular space invasion (involvement)	
LVSP	left ventricular systolic pressure	
LVSW	left ventricular stroke work	
LVSWI	left ventricular stroke work index	M	male
LVT	levetiracetam (Keppra)		manual
LVV	left ventricular volume		marital
	live varicella vaccine		married
LVW	left ventricular wall		masked (audiology)
LVWI	left ventricular work index		mass
LVWMA	left ventricular wall motion abnormality		medial
			memory
LVWMI	left ventricular wall motion index		mesial
			meta
LVWT	left ventricular wall thickness		meter (m)
			mild
LW	lacerating wound		million
	living will		minimum
L & W	Lee and White (coagulation)		molar
			Monday
	living and well		monocytes
LWAQ	Living with Asthma Questionnaire		mother
			mouth
LWCT	Lee-White clotting time		murmur
LWBS	left without being seen		muscle
LWC	leave without consent		*Mycobacterium*
LWCT	left without completing treatment		*Mycoplasma*
			myopia
LWOP	leave without pay		myopic
LWOT	left without treatment	Ⓜ	thousand
		M₁	murmur
LWP	large whirlpool	M₁	first mitral sound
LX	larynx local irradiation	M1	left mastoid
	lower extremity		tropicamide 1% ophthalmic solution (Mydriacyl)
LXC	laxative of choice		
LXT	left exotropia		
LYCD	live-yeast cell derivative	M1 to M7	categories of acute nonlymphoblastic leukemia
LYEL	lost-years of expected life		
LYG	lymphomatoid granulomatosis	M₂	second mitral sound
LYM	Lyme disease vaccine	m²	square meters (body surface)
	lymphocytes		
lymphs	lymphocytes	M2	right mastoid
LYS	large yellow soft (stools)	M-2	vincristine, carmustine, cyclophosphamide, melphalan, and prednisone
	life-year saved (cost of)		
	lysine		
lytes	electrolytes (Na, K, Cl, etc.)		
		M₃	third mitral sound
	electrolyte panel (see page 392)	M-3	medical student 3rd year
LZ	landing zone	3M	mitomycin, mitoxantrone, and methotrexate
LZP	lorazepam (Ativan)		

L

M-3+7	mitoxantrone and cytarabine		mid-arm circumference
			minimum alveolar concentration
M-4	medical student 4th year		monitored anesthesia care
MA	machine		multi-access catheter
	Master of Arts		*Mycobacterium avium* complex
	mean arterial (blood pressure)	MACC	methotrexate, doxorubicin, (Adriamycin)
	medical assistance		cyclophosphamide, and
	medical authorization		lomustine (Cee Nu)
	megestrol acetate	MACCC	Master Arts, Certified
	menstrual age		Clinical Competence
	mental age	MACE	major adverse cardiac
	meter angle		(cardiovascular) event(s)
	Mexican American		Malon antegrade
	microalbuminuria		continence (colonic)
	metabolic acidosis		enema
	microaneurysms	MACOP-B	methotrexate, doxorubicin,
	Miller-Abbott (tube)		(Adriamycin) cyclophos-
	milliamps		phamide, vincristine
	monoclonal antibodies		(Oncovin), prednisone,
	motorcycle accident		and bleomycin with
M/A	mood and/or affect		leucovorin rescue
MA-1	Bennett volume ventilator	MACRO	macrocytes
MAA	macroaggregates of albumin	MACS	magnetic activated cell sorting
	Marketing Authorization	MACs	malignancy-associated
	Application (European		changes
	Union)	MACTAR	McMaster-Toronto
MAARI	medically attended acute respiratory illness		Arthritis Patient Reference (Disability
MAAS	Motor Activity Assessment Scale		Questionnaire)
MAB	Massachusetts Biologic	MAD	major affective disorder
	Laboratories		mandibular advancement
	maximum androgen blockade		device
			mind altering drugs
Mab	monoclonal antibody		moderate atopic dermatitis
MABP	mean arterial blood pressure	MADD	Mothers Against Drunk Driving
MAC	macrocytic erythrocytes		multiple acyl-CoA
	macrophage		dehydrogenase
	macula		deficiency
	maximal allowable concentration	MADL	mobility activities of daily living
	medial arterial calcification	MADRS	Montgomery-Åsburg Depression Rating
	membrane attack complex		Scale
	Mental Adjustment to Cancer (scale)	MAE	medical air evacuation moves all extremities
	methotrexate, dactinomycin	MAES	moves all extremities slowly
	(Actinomycin D), and cyclophosphamide		

M

MAEEW	moves all extremities equally well
MAEW	moves all extremities well
MAF	malignant ascites fluid
	metabolic activity factor
	Mexican-American female
MAFAs	movement-associated fetal (heart rate) accelerations
MAFO	molded ankle/foot orthosis
MAFP	maternal alpha-fetoprotein
MAG	medication administration guideline (record)
mag cit	magnesium citrate
MAGP	meatal advancement glandulophaleoplasty
mag sulf	magnesium sulfate
MAHA	macroangiopathic hemolytic anemia
MAI	maximal aggregation index
	Medication Appropriateness Index
	minor acute illness
	Mycobacterium avium-intracellulare
MAID	mesna, doxorubicin (Adriamycin), ifosfamide, and dacarbazine
MAIR	metabolic acidosis-induced retinopathy
MAL	malaria vaccine
	malignant
	methyl aminolevulinate
	midaxillary line
	Motor Activity Log
MALDI	matrix-assisted laser desorption ionization
MALDI-TOFMS	matrix-assisted laser desorption ionization-time-of-flight mass spectrometry
MALG	Minnesota antilymphoblast globulin
malig	malignant
MALT	mucosa-associated lymphoid tissue
MALToma	lymphoma of mucosa-associated lymphoid tissue

MAM	mammogram
	Mexican-American male
	monitored administration of medication
MAMC	mid-arm muscle circumference
Mammo	mammography
MAMP	milliampere
m-AMSA	amsacrine
MAMTT	minimal active muscle tendon tension
MAN	malignancy associated neutropenia
Mand	mandibular
MANE	Morrow Assessment of Nausea and Emesis
MANOVA	multivariate analysis of variance
MAO	maximum acid output
MAO-A	monoamine oxidase type A
MAO-B	monoamine oxidase type B
MAOI	monoamine oxidase inhibitor
MAOP	Mid-Atlantic Oncology Program
MAP	magnesium, ammonium, and phosphate (Struvite stones)
	mean airway pressure
	mean arterial pressure
	Medical Assistance Program
	megaloblastic anemia of pregnancy
	Miller Assessment for Preschoolers (test for developmental delays)
	mitogen-activated protein
	mitomycin, doxorubicin (Adriamycin), and cisplatin (Platinol)
	morning after pill (oral contraceptives)
	muscle-action potential
	Mycobacterium avium subspecies *paratuberculosis*
MAPC	multipotent adult progenitor cell
MAPI	Millon Adolescent Personality Inventory

MAPS	Make a Picture Story	MATHS	muscle pain, allergy, tachycardia and tiredness, and headache syndrome
MAR	marital		
	medication administration record		
	melanoma-associated retinopathy	MAU	microalbuminuria
		MAVR	mitral and aortic valve replacement
	mineral apposition rates		
MARE	manual active-resistive exercise	max	maxillary
			maximal
MARSA	methicillin-aminoglycoside-resistant *Staphylococcus aureus*	MAX A	maximum assistance (assist)
		MAXCONT	maximum contrast method
		MAxL	midaxillary line
MAS	macrophage activation syndrome	MAYO	mayonnaise
		MB	buccal margin
	McClune-Albright syndrome		mandible
			Mallory body
	meconium aspiration syndrome		Medical Board
			medulloblastoma
	Memory Assessment Scale		mesiobuccal
			methylene blue
	minimum-access surgery		myocardial bands
	mobile arm support	M/B	mother/baby
	Modified Ashworth Scale	MBA	Master of Business Administration
MASA	mutant allele-specific amplification		
MASDA^{SM}	Multiple-Allele-Specific Diagnostic Assay	M-BACOD	methotrexate (high-dose), bleomycin, doxorubicin (Adriamycin), cyclophosphamide, vincristine (Oncovin), and dexamethasone with leucovorin rescue
MASER	microwave amplification (application) by stimulated emission of radiation		
MASH POT	mashed potatoes	MBC	male breast cancer
			maximum bladder capacity
MAST	mastectomy		maximum breathing capacity
	medical antishock trousers		
	Michigan Alcoholism Screening Test		metastatic breast cancer
			methotrexate, bleomycin, and cisplatin
	military antishock trousers		
MAT	manual arts therapy		minimal bactericidal concentration
	maternal		
	maternity	MB-CK	a creatinine kinase isoenzyme
	mature		
	medication administration team	MBD	metabolic bone disease
			metastatic bone disease
	metabolic activation therapy		methylene blue dye
			minimal brain damage
	microscopic agglutination test		minimal brain dysfunction
		MBE	may be elevated
	Miller-Abbott tube		medium below elbow
	multifocal atrial tachycardia	MBF	meat-base formula
			myocardial blood flow

M

219

MBFC	medial brachial fascial compartment	MCA	Medicines Control Agency (United Kingdom)
MBEST	modulus blipped echo-planar single-pulse technique		megestrol, cyclophosphamide, and doxorubicin (Adriamycin)
MBHI	Millon Behavioral Health Inventory		metacarpal amputation
MBI	methylene blue installation		micrometastases clonogenic assay
MBL	mannose-binding lectin		middle cerebral aneurysm
	menstrual blood loss		middle cerebral artery
MBM	mind-body medicine		monoclonal antibodies
	mother's breast milk		motorcycle accident
MBNW	multiple-breath nitrogen washout		multichannel analyzer
MBO	mesiobuccal occulsion		multiple congenital anomalies
MBOT	mucinous borderline ovarian tumors	2-MCA	2-methyl citric acid
MBP	malignant brachial plexopathy	MCAD	medium-chain acyl-CoA dehydrogenase
	mannan-binding protein	MCAF	monocyte chemoattractant and activity factor
	mannose-binding protein		
	medullary bone pain	MCAO	middle cerebral artery occlusion
	mesiobuccopulpal		
	myelin basic protein	MCAP	middle cerebral artery pressure
MBq	megabecquerels		
MBR	major breakpoint region	McAS	McCune-Albright syndrome
MBS	modified barium swallow	MCAT	Medical College Admission Test
MBT	maternal blood type	MCB	Medicines Control Board (United Kingdom's equivalent to the United States Food and Drug Administration)
	multiple blunt trauma		
MBTS	modified Blalock-Taussig shunt		
MC	male child		
	medium-chain (triglycerides)		midcycle bleeding
	metacarpal		middle chamber bubbling
	metatarso - cuneiform	MCBDD	National Center on Birth Defects and Developmental Disabilities
	microcalcifications (breast)		
	mini-laparotomy cholecystectomy	McB pt	McBurney point
	mitoxantrone and cytarabine	MCBS	Medicare Current Beneficiary Survey
	mitral commissurotomy	MCC	meningococcal serogroup C conjugate
	mixed cellularity		
	molluscum contagiosum		Merkel cell carcinoma
	monocomponent highly purified pork insulin		microcrystalline cellulose
	Moraxella catarrhalis		midstream clean-catch
	mouth care	MCCU	mobile coronary care unit
	myocarditis	MCD	malformation of cortical development
m + c	morphine and cocaine		mean cell diameter

	Medicaid	MCN	minimal change
	minimal-change disease		nephropathy
	multicystic dysplasia	MCNS	minimal change nephrotic
MCDK	multicystic dysplasia of		syndrome
	the kidney	MCO	managed care organization
MCDT	mast cell degranulation		mupirocin calcium
	test		ointment (Bactroban
MCE	major coronary event		Nasal)
MCF	multicentric foci	MCP	mean carotid pressure
MCFA	medium-chain fatty acid		metacarpophalangeal joint
mcg	microgram (1,000 mcg =		metoclopramide (Reglan)
	1 milligram) (do not		monocyte chemotactic
	hand write μg, as it is		protein
	mistakenly read as	MCR	Medicare
	milligram [mg])		metabolic clearance rate
MCG	magnetocardiogram		minor cluster region
	magnetocardiography		myocardial
MCGN	minimal-change		revascularization
	glomerular nephritis	MC=R	moderately constricted
MCH	mean corpuscular		and equally reactive
	hemoglobin	MCRC	metastatic colorectal
	microfibrillar collagen		cancer
	hemostat	MCS	manufacturer cannot
	muscle contraction		supply
	headache		mental component
MCHC	mean corpuscular		summary
	hemoglobin		microculture and sensitivity
	concentration		moderate constant suction
MCHL	medial head of the		multiple chemical
	coracohumeral ligament		sensitivity
MCI	mild cognitive impairment		myocardial contractile
mCi	millicurie		state
MCID	minimum clinically	MCSA	minimal cross-sectional
	important difference(s)		area
mckat	microkatal (1 millionth	M-CSF	macrophage colony-
	$[10^{-6}]$ of a katal)		stimulating factor
MCL	mantle cell lymphoma	MC-SR	moderately constricted
	maximum comfort level		and slightly reactive
	medial collateral ligament	MCT	manual cervical traction
	midclavicular line		mean circulation time
	midcostal line		medial canthal tendon
	modified chest lead		medium chain triglyceride
	most comfortable level		medullary carcinoma of
mcL	microliter (1/1,000 of an		the thyroid
	mL)		microwave coagulation
MCLL	most comfortable		therapy
	listening level	MCTC	metrizamide computed
MCLNS	mucocutaneous lymph		tomography
	node syndrome		cisternogram
MCMI	Millon Clinical Multiaxial	MCTD	mixed connective tissue
	Inventory		disease
mcmol	micromoles (one millionth	MCTZ	methyclothiazide
	$[10^{-6}]$ of a mole)		(Enduron)

MCU	micturating cystourethrogram		medial dorsal cutaneous (nerve)
MCV	mean corpuscular volume	MDCM	mildly dilated congestive cardiomyopathy
MCVRI	minimal coronary vascular resistance index	MDCT	multidetector-row computed tomography
MCYLS	marginal cost per year of life saved	MDD	major depressive disorder
MD	macula degeneration		manic-depressive disorder
	maintenance dialysis		
	maintenance dose	MDE	major depressive episode
	major depression	MDF	myocardial depressant factor
	mammary dysplasia		
	manic depression	MDGF	macrophage-derived growth factor
	mean deviation		
	medical doctor	MDGs	Millennium Development Goals
	mediodorsal		
	Menière disease	MDI	manic-depressive illness
	mental deficiency		mental developmental index
	mesiodistal		
	movement disorder		metered-dose inhaler
	multiple dose		methylenedioxyindenes
	muscular dystrophy		multiple daily injection
	myocardial damage		multiple dosage insulin
MD-50®	diatrizoate sodium injection 50%	MDIA	Mental Development Index, Adjusted
MDA	malondialdehyde	MDII	multiple daily insulin injection
	manual dilation of the anus		
	mass drug administrations (diethylcarbamazine plus albendazole to stop transmission of filariasis)	MDIS	metered-dose inhaler-spacer (device)
		MDiv	Master of Divinity
		MDM	mid-diastolic murmur
			minor determinant mix (of penicillin)
	Medical Devises Agency (United Kingdom)	MDMA	methylenedioxy-methamphetamine (ecstasy)
	methylenedioxyamphet-amine		
		MDNT	midnight
	micrometastases detection assay	MDO	mentally disordered offender
	motor discriminative acuity	MDOT	modified directly observed therapy
	Multichannel Discrete Analyzer	MDP	methylene diphosphonate
MDAC	multiple-dose activated charcoal	MDPH	Michigan Department of Public Health
MDACC	MD Anderson Cancer Center	MDPI	maximum daily permissible intake
MDA LDL	malondialdehydeconju-gated low-density lipoprotein	MDR	Medical Device Reporting (regulation)
			minimum daily requirement
MDASI	MD Anderson Symptom Inventory		multidrug resistance
MDC	Major Diagnostic Category	MD=R	moderately dilated and equally reactive

MDR-1	multidrug resistance gene		monitor and evaluate
MDRE	multiple-drug-resistant enterococci		myeloid-erythroid (ratio)
		M&E	Mecholyl and Eserine
MDREF	multidrug resistant enteric fever		mucositis and enteritis
		MEA	microwave endometrial ablation
MDRO	multidrug resistant organism		measles virus vaccine
MDRSP	multidrug resistant *Streptococcus pneumoniae*	MEA-I	multiple endocrine adenomatosis type I
		MEB	Medical Evaluation Board
MDRT	multiple-drug rescue therapy		methylene blue
		MEC	meconium
MDRTB	multidrug resistant tuberculosis		middle ear canal(s)
			mitoxantrone, etoposide, and cytarabine
MDS	maternal deprivation syndrome	MeCCNU	semustine
	Miller-Dieker syndrome	MECG	maternal electrocardiogram
	Minimum Data Set		
	myelodysplastic syndromes	MeCP	semustine (methyl CCNU) cyclophosphamide, and prednisone
MD-SR	moderately dilated and slightly reactive	MED	male erectile dysfunction
MDSU	medical day stay unit		maximal (maximum) economic dose
MDT	maggot debridement therapy		medial
	Mechanical Diagnostic Therapist		median erythrocyte diameter
	motion detection threshold		medical
			medication
	multidisciplinary team		medicine
	multidrug therapy		medium
MDTM	multidisciplinary team meeting		medulloblastoma
			minimal erythema dose
MDTP	multidisciplinary treatment plan		minimum effective dose
MDU	maintenance dialysis unit		multiple epiphyseal dysplasia
	microvascular Doppler ultrasonography	MEd	Master of Education
MDUO	myocardial disease of unknown origin	MEDAC	multiple endocrine deficiency Addison disease (autoimmune) candidiasis
MDV	Marek disease virus		
	multiple dose vial	MEDCO	Medcosonolator
MDY	month, date, and year	MedDRA	Medical Dictionary for Regulatory Activities
ME	macular edema	MEDEX	medication administration record
	manic episode		
	medical events	MED-LARS	Medical Literature Analysis and Retrieval System
	medical evidence		
	medical examiner		
	mestranol	MEDLINE	National Library of Medicine medical database
	Methodist		
	middle ear		
	myalgic encephalomyelitis		
M/E	metabolic/endocrine		

MED NEC	medically necessary
MedPAR	Medicare Provider Analysis Review File
MEDS	medications
MEE	maintenance energy expenditure
	measured energy expenditure
	middle ear effusion
MEE/OC	middle ear exploration with ossicular chain reconstruction
MEF	maximum expired flow rate
	middle ear fluid
MEFR	mid expiratory flow rate
MEFV	maximum expiratory flow-volume
MEG	magnetoencephalogram
	magnetoencephalography
Meg-CSF	megakaryocytic colony-stimulating factor
MEGX	monoethylglycinexylidide
MeHg	methylmercury
MEI	magnetic endoscope imaging
	medical economic index
MEIA	microparticle enzyme immunoassay
MEKC	micellar electrokinetic chromatography
MEL	maximum exposure limit
	melatonin
MELAS	mitochondrial encephalo-myopathy with lactic acidosis, and stroke-like episodes (syndrome)
MEL B	melarsoprol (Arsobal)
MELD	Model for End-Stage Liver Disease (score)
MEM	memory
	monocular estimate method (near retinoscopy)
MEMB	modified eosin-methylene blue (agar)
MEN	meningeal
	meninges
	meningitis
	meningococcal (*Neisseria meningitidis*) (sero-groups unspecified) vaccine

MEN (II)	multiple endocrine neoplasia (type II)
MEN$_{cn-AC}$	meningococcal (*Neisseria meningitidis*) serogroups A, C conjugate vaccine
MEN$_{cn-B}$	meningococcal (*Neisseria meningitidis*) serogroup B conjugate vaccine
MEN$_{ps}$	meningococcal (*Neisseria meningitidis*) polysaccharide vaccine, not otherwise specified
MEN$_{ps-ACYW}$	meningococcal (*Neisseria meningitidis*) serogroups A, C, Y, W-135 polysaccharide vaccine
MEN$_{ps-B}$	meningococcal (*Neisseria meningitidis*) serogroup B polysaccharide vaccine
MENS	microcurrent electrical neuromuscular stimulation
	mini-electrical nerve stimulator
MEO	malignant external otitis
MeOH	methyl alcohol
MEOS	microsomal ethanol oxidizing system
MEP	maximal expiratory pressure
	meperidine (Demerol)
	motor-evoked potential
	multimodality-evoked potential
MEPA	Medication Error Prevention Analysis (FDA)
MEPS	Medical Expenditure Panel Survey
mEq	milliequivalent
mEq/24 H	milliequivalents per 24 hours
mEq/L	milliequivalents per liter
MER	medical evidence of record
	methanol-extracted residue (of phenol-treated BCG)
M/E ratio	myeloid/erythroid ratio

MERRF	myoclonic epilepsy and ragged red fibers		middle finger
MES	maximal electroshock		midforceps
	mesial		mother and father
MESA	microsurgical epididymal sperm aspiration		mycosis fungoides
			myelofibrosis
			myocardial fibrosis
MeSH	Medical Subject Headings of the National Library of Medicine	M/F	male-female ratio
		M & F	male and female
			mother and father
MESS	Mangled Extremity Severe Score	MFA	malaise, fatigue, and anorexia
MEST	mesodermal specific transcript (gene)	MFAT	multifocal atrial tachycardia
MET	medical emergency treatment	MFB	metallic foreign body multiple-frequency bioimpedance
	metabolic		
	metamyelocytes	MFC	medial femoral condyle
	metastasis	MfC	*Medicines for Children*
	metronidazole	MFCU	Medicaid Fraud Control Unit
meT	methyltestosterone		
META	metamyelocytes	MFD	Memory for Designs
METH	methicillin		midforceps delivery
MetHb	methemoglobin		milk-free diet
	methemoglobinemia		multiple fractions per day
methyl CCNU	semustine	MFEM	maximal forced expiratory maneuver
methyl G	mitroguazone dihydrochloride (Zyrkamine)	MFFT	Matching Familiar Figures Test
		MFH	malignant fibrous histiocytoma
methyl GAG	mitroguazone dihydrochloride (Zyrkamine)	MFI	mean fluorescent intensity Multidimensional Fatigue Inventory
METS	metabolic equivalents (multiples of resting oxygen uptake)	MFM	multifidus muscle
		MFNS	mometasone furoate nasal spray (Nasonex)
	metastases		
METT	maximum exercise tolerance test	MFPS	myofascial pain syndrome
		MFR	mid-forceps rotation
MEV	million electron volts		myofascial release
MEWDS	multifocal evanescent white dot syndrome	MFS	Marfan syndrome maternal-fetal surgery
MEX	Mexican		metastases free survival
MF	Malassezia folliculitis		Miller-Fisher syndrome
	Malassezia furfur		mitral first sound
	masculinity/femininity		monofixation syndrome
	meat-free	MFT	muscle function test
	median frequency (anesthesia-depth monitor)	MFU	medical follow-up
		MFVNS	middle fossa vestibular nerve section
	mesial facial	MFVPT	Motor Free Visual Perception Test
	methotrexate and fluorouracil	MFVR	minimal forearm vascular resistance
	midcavity forceps		

MG	Marcus Gunn	MgO	magnesium oxide
	Michaelis-Gutmann (bodies)	MG/OL	molecular genetics/oncology laboratory
	milligram (mg)		
	myasthenia gravis	MGP	Marcus Gunn pupil
mg	milligram (1,000 mg = 1 gram)		medical group practice
		MGR	murmurs, gallops, or rubs
Mg	magnesium	MGS	magnetic guidance system
mG	milligauss	MGS	malignant glandular schwannoma
μg	microgram (1/1000 of a milligram) (This is a dangerous abbreviation when hand written, as it is read as mg. Use mcg)	MgSO₄	magnesium sulfate (Epsom salt) (this is dangerous terminology as it can be interpreted as morphine sulfate)
M&G	myringotomy and grommets	MGT	management
		mgtt	minidrop (60 minidrops = 1 mL)
mg%	milligrams per 100 milliliters	MGUS	monoclonal gammopathy of undetermined significance
MGBG	mitoguazone (Zyrkamine)		
MGCT	malignant glandular cell tumor	MGW	multiple gunshot wound
MGD	meibomian gland dysfunction	MGW enema	magnesium sulfate, glycerin, and water enema
MGd	motexafin gadolinium (Xcytrin)	M-GXT	multistage graded exercise test
MGDF	megakaryocyte growth and development factor	mGy	milligray (radiation unit)
mg/dl	milligrams per 100 milliliters	MH	macular hemorrhage
			malignant hyperthermia
MGF	macrophage growth factor		marital history
			medical history
	mast cell growth factor		menstrual history
	maternal grandfather		mental health
MGG	May-Grünwald-Giemsa (stain)		moist heat
MGGM	maternal great grandmother	MHA	Mental Health Assistant
			methotrexate, hydrocortisone, and cytarabine (ara-C)
MGHL	middle glenohumeral ligament		
mg/kg	milligram per kilogram		microangiopathic hemolytic anemia
mg/kg/d	milligram per kilogram per day		microhemagglutination
mg/kg/hr	milligram per kilogram per hour		migraine headache
		MHA-TP	microhemagglutination-*Treponema pallidum*
MGM	maternal grandmother		
	milligram (mg is correct)	MHB	maximum hospital benefits
MGMA	Medical Group Management Association		
		MHb	methemoglobin
		MHBSS	modified Hank balanced salt solution
MGN	membranous glomerulonephritis	MHC	major histocompatibility complex
MGO	methylglyoxal		

	mental health center (clinic)	**M**
	mental health counselor	
M/hct	microhematocrit	
MHD	10-hydroxycarbazepine (oxcarbazepine metabolite)	
	maintenance hemodialysis	
	maximum heart distance (radiation therapy)	
mHg	millimeters of mercury	
MHH	mental health hold	
MHI	Mental Health Index (information)	
MHL	maximum heart length (radiation therapy)	
	mesenchymal hamartoma of the liver	
MHIP	mental health inpatient	
MH/MR	mental health and mental retardation	
MHN	massive hepatic necrosis	
MHO	medical house officer	
MHP	moist heat packs	
MHRI	Mental Health Research Institute	
MHS	major histocompatibility system	
	malignant hyperthermia susceptible	
	monomethyl hydrogen sulfate	
	multihospital system	
MHT	malignant hypertension	
	mental health team	
	Mental Health Technician	
MHTAP	microhemagglutination assay for antibody to *Treponema pallidum*	
MHV	mechanical heart valves	
	middle hepatic vein	
MHW	medial heel wedge	
	mental health worker	
MHX	methohexital sodium	
MHx	medical history	
MHxR	medical history review	
MHz	megahertz	
MI	membrane intact	
	mental illness	
	mental institution	
	mesial incisal	
	mitral insufficiency	
	myocardial infarction	

MIA	medically indigent adult	
	missing in action	
MIBE	measles inclusion body encephalitis	
MIBI	technetium Tc99m sestamibi (a myocardial perfusion agent; Cardiolite)	
MIBG	iobenguane sulfate I 123 (meta-iodobenzyl guanidine I 123)	
MIBK	methylisobutylketone	
MIC	maternal and infant care	
	methacholine inhalation challenge	
	medical intensive care	
	microscope	
	microcytic erythrocytes	
	minimum inhibitory concentration	
MICA	mentally ill, chemical abuser	
MICAR	Mortality Medical Indexing, Classification, and Retrieval	
MICE	mesna, ifosfamide, carboplatin, and etoposide	
MICN	mobile intensive care nurse	
MICR	methacholine inhalation challenge response	
MICRO	microcytes	
MICS	minimally invasive cardiac surgery	
MICU	medical intensive care unit	
	mobile intensive care unit	
MID	mesioincisodistal	
	microvillus inclusion disease	
	minimal ineffective dose	
	multi-infarct dementia	
MIDAS	migraine disability assessment scale	
MIDCAB	minimally invasive direct coronary artery bypass	
MIDD	maternally inherited diabetes and deafness	
MID EPIS	midline episiotomy	
Mid I	middle insomnia	
MIE	maximim inspiratory effort	

	meconium ileus equivalent (cystic fibrosis)	MIO	minimum identifiable odor
	medical improvement		monocular indirect ophthalmoscopy
	expected	MIP	macrophage inflammatory
MIEI	medication-induced esophageal injury		protein
MIF	Merthiolate, iodine, and formalin		maximum inspiratory pressure
	mifepristone (RU 486; Mifeprex)		maximum-intensity projection (radiology)
	migration inhibitory factor		mean intrathoracic pressure
MIFR	midinspiratory flow rate		mean intravascular
MIF 50% VC	midinspiratory flow at 50% of vital capacity		pressure
MIG	measles immune globulin		medical improvement possible
MIGET	multiple inert gas elimination technique		metacarpointerphalangeal
			Michigan Biologic
MIH	medication-induced headache	MIRD	Products Institute
	migraine with		medical internal radiation dose
	interparoxysmal headache	MIRP	myocardial infarction rehabilitation program
	myointimal hyperplasia	MIRS	Medical Improvement
MIL	military		Review Standard
	mesial incisal lingual (surface)	MIS	management information systems
	mother-in-law		minimally invasive surgery
MIMCU	medical intermediate care unit		mitral insufficiency
MIN	mammary intraepithelial		moderate intermittent suction
	neoplasia	MISA	mentally ill and substance
	melanocytic		abusing
	intraepidermal	MISC	miscarriage
	neoplasia		miscellaneous
	mineral	M Isch	myocardial ischemia
	minimum	MISH	multiple *in situ*
	minor		hybridization
	minute (min)	MISO	misonidazole
MIN A	minimal assistance (assist)	MISS	minimally invasive spine
MIME	mitoguazone, ifosfamide,		surgery
	methotrexate, and		Modified Injury Severity
	etoposide with mesna		Score (Scale)
MINE	Medical Information		Mothers in Sympathy and
	Network of Europe		Support
	mesna, ifosfamide,	MIT	meconium in trachea
	mitoxantrone		miracidia immobilization
	(Novantrone), and		test
	etoposide		mono-iodotyrosine
	medical improvement not		multiple injection therapy
	expected		(of insulin)
MINI	Mini International	MITO-C	mitomycin (Mutamycin)
	Neuropsychiatric	MITOX	mitoxantrone
	Interview		(Novantrone)

MIU	million international units		myelomonocytic
	minor injury unit		leukemia, chronic
mIU	milli-international unit	MLD	manual lymph drainage
	(one-thousandth of an		masking level difference
	International unit)		melioidosis (*Pseudomonas*
MIVA	mivacurium (Mivacron)		*pseudomallei*) vaccine
MIVE	maximum isometric		metachromatic
	voluntary extension		leukodystrophy
MIVF	maximum isometric		microlumbar diskectomy
	voluntary flexion		microsurgical lumbar
MIW	mental inquest warrant		diskectomy
mix mon	mixed monitor		minimal lethal dose
MJ	marijuana	MLDT	Manual Lymph Drainage
	megajoule		Therapist
MJD	Machado-Joseph Disease	MLE	maximum likelihood
MJL	medial joint line		estimation
MJS	medial joint space		midline (medial)
MJT	Mead Johnson tube		episiotomy
μkat	microkatal (micro-	MLF	median longitudinal
	moles/sec)		fasciculus
MKAB	may keep at bedside	MLN	manifest latent nystagmus
MKB	married, keeping baby		mediastinal lymph node
MK-CSF	megakaryocyte colony-		melanoma vaccine
	stimulating factor		mesenteric lymph node
MKI	mitotic-karyorrhectic	MLNS	minimal lesions nephrotic
	index		syndrome
MKM	Mehrkoordinaten		mucocutaneous lymph
	Manipulator		node syndrome
	microgram per kilogram		(Kawasaki syndrome)
	per minute	MLO	mesiolinguo-occlusal
ML	malignant lymphoma	MLP	mento-laeva posterior
	mediolateral		mesiolinguopulpal
	middle lobe		midlevel provider
	midline	MLPN	Medical Licensed
	mucosal leishmaniasis		Practical Nurse
mL	milliliter (1,000 mL =	MLPP	maximum loose-packed
	1 liter)		position
M/L	monocyte to lymphocyte	MLR	middle latency response
	(ratio)		mixed lymphocyte
	mother-in-law		reaction
MLA	medical laboratory assay		multiple logistic
	mento-laeva anterior		regression
MLAC	minimum local analgesic	MLRA	multiple linear-regression
	concentration		analysis
MLAP	mean left atrial pressure	MLS	macrolides, lincosamides,
MLBW	moderately low birth		and streptogramins
	weight		Maroteaux-Lamy
MLC	metastatic liver cancer		syndrome
	minimal lethal		maximum likelihood score
	concentration		mediastinal B-cell
	mixed lymphocyte culture		lymphoma with sclerosis
	multilevel care	MLT	melatonin
	multilumen catheter		mento-laeva transversa

MLU	mean length of utterance	MMFR	maximal mid-expiratory flow rate
MLV	monitored live voice		
MLWHF	Minnesota Living with Heart Failure (questionnaire)	MMG	mammography mechanomyography
		mm Hg	millimeters of mercury
MM	major medical (insurance)	MMI	maximal medical improvement
	malignant melanoma		
	malignant mesothelioma	MMK	Marshall-Marchetti-Krantz (cystourethropexy)
	Marshall-Marchetti		
	medial malleolus	MML	minimal masking level (audiology)
	medication management		
	member months	MMM	metastatic malignant melanoma
	meningococcic meningitis		
	mercaptopurine and methotrexate		mitoxantrone, methotrexate, and mitomycin
	methadone maintenance		mucous membrane moist
	micrometastases		
	millimeter (mm)		
	mismatch (ing)		myelofibrosis with myeloid metaplasia
	mist mask		
	morbidity and mortality	mMMSE	modified version of the mini mental status examination
	motor meal		
	mucous membrane		
	multiple myeloma	MMMT	malignant mixed mesodermal tumor
	muscle movement		
	myelomeningocele		metastatic mixed müllerian tumor
mM.	millimole (mmol)		
mm	millimeter	MMN	mismatch negativity
M&M	milk and molasses		multifocal motor neuropathy
	morbidity and mortality		
MMA	methylmalonic acid	MMOA	maxillary mandibular odontectomy alveolectomy
	methylmethacrylate		
	middle meningeal artery		
MMC	mitomycin (mitomycin C)	mmol	millimole
	myelomeningocele	μmol	micromole
MMCT	mitomycin C trabeculectomy	MMP	matrix metalloproteinase mitochondrial myopathy
MMD	malignant metastatic disease		multiple medical problems
	moyamoya disease		multiplexed molecular profiling (system)
	mucus membranes dry		
	myotonic muscular dystrophy	MMP-8	metalloproteinase-8
		MMPI	matrix metalloproteinase inhibitor
MME	membrane metalloendopeptidase		Minnesota Multiphasic Personality Inventory
MMECT	multiple monitor electroconvulsive therapy	MMPI-D	Minnesota Multiphasic Personality Inventory-Depression Scale
MMEFR	maximal mid-expiratory flow rate	6-MMPR	6-methylmercaptopurine riboside
MMF	mean maximum flow	MMPs	membership medical practices
	mycophenolate mofetil (CellCept)		

230

MMR	measles, mumps, and rubella		mononuclear leukocytes
	midline malignant reticulosis	MNCV	motor nerve conduction velocity
	mild mental retardation	MND	minor neurological dysfunction
	mismatch repair		modified neck dissection
MMRISK	a skin cancer mnemonic; **m**oles that are atypical, **m**oles that are many in number, **r**ed hair or freckles, **i**nability to tan, **s**unburn, **k**indred		motor neuron disease
		MNF	myelinated nerve fibers
		MNG	multinodular goiter
		MNM	mononeuritis multiplex
		MNMCB	motor neuropathy with multifocal conduction block
MMRS	Metropolitan Medical Response System		
MMR-VAR	measles virus, mumps virus, rubella virus, and varicella virus vaccine	MNNB	Monas-Nitz Neuropsychological Battery
		MNPRT	mixed neutron and photon radiotherapy
MMS	Medication Management Standards	MNR	marrow neutrophil reserve
	Mini-Mental State (examination)	MNS	mean nocturnal saturation
		MNSc	Master of Nursing Science
	Mohs micrographic surgery	MnSOD	manganese superoxide dismutase
MMSE	Mini-Mental State Examination	Mn SSEPS	median-nerve somatosensory-evoked potentials
MMT	malignant mesenchymal tumors		
	manual muscle test	MNTB	medial nucleus of the trapezoid body
	meal-tolerance test	MNX	meniscectomy
	medial meniscal tear	MNZ	metronidazole (Flagyl)
	methadone maintenance treatment	MO	medial oblique (x-ray view)
	Mini Mental Test		menhaden oil
	mixed müllerian tumors		mesio-occlusal
MMTP	Methadone Maintenance Treatment Program		mineral oil
			month (mo)
MMTV	malignant mesothelioma of the tunica vaginalis		months old
			morbidly obese
	monomorphic ventricular tachycardia		mother
			myositis ossificans
	mouse mammary tumor virus	Mo	molybdenum
MMV	mandatory minute volume	M/O	morning of
MMWR	*Morbidity and Mortality Weekly Report*	MOA	mechanism of action
			metronidazole, omeprazole, and amoxicillin
MN	midnight		
	mononuclear	MoAb	monoclonal antibody
Mn	manganese	MOAHI	mixed obstructive apnea and hypopnea index
M&N	morning and night		
	Mydriacyl and Neo-Synephrine	MOB	medical office building
MNC	monomicrobial necrotizing cellulitis		mobility
			mobilization

MOB-PT	mitomycin, vincristine (Oncovin), bleomycin, and cisplatin (Platinol AQ)
MOC	medial olivocochlear
	Medical Officer on Call
	metronidazole, omeprazole, and clarithromycin
	mother of child
MOCI	Maudsley Obsessive-Compulsive Inventory
MOD	maturity onset diabetes
	medical officer of the day
	mesio-occlusodistal
	moderate
	mode of death
	moment of death
	multiorgan dysfunction
MOD A	moderate assistance (assist)
MODEMS	Musculoskeletal Outcomes Data Evaluation and Management Scale
MOD I	modified independent (for example, a patient who is independent, but requires a walker)
MODM	mature-onset diabetes mellitus
MODS	multiple-organ dysfunction syndrome
MODY	maturity-onset diabetes of youth
MOE	movement of extremities
MOEMs	micro-opto-electro-mechanical systems
MOF	mesial occlusal facial
	methotrexate, vincristine (Oncovin), and fluorouracil
	methoxyflurane (Penthrane)
	multiple-organ failure
MOFS	multiple-organ failure syndrome
MOG	myelin oligodendrocyte glycoprotein
MOH	medication overuse headache
	Ministry of Health

MoH	Ministry of Health (Canada)
Mohs	Mohs technique; serial excision and microscopic examination of skin cancers
MOI	mechanism of injury
	multiplicity of infection
MoICU	mobile intensive care unit
MOJAC	mood orientation, judgement, affect, and content
MOL	method of limits
MOM	milk of magnesia
	mother
	mucoid otitis media
MoM	multiples of the median
MOMP	major outer membrane protein
MON	maximum observation nursery
	monitor
MONO	infectious mononucleosis
	monocyte
	monospot
mono, di	monochorionic, diamniotic
mono, mono	monochorionic, monoamniotic
MOP	medical outpatient
8 MOP	methoxsalen (Oxsorlen)
MOPP	mechlorethamine, vincristine (Oncovin), procarbazine, and prednisone
MOPV	monovalent oral poliovirus vaccine
MOR	morphine (This is a dangerous abbreviation)
MOS	Medical Outcome Study
	mirror optical system
	months
MOSES	Multidimensional Observational Scale for Elderly Subjects
MOSF	multiple-organ system failure
MOS sf-20	Medical Outcomes Study, short form 20 items
MOS sf-36	Medical Outcomes Study, short form, 36 items
mOsm	milliosmole
mOsmol	milliosmole

MOT	motility examination	MPB	male-pattern baldness
MOTA	Method Other Than Acceleration		mephobarbital
		MPBFV	mean pulmonary-blood-flow velocity
MOTS	mucosal oral therapeutic system	MPBNS	modified Peyronie bladder neck suspension
MOTT	mycobacteria other than tubercle	MPC	meperidine, promethazine, and chlorpromazine
MOU	medical oncology unit		mucopurulent cervicitis
	memorandum of understanding	MPCC	Medical Policy Coordinating Committee
MOUS	multiple occurrences of unexplained symptoms	MPCN	microscopically positive and culturally negative
MOV	minimum obstructive volume	M-PCR	multiplex polymerase chain reaction
	multiple oral vitamin	MPCU	medical progressive care unit
MOW	Meals on Wheels	MPD	maximum permissable dose
MP	malignant pyoderma		
	melphalan and prednisone		methylphenidate (Ritalin)
	menstrual period		moisture permeable dressing
	mercaptopurine (Purinethol)		multiple personality disorder
	metacarpal phalangeal joint		myeloproliferative disorder
	mitoxantrone and prednisone		myofascial pain dysfunction (syndrome)
	moist park	mPD	minimal peripheral dose
	monitor pattern		
	monophasic	MPE	malignant pleural effusion
	motor potential		massive pulmonary embolism
	mouthpiece		mean prediction error
	myocardial perfusion		multiphoton excitation
M & P	Millipore and phase	MPEC	multipolar electrocoagulation
4 MP	methylpyrazole (fomepizole; Antizol)	MPEG	methoxypolyethylene glycol
6-MP	mercaptopurine (Purenthol)	MPF	methylparaben free
MPA	main pulmonary artery	m-PFL	methotrexate, cisplatin (Platinol), fluorouracil, and leucovorin
	Medical Products Agency (Sweden)	MPGN	membranoproliferative glomerulonephritis
	medroxyprogesterone acetate	MPH	massive pulmonary hemorrhage
MPa	megapascal		Master of Public Health
MPAC	Memorial Pain Assessment Card		methylphenidate (Ritalin)
MPA/E$_2$C	medroxyprogesterone acetate; estradiol cypionate (Lunelle)		miles per hour
MPAP	mean pulmonary artery pressure	MPHD	multiple pituitary hormone deficiencies
MPAQ	McGill Pain Assessment Questionnaire	MPI	master patient index
MPAS	Masters of Physician Assistant Studies		

	Maudsley Personality Inventory	MPTRD	motor, pain, touch, and reflex deficit
	milk-product intolerance	MPU	maternal pediatric unit
	myocardial perfusion imaging	MPV	mean platelet volume
MPIF-1	myeloid progenitor inhibitory factor-1	MQ	mefloquine (Lariam) memory quotient
MPJ	metacarpophalangeal joint	MQOL	McGill Quality of Life Questionnaire
MPK	milligram per kilogram	MR	Maddox rod
MPL	maximum permissable level		magnetic resonance manifest refraction
	mesiopulpolingual		may repeat
MPL®	monophosphoryl lipid A		measles-rubella
MPLC	medium pressure liquid chromatography		medial rectus medical record
MPM	malignant peritoneal mesothelioma		mental retardation milliroentgen
	malignant pleural mesothelioma		mitral regurgitation moderate resistance
	Mortality Prediction Model	M&R	measure and record
MPN	monthly progress note	MR × 1	may repeat times one (once)
	most probable number		
	multiple primary neoplasms	MRA	magnetic resonance angiography
MPO	male-pattern obesity		main renal artery
	myeloperoxidase		medical record administrator
MPOA	medial preoptic area		
MPP	massive periretinal proliferation		medical research associate midright atrium
	maximum pressure picture		multivariate regression analysis
MPP	multiple presentation phenotype	mrad	millirad
MPQ	McGill Pain Questionnaire	MRAN	medical resident admitting note
MPPT	methylprednisolone pulse therapy	MRAP	mean right atrial pressure
MPR	massive periretinal retraction	MRAS	main renal artery stenosis
	multiplanar reconstruction	MRC	Master of Rehabilitation Counseling
MPS	Maternal Perinatal Scale	MRCA	magnetic resonance coronary angiography
	mean particle size		
	mononuclear phagocyte system	MRCC	metastatic renal cell carcinoma
	mucopolysaccharidosis	MRCP	magnetic resonance cholangiopancreatography
	multiphasic screening		
MPS-1	mucopolysaccharidosis I		Member of the Royal College of Physicians
MPS-II	mucopolysaccharidosis II (Hunter syndrome)		mental retardation, cerebral palsy
MPSS	massively parallel signature sequencing	MRCPs	movement-related cortical potentials
	methylprednisolone sodium succinate	MRCS	Member of the Royal College of Surgeons
MPT	multiple parameter telemetry	MRD	margin reflex distance

	Medical Records Department	MROU	medial rectus, both eyes
	Minimal Record of Disability	MRP	multidrug resistance-associated protein
	minimal residual disease	MP-RAGE	magnetization prepared rapid acquisition gradient-echo
MRDD	maximum recommended daily dose		
	Mental Retardation and Development Disabilities	MRPN	medical resident progress note
	mentally retarded and developmentally disabled	MRPs	medication-related problems
		MRR	medical record review
MRDM	malnutrition-related diabetes mellitus	MRS	magnetic resonance spectroscopy
MRDSA	magnetic resonance digital subtraction angiography		mental retardation syndrome
			methicillin-resistant *Staphylococcus aureus*
MRE	manual resistance exercise	MRSA	methicillin-resistant *Staphylococcus aureus*
	most recent episode		
MRFC	mouse rosette-forming cells	MRSE	methicillin-resistant *Staphylococcus epidermidis*
MR FIT	Multiple Risk Factor Intervention Trial		
		MRSI	magnetic resonance spectroscopic imaging
MRG	mortality reference group		
	murmurs, rubs, and gallops	MRSS	methicillin-resistant *Staphylococcus* species
MRH	Maddox rod hyperphoria		modified Rodnan skin-thickness score
MRHD	maximum recommended human dose		
		MRT	magnetic resonance tomography
MRHT	modified rhyme hearing test		malignant rhabdoid tumor
MRI	magnetic resonance imaging		mean response time
			modified rhyme test
M & R I & O	measure and record input and output	MRTA	magnetic resonance tomographic angiography
MRK	Merck & Co., Inc.		
MRL	minimal response level	MRU	medical resource utilization
	moderate rubra lochia		
MRLVD	maximum residue limits of veterinary drugs	MRV(r)	mixed respiratory vaccine
		MRX	*Moraxella catarrhalis* vaccine
MRLT	mesalamine-related lung toxicity		
		MR × 1	may repeat once
MRM	modified radical mastectomy	MS	mass spectroscopy
			Master of Science
MRN	magnetic resonance neurography		median sternotomy
	malignant renal neoplasm		medical student
	medical record number		mental status
	medical resident's note		milk shake
mRNA	messenger ribonucleic acid		minimal support
			mitral sounds
MRO	multidrug resistant organism(s)		mitral stenosis
			moderately susceptible
			morning stiffness

morphine sulfate (This is a dangerous abbreviation)
motile sperm
multiple sclerosis
muscle spasm
muscle strength
musculoskeletal

M & S microculture and sensitivity

3MS Modified Mini-Mental Status (examination)

MS III third-year medical student

MSA Medical Savings Accounts
membrane-stabilizing activity
methane sulfonic acid
metropolitan statistical area
microsomal autoantibodies
multiple system atrophy

MSAF meconium-stained amniotic fluid

MSAFP maternal serum alpha-fetoprotein

MSAP mean systemic arterial pressure

MSAS Mandel Social Adjustment Scale

MSAS-SF Memorial Symptom Assessment Scale–short form

MSB mainstem bronchus

MSBOS maximum surgical blood order schedule

MSBP Munchausen syndrome by proxy

MSC major symptom complex
Medical Service Corps
mesenchymal stromal cells
midsystolic click
MS Contin®

MSCA McCarthy Scales of Children's Abilities

MSCC malignant spinal cord compression
midstream clean-catch (urine culture)

MSCCC Master Sciences, Certified Clinical Competence

MSCR-AMMS microbial surface component reacting with adhesive matrix molecules

MSCs mesenchymal stem cells

MSCT multislice computed tomography

MSCU medical special care unit

MSCWP musculoskeletal chest wall pain

MSD male sexual dysfunction
microsurgical diskectomy
midsleep disturbance
musculoskeletal disorder

MSDBP mean sitting diastolic blood pressure

MSDS material safety data sheet

MSE Mental Status Examination

msec milliseconds

MSEL myasthenic syndrome of Eaton-Lambert

MSER mean systolic ejection rate
Mental Status Examination Record

MSF meconium-stained fluid
Médicins Sans Frontières (Doctors Without Borders)
Mediterranean spotted fever
megakaryocyte stimulating factor

MSG massage
methysergide (Sansert)
monosodium glutamate

MSH melanocyte-stimulating hormone

MSHA mannose-sensitive hemagglutinin

MSI magnetic source imaging
mass sociogenic illness
microsatellite instability
multiple subcortical infarction
musculoskeletal impairment

MSIA mass spectrometric immunoassay

MSIR® morphine sulfate immediate release tablets

MSIS	Multiple Severity of Illness System	MSSP	Maternal Support Services Program
MSK	medullary sponge kidney musculoskeletal	MSSU	midstream specimen of urine
MSKCC	Memorial Sloan-Kettering Cancer Center	MST	maladies sexuellement transmissibles (French for sexually transmitted diseases)
MSL	midsternal line multiple symmetrical lipomatosis		mean survival time
MSLT	multiple sleep latency test		median survival time
MSM	magnetic starch microspheres		mental stress test multiple subpial transection
	men who have sex with men	MSTA®	mumps skin test antigen
	methsuximide (Celontin)	MSTI	multiple soft tissue injuries
	methylsulfonylmethane		
	midsystolic murmur	MSTS	American Musculoskeletal Tumor Society (functional rating system)
MSN	Master of Science in Nursing		
MSNA	muscle sympathetic nerve activity	MSU	maple-syrup urine midstream urine
MSO	managed services organization		monosodium urate
		MSUD	maple-syrup urine disease
	mentally stable and oriented	MSUS	musculoskeletal ultrasound
	mental status, oriented most significant other	MSUs	midstream specimens of urine
MSO₄	morphine sulfate (this is a dangerous abbreviation)	mSv	millisievert (radiation unit)
		MSW	Master of Social Work
MSOD	multisystem organ dysfunction		multiple stab wounds
MSOF	multisystem organ failure	MT	empty
MS-PCR	methylation-specific polymerase chain reaction		macular target maggot therapy
			maintenance therapy
MSPN	medical student progress notes		malaria therapy malignant teratoma
MSPU	medical short procedure unit		Medical Technologist metatarsal
MSQ	Mental Status Questionnaire		middle turbinate
	meters squared		monitor technician mucosal thickening
MSR	muscle stretch reflexes		muscles and tendons
MSRPP	Multidimensional Scale for Rating Psychiatric Patients		muscle tone
			music therapy (Therapist)
			myringotomy tube(s)
MSS	Marital Satisfaction Scale	M/T	masses of tenderness
	mean sac size		myringotomy with tubes
	microsatellite stable	M & T	Monilia and Trichomonas
	minor surgery suite		muscles and tendons
MSSA	methicillin-susceptible Staphylococcus aureus		myringotomy and tubes
		MTA	Medical Technical Assistant
MSS-CR	mean sac size and crown-rump length		metatarsal adduction

M

multi-targeted antifolate (pemetrexed disodium [Alimta])

MTAD tympanic membrane of the right ear

MT/AK music therapy/audiokinetics

MTAS tympanic membrane of the left ear

MTAU tympanic membranes of both ears

MTB *Mycobacterium tuberculosis*

MTBC Music Therapist-Board Certified

MTBE methyl tert-butyl ether

MTC magnetization transfer contrast (radiology)
medullary thyroid carcinoma
metoclopramide
mitomycin (Mutamycin)

MTCSA mid-thigh muscle cross-sectional area

MTCT mother-to-child transmission

MTD maximum tolerated dose
metastatic trophoblastic disease
Monroe tidal drainage
Mycobacterium tuberculosis direct (test)

MTDDA Minnesota Test for Differential Diagnosis of Aphasia

MTDI maximum tolerable daily intake

MTDT *Mycobacterium tuberculosis* direct test

MTE multiple trace elements

MTE-4® trace metal elements injection (there is also a #5, #6, and #7)

MTET modified treadmill exercise testing

MTF medical treatment facility

MTG middle temporal gyrus (gyri)
midthigh girth

MTHFR methylene tetrahydrofolate reductase

MTI magnetization transfer imaging

malignant teratoma intermediate

MTJ midtarsal joint

MTL medial temporal lobe
Metropolitan Life (Insurance Company)
Table (for desirable weight)

MTLE medial (mesial) temporal-lobe epilepsy

MTM modified Thayer-Martin medium
mouth-to-mouth (resuscitation)

MTNX methylnaltrexone

mTOR mammalian target of rapamycin

MTP master treatment plan
medical termination of pregnancy
metatarsophalangeal
microsomal triglyceride transfer protein

MTPJ metatarsophalangeal joint

MTR mother

MTR-O no masses, tenderness, or rebound

MTRS Licensed Master Therapeutic Recreation Specialist

MTS mesial temporal sclerosis

MTST maximal treadmill stress test

MTT mamillothalamic tract
mean transit time
methylthiotetrazole

MTU malignant teratoma undifferentiated
methylthiouracil

MTX methotrexate

MTZ mirtazapine (Remeron)
mitoxantrone (Novantrone)

MU million units
Murphy unit

mU milliunits

MUA manipulation under anesthesia

MUAC middle upper arm circumference

MUAP motor unit action potential

MUD matched-unrelated donor

MUDDLES miosis, urination, diarrhea, diaphoresis, lacrimation, excitation of central nervous system, and salivation (effects of cholinesterase inhibitors)

MUDPILES methanol, metformin; uremia; diabetic ketoacidosis; phenformin, paraldehyde; iron, isoniazid, ibuprofen; lactic acidosis; ethanol, ethylene glycol; and salicylates, sepsis (causes of metabolic acidosis)

MUE medication use evaluation

MUFA monounsaturated fatty acid

MUGA multigated (radionuclide) angiogram
multiple gated acquisition (scan)

MUGX multiple gated acquisition exercise

MULE microcomputer upper limb exerciser

MuLV murine leukemia virus

MUM mumps virus vaccine

MUNE motor unit estimates

MUNSH Memorial University of Newfoundland Scale of Happiness

MUO metastasis of unknown origin

MUPAT multiple-site perineal applicator technique

MUSE® Medicated Urethral System for Erection (alprostadil urethral suppository)

mus-lig musculoligamentous

MUU mouse uterine units

MV manual ventilation
mechanical ventilation
millivolts
minute volume
mitoxantrone and etoposide (VePesid)
mitral valve
mixed venous
multivesicular

MVA malignant vertricular arrhythmias
manual vacuum aspiration
mitral valve area
motor vehicle accident

M-VAC methotrexate, vinblastine doxorubicin (Adriamycin), and cisplatin

MVB methotrexate and vinblastine
mixed venous blood

MVC maximal voluntary contraction
motor vehicle collision (crash)

MVc mitral valve closure

MVD microvascular decompression
microvessel density
mitral valve disease
multivessel disease

MVE mitral valve (leaflet) excursion
Murray Valley encephalitis

MV Grad mitral valve gradient

MVI malignant vascular injury
multiple vitamin injection

MVI® brand name for parenteral multivitamins

MVI 12® brand name for parenteral multivitamins

MVIC maximum voluntary isometric contractions

MVID microvillus inclusion disease

MVO mixed venous oxygen saturation

MVO$_2$ myocardial oxygen consumption

MVP mean venous pressure
mitomycin, vinblastine, and cisplatin (Platinol AQ)
mitral valve prolapse

MVPA moderate-to-vigorous physical activity

MVPP	mechlorethamine, vinblastine, procarbazine, and prednisone		movement myringotomy
		My	myopia
MVPS	mitral valve prolapse syndrome	MYD	mydriatic
		myelo	myelocytes myelogram
MVR	massive vitreous retraction	MyG	myasthenia gravis
	micro-vitreoretinal (blade)	MYOP	myopia
	mitral valve regurgitation	MYR	myringotomy
	mitral valve replacement	MYS	medium yellow soft (stools)
MVRI	mixed vaccine respiratory infections	MZ	monozygotic
		M/Z	mass/charge
MVS	mitral valve stenosis	MZL	marginal zone lymphocyte
	motor, vascular, and sensory	MZT	monozygotic twins
MVT	movement multiform ventricular tachycardia multivitamin		
MVU	Montevideo units		
MVV	maximum ventilatory volume maximum voluntary ventilation mixed vespid venom		
6-MW	6-minute walk (test)		
12-MW	12-minute walk (test)		
MWB	minimal weight bearing		
MWC	major wound complications		
MWCO	molecular weight cutoff		
MWD	maximum walking distance microwave diathermy		
6-MWD	6-minute walking distance		
M-W-F	Monday-Wednesday-Friday		
MWI	Medical Walk-In (Clinic)		
MWOA	migraine without aura		
MWS	Mickety-Wilson syndrome		
MWT	maintenance of wakefulness test Mallory-Weiss tear malpositioned wisdom teeth maximal walking time		
6-MWT	6-minute walk test		
MWTP	municipal wastewater treatment plants		
Mx	manifest refraction mastectomy maxilla		

N

			Nurse Anesthetist
			nursing assistant
	Na		sodium
	Na$^+$		sodium
	N & A		normal and active
N	nausea	NAA	*N*-acetylaspartate
	negative		National Average
	Negro		Allowance (federal
	Neisseria		physician office visit
	nerve		cost guide)
	neutrophil		neutron activation analysis
	never		no apparent abnormalities
	newton		nucleic acid amplification
	night	NAAC	no apparent anesthesia
	nipple		complications
	nitrogen	NAA/Cr	N-acetylaspartate/creatine
	no		ratio
	nodes	NAAT	nucleic acid amplification
	nonalcoholic		techniques (testing)
	none	NAATPT	not available at the
	normal		present time
	North (as in the location	NAB	not at bedside
	2N, would be second	NABS	normoactive bowel sounds
	floor, North wing)	NAbs	neutralizing antibodies
	not	NABT	normal-appearing brain
	notified		tissue
	noun	NABTC	North American Brain
	NPH insulin		Tumor Consortium
	size of sample	NABX	needle aspiration biopsy
N1	study night 1	NAC	acetylcysteine (N-
N I....	first through twelfth		acetylcysteine;
N XII	cranial nerves		Mucomyst)
O.1 N	tenth-normal		neoadjuvant chemotherapy
N$_2$	nitrogen		nipple-areola complex
N 2.5	phenylephrine HCl 2.5%		no acute changes
	ophthalmic solution		no anesthesia
	(Neo-Synephrine)		complications
n-3	omega-3	NACD	no anatomical cause of
5′-N	5′-nucleotidase		death
N-9	nonoxynol 9	NaClO	sodium hypochlorite
NA	Narcotics Anonymous	NaCl	sodium chloride (salt)
	Native American	NaCMC	sodium carboxymethyl
	Negro adult		cellulose
	new admission	NACS	Neurologic and Adaptive
	nicotinic acid		Capacity Score
	nonalcoholic	NACT	neoadjuvant chemotherapy
	norethindrone acetate	NAD	nicotinamide adenine
	normal axis		dinucleotide
	not admitted		no active disease
	not applicable		no acute distress
	not available		no apparent distress
	nurse aide		no appreciable disease
	nurse's aid		normal axis deviation

nothing abnormal detected

NADA — New Animal Drug Application

NADase — nicotinamide adenine dinucleotide glycohydrolase

NADE — New Animal Drug Evaluation

NADPH — nicotinamide adenine dinucleotide phosphate

NADSIC — no apparent disease seen in chest

NaE — exchangeable sodium

NAF — nafcillin
Native-American female
Negro adult female
normal adult female
Notice of Adverse Findings (FDA post-audit letter)

NaF — sodium fluoride

NAFLD — nonalcoholic fatty liver disease

NAG — narrow angle glaucoma

NaHCO$_3$ — sodium bicarbonate

NAHI — nonaccidental head injury

NAI — no action indicated
no acute inflammation
nonaccidental injury
Nuremberg Aging Inventory

NaI — sodium iodide

NAION — nonarteritic ischemic optic neuropathy

NAIT — neonatal alloimmune thrombocytopenia

NAL — nasal angiocentric lymphoma

NAM — nail-apparatus melanoma
Native-American male
no abnormal masses
normal adult male

nAMD — neovascular age-related macular degeneration

NANB — non-A, non-B (hepatitis) (hepatitis C)

NANBH — non-A, non-B hepatitis (hepatitis C)

NANC — nonadrenergic, noncholinergic

NANDA — North American Nursing Diagnosis Association (taxonomy)

NaNP — sodium nitroprusside (Nipride)

NANSAIDs — nonaspirin, nonsteroidal anti-inflammatory drugs

NaOCl — sodium hypochlorite

NaOH — sodium hydroxide

NAP — narrative, assessment, and plan
nosocomial acquired pneumonia

NAPA — N-acetyl procainamide

NAPD — no active pulmonary disease

Na Pent — Pentothal Sodium

NAR — nasal airflow resistance
no action required
no adverse reaction
nonambulatory restraint
not at risk

NARC — narcotic(s)

NaRI — noradrenaline reuptake inhibitor

NART — National Adult Reading Test (United Kingdom)

NAS — nasal
neonatal abstinence syndrome
no abnormality seen
no added salt

NASBA — nucleic-acid sequencing based amplification

NaSCN — sodium thiocyanate

NASH — nonalcoholic steatohepatitis

NAS-NRC — National Academy of Sciences – National Research Council

NaSSA — noradrenergic and specific serotonergic antidepresssant

NASTT — nonspecific abnormality of ST segment and T wave

NAT — N-acetyltransferase
no action taken
no acute trauma
nonaccidental trauma
nonspecific abnormality of T wave
nucleic acid test (testing)

Na^{99m}TcO$_4{}^-$ — sodium pertechnetate Tc 99m

NAUC	normalized area under the curve	NBTE	nonbacterial thrombotic endocarditis
NAUTI	nosocomially-associated urinary tract infections	NBTNF	newborn, term, normal female
NAW	nasal antral window	NBTNM	newborn, term, normal, male
NAWM	normal-appearing white matter	NBW	normal birth weight (2,500–3,999 g)
NB	nail bed	NC	nasal cannula
	needle biopsy		Negro child
	neuroblastomas		neurologic check
	newborn		no change
	nitrogen balance		no charge
	note well		no complaints
NBC	newborn center		noncontributory
	nonbed care		normocephalic
	nuclear, biological, and chemical		nose clamp
			nose clips
NBCCS	nevoid basal-cell carcinoma syndrome		not classified
			not completed
NBD	neurologic bladder dysfunction		not cultured
		9 NC	rubitecan (9-nitrocamptothecin; Orathecin)
	no brain damage		
NBF	not breast fed		
NBH	new bag (bottle) hung	NCA	neurocirculatory asthenia
NBHH	newborn helpful hints		
NBI	no bone injury		no congenital abnormalities
NBICU	newborn intensive care unit		
		N/CAN	nasal cannula
nBiPAP	nasal bilevel (biphasic) positive airway pressure	NCAP	nasal continuous airway pressure
NBIs	nosocomial bloodstream infections	NCAS	zinostatin (neocarzinostatin)
NBL/OM	neuroblastoma and opsoclonus-myoclonus	NC/AT	normocephalic atraumatic
NBM	no bowel movement	NCB	natural childbirth
	normal bone marrow		no code blue
	normal bowel movement	NCBI	National Center for Biotechnology Information (NIH)
	nothing by mouth		
NBN	newborn nursery		
NBP	needle biopsy of prostate	NCC	neurocysticercosis
	no bone pathology		no concentrated carbohydrates
NBQC	narrow base quad cane		
NBR	no blood return		nursing care card
NBS	newborn screen (serum thyroxine and phenylketonuria)	NCCAM	National Center for Complementary and Alternative Medicine (NIH)
	Nijmegen breakage syndrome	NCCDPHP	National Center for Chronic Disease and Prevention and Health Promotion (CDC)
	no bacteria seen		
	normal bowel sounds		
NBT	nitroblue tetrazolium reduction (tests)	NCCI	National Correct Coding Initiative
	normal breast tissue		

NCCLS	National Committee for Clinical Laboratory Standards	NCJ	needle catheter jejunostomy
NCCN	National Comprehensive Cancer Network	NCL	neuronal ceroid lipofuscinosis
NCCP	noncardiac chest pain		no cautionary labels
NCCTG	North Central Cancer Treatment Group		nuclear cardiology laboratory
NCCU	neurosurgical continuous care unit	NCLD	neonatal chronic lung disease
NCD	neck-capsule distance	NCM	nailfold capillary microscope
	no congenital deformities		nonclinical manager
	normal childhood diseases	NCNC	normochromic,
	not considered disabling		normocytic
	not considered disqualifying	NCNR	National Center for Nursing
	Nursing-Care Dependency (scale)		Research (NIH)
NCDB	National Cancer Data Base	NCO	no complaints offered noncommissioned officer
NCE	new chemical entity	NCOG	North California Oncology Group
NCEH	National Center for Environmental Health (CDC)	NCP	no caffeine or pepper nursing care plan
NCEP	National Cholesterol Education Program	NCPAP	nasal continuous positive airway pressure
NCF	neutrophilic chemotactic factor	NCPB	neurolytic celiac plexus block
	no cold fluids	NcpPCu	nonceruloplasmin plasma copper
NCHGR	National Center for Human Genome Research (NIH)	NCPR	no cardiopulmonary resuscitation
NCHS	National Center for Health Statistics	NCQA	National Commission for Quality Assurance
NCI	National Cancer Institute	nCR	nodular complete response
NCIC	National Cancer Institute of Canada	NCRA	National Cancer Registrars Association
NCI-CTC	National Cancer Institute Common Toxicity Criteria	NCRC	nonchild-resistant container
NCIC-CTG	National Cancer Institute of Canada Clinical Trials Group	NCRR	National Center for Research Resources (NIH)
NCID	National Center for Infectious Diseases (CDC)	NCS	nerve conduction studies no concentrated sweets noncontact supervision not clinically significant zinostatin (neocarzinostatin)
NCIPC	National Center for Injury Prevention and Control (CDC)	NCSE	nonconvulsive status epilepticus
NCIS	nursing care information sheet	NCT	neoadjuvant chemotherapy neutron capture therapy
NCIT	Nursing Care Intervention Tool		noncontact tonometry

	Nursing Care Technician	NDIRS	nondispersive infrared
NCTR	National Center for		spectrometer
	Toxicological Research	NDM	neonatal diabetes mellitus
NCV	nerve conduction velocity	NDMS	National Disaster Medical
	nuclear venogram		System
NCVHS	National Committee on	Nd/NT	nondistended, nontender
	Vital and Health	NDO	neurogenic detrusor
	Statistics		overactivity
NCX	sodium-calcium exchanger	NDP	nedaplatin
ND	Doctor of Naturopathy		net dietary protein
	(Naturopathic		Nurse Discharge Planner
	Physician)	NDR	neurotic depressive
	nasal deformity		reaction
	nasal discharge		normal detrusor reflex
	nasoduodenal	NDRI	norepinephrine and
	natural death		dopamine reuptake
	neck dissection		inhibitor
	neonatal death	NDS	Neurologic Disability
	neurological development		Score
	neurotic depression		neuropathy disability score
	Newcastle disease		New Drug Submission
	no data	NDSO	nasolacrimal drainage
	no disease		system obstruction
	nondisabling	NDST	neurodevelopmental
	nondistended		screening test
	none detectable	NDT	nasal duodenostomy tube
	normal delivery		Neurocognitive Driving
	normal development		Test
	nose drops		neurodevelopmental
	not detected		techniques
	not diagnosed		neurodevelopmental
	not done		treatment
	nothing done		noise detection threshold
	Nursing Doctorate	NDV	Newcastle disease virus
N&D	nodular and diffuse	Nd:YAG	neodymium:yttrium-
Nd	neodymium		aluminum-garnet (laser)
NDA	New Drug Application	Nd:YLF	neodymium: yttrium-
	no data available		lithium-fluoride (laser)
	no demonstrable	NE	nasoenteric
	antibodies		nausea and emesis
	no detectable activity		nephropathica epidemica
NDC	National Drug Code		neurological examination
NDD	no dialysis days		never exposed
NDE	near-death experience		no effect
NDEA	no deviation of electrical		no enlargement
	axis		norethindrone
NDF	neutral density filter (test)		norepinephrine
	no disease found		not elevated
NDGA	nordihydroguaiaretic acid		not examined
NDI	National Death Index	NEAA	nonessential amino acids
	nephrogenic diabetes	NEAC	norethindrone acetate
	insipidus	NEAD	nonepileptic attack
NDIR	nondispersive infrared		disorder

NEAT	nonexercise activity thermogenesis
NEB	hand-held nebulizer
NEC	necrotizing entercolitis
	noise equivalent counts
	nonesterified cholesterol
	not elsewhere classified
NECT	nonenhanced computed tomography (scan)
NED	no evidence of disease
NEDSS	National Electronic Disease Surveillance System
NEE	neonatal epileptic encephalopathy
NEEG	normal electroencephalogram
NEEP	negative end-expiratory pressure
NEF	negative expiratory force
NEFA	nonesterified fatty acid(s)
NEFG	normal external female genitalia
NEFT	nasoenteric feeding tube
NEG	negative
	neglect
NEI	National Eye Institute (NIH)
NEJM	*New England Journal of Medicine*
NEM	neurotrophic enhancing molecule
	no evidence of malignancy
NEMD	nonexudative macular degeneration
	nonspecific esophageal motility disorder
NENT	nasal endotracheal tube
NEO	necrotizing external otitis
NEOH	neonatal high risk
NEOM	neonatal medium risk
NEP	needle-exchange program
	neutral endopeptidase
	no evidence of pathology
NEPD	no evidence of pulmonary disease
NEPHRO	nephrogram
NEPPK	nonepidermolytic palmoplantar keratoderma
NER	no evidence of recurrence
NERD	no evidence of recurrent disease

	nonerosive reflux disease
NES	nonepileptic seizure
	nonstandard electrolyte solution
	not elsewhere specified
NESP	novel erythropoiesis stimulating protein (darbepoetin [Aranesp])
NET	choroidal or subretinal neovascularization
	Internet
	naso-endotracheal tube
	neuroectodermal tumor
NETA	norethindrone acetate (Aygestin)
NETSS	National Electronic Telecommunications System for Surveillance
NETT	nasal endotracheal tube
NEVA	nocturnal electrobioimpedance volumetric assessment (penile measurement)
NEX	nose-to-ear-to-xiphoid
	number of excitations (radiology)
NETZ	needle (diathermy) excision of the transformation zone
NF	necrotizing fasciitis
	Negro female
	neurofibromatosis
	night frequency (of voiding)
	none found
	not found
	nursed fair
	nursing facility
Nf	*Naegleria fowleri*
NF1	neurofibromatosis type 1
NF2	neurofibromatosis type 2
NFA	Nerve Fiber Analyzer®
NFALO	Nerve Fiber Analyzer laser oththalmoscope
NFAP	nursing facility-acquired pneumonia
NFAR	no further action required
NFCS	Neonatal Facial Coding System
NFD	no family doctor
NFFD	not fit for duty
NFI	nerve-function impairment
	no-fault insurance

	no further information	NHBD	nonheart-beating donor
	normal female infant	NHC	neighborhood health center
NFL	nerve fiber layer		neonatal hypocalcemia
	Novantrone (mitoxantrone), fluorouracil, and leucovorin		nursing home care
		NH_3	ammonia
		NH_4Cl	ammonium chloride
NFLX	norfloxacin (Noroxin)	NHCU	nursing home care unit
NFP	natural family planning	NHD	nocturnal hemodialysis
	no family physician		normal hair distribution
	not for publication	NHE	sodium/hydrogen exchanger
NFT	no further treatment		
NFTD	normal full-term delivery	NHEJ	nonhomologous end-joining
NFTE	not found this examination	NHGRI	National Human Genome Research Institute (NIH)
NFTs	neurofibrillary tangles		
NFTSD	normal full-term spontaneous delivery	NHL	nodular histiocytic lymphoma
NFTT	nonorganic failure to thrive		non-Hodgkin lymphomas
		nHL	normalized hearing level
NFV	nelfinavir (Viracept)	NHLBI	National Heart, Lung, and Blood Institute (NIH)
NFW	nursed fairly well		
NG	nanogram (ng) (10^{-9} gram)		
		NHLPP	hereditary neuropathy with liability for pressure palsy
	nasogastric		
	night guard		
	nitroglycerin	NHM	no heroic measures
	no growth	NHO	notify house officer
	norgestrel	NHP	Nottingham Health Profile
ng	nanogram		nursing home placement
NGB	neurogenic bladder	NHPs	natural health products
NGF	nerve growth factor	NHPT	nine-hole peg test
n giv	not given	NHS	National Health Service (UK)
NGJ	nasogastro-jejunostomy		
NGM	norgestimate	NHT	neoadjuvant hormonal therapy
NGO	nongovernmental organization		
			nursing home transfer
NGOs	nongovernmental organizations	NHTR	nonhemolytic transfusion reaction
NGR	nasogastric replacement	NHW	nonhealing wound
NGRI	not guilty by reason of insanity	NI	neurological improvement
			no improvement
NGSF	nothing grown so far		no information
NGT	nasogastric tube		none indicated
	normal glucose tolerance		not identified
NgTD	negative to date		not isolated
NGU	nongonococcal urethritis	NIA	National Institute on Aging (NIH)
NH	normal-hearing		
	nursing home		no information available
NHA	no histologic abnormalities	NIAAA	National Institute on Alcohol Abuse and Alcoholism (NIH)
NHB	nonheart-beating (donor)		

NIADDK	National Institute of Arthritis, Diabetes, and Digestive and Kidney Diseases (NIH)	NIDCD	National Institute of Deafness and other Communication Disorders (NIH)
NIAID	National Institute of Allergy and Infectious Diseases (NIH)	NIDCR	National Institute of Dental and Craniofacial Research (NIH)
NIAL	not in active labor	NIDD	noninsulin-dependent diabetes
NIAMS	National Institute of Arthritis and Musculoskeletal and Skin Diseases (NIH)	NIDDK	National Institute of Diabetes and Digestive and Kidney Diseases (NIH)
NIA-RI	National Institute on Aging–Reagan Institute	NIDDM	noninsulin-dependent diabetes mellitus
NIBP	noninvasive blood pressure	NIDR	National Institute of Dental Research (NIH)
NIBPM	noninvasive blood pressure measurement	NIEHS	National Institute of Environmental Health Sciences (NIH)
NIC	Nursing Intervention Classification	NIF	negative inspiratory force neutrophil inhibitory factor not in file
NICC	neonatal intensive care center noninfectious chronic cystitis	NIFS	noninvasive flow studies
NICE	National Institute for Clinical Excellence (United Kingdom) new, interesting, and challenging experiences	NIG	NSAIA (nonsteroidal anti-inflamatory agent) induced gastropathy
		NIGMS	National Institute of General Medical Sciences (NIH)
NICHD	National Institute of Child Health and Human Development (NIH)	NIH	National Institutes of Health
NICO	neuralgia-inducing cavitational osteonecrosis	NIHD	noise-induced hearing damage
	noninvasive cardiac output (monitor)	NIHL	noise-induced hearing loss
NICS	noninvasive carotid studies	NIHSS	National Institutes of Health Stroke Scale
NICU	neonatal intensive care unit neurosurgical intensive care unit	NIID	neuronal intranuclear inclusion disease
		NIL	not in labor
NID	no identifiable disease not in distress	NIMAs	noninherited maternal antigens
NIDA	National Institute of Drug Abuse (NIH)	NIMH	National Institute of Mental Health (NIH)
NIDA five	National Institute on Drug Abuse screen for cannabinoids, cocaine metabolite, amphetamine/metham-phetamine, opiates, and phencyclidine	NIMHDIS	National Institute for Mental Health Diagnostic Interview Schedule (NIH)
		NIMR	National Institute of Medical Research (United Kingdom)

NINDS	National Institute of Neurological Disorders and Stroke (NIH)	NJ	nasojejunal
		NK	natural killer (cells)
			not known
NINR	National Institute for Nursing Research (NIH)	NK_1	neurokinin 1
		NKA	no known allergies
NINU	neuro intermediate nursing unit	nkat	nanokatal (nanomole/sec)
		NKB	no known basis
NINVS	noninvasive neurovascular studies		not keeping baby
			neurokinin B
NIOPCs	no intraoperative complications	NKC	nonketotic coma
		NKD	no known diseases
NIOSH	National Institute of Occupational Safety and Health (NIH)	NKDA	no known drug allergies
		NKFA	no known food allergies
		NKH	nonketotic hyperglycemia
NIP	catnip	NKHA	nonketotic hyperosmolar acidosis
	National Immunization Program	NKHHC	nonketotic hyperglycemic-hyperosmolar coma
	no infection present		
	no inflammation present	NKHOC	nonketotic hyperosmolar coma
NIPAs	noninherited paternal antigens	NKHS	nonketotic hyperosmolar syndrome
NIPD	nocturnal intermittent peritoneal dialysis	NKMA	no known medication (medical) allergies
NIPPV	noninvasive positive-pressure ventilation	NL	nasolacrimal
			nonlatex
NIPS	Neonatal Infant Pain Scale		normal
NIP/S	noninvasive programming stimulation		normal libido
		NLB	needle liver biopsy
NIPSV	noninvasive pressure support ventilation	NLC	nocturnal leg cramps
		NLC & C	normal libido, coitus, and climax
NIR	near infrared	NLD	nasolacrimal duct
	nitroprusside-induced relaxation		necrobiosis lipoidica diabeticorum
NIRCA	nonisotopic RNase cleavage assay		no local doctor
NISH	nonradioactive *in situ* hybridization	NLDO	nasolacrimal duct obstruction
NISS	New Injury Severity Score	NLE	neonatal lupus erythematosus
NISs	no-impact sports		nursing late entry
NIST	National Institute of Standards and Technology	NLEA	Nutrition Labeling and Education Act of 1990
NISV	nonionic surfactant vesicle	NLF	nasolabial fold
NITD	neuroleptic-induced tardive dyskinesia		nelfinavir (Viracept)
Nitro	nitroglycerin (this is a dangerous abbreviation)	NLFGNR	nonlactose fermenting gram-negative rod
	sodium nitroprusside (this is a dangerous abbreviation)	NLM	National Library of Medicine
			no limitation of motion
NIV	noninvasive ventilation		
NIVLS	noninvasive vascular laboratory studies	NLMC	nocturnal leg muscle cramp

NLN	National League for Nursing		no more information
			normal male infant
	no longer needed	NMJ	neuromuscular junction
NLO	nasolacrimal occlusion	NML	normal
NLP	natural language processing	NMKB	not married, keeping baby
		NMM	nodular malignant melanoma
	nodular liquifying panniculitis		
		NMN	no middle name
	no light perception	NMNKB	not married, not keeping baby
NLS	neonatal lupus syndrome		
NLs	neuroimmunophilin ligands	nmol	nanomole (one billionth $[10^{-9}]$ of a mole)
NLT	not later than		
	not less than	NMOH	no medical ocular history
NLV	nelfinavir (Viracept)	NMP	normal menstrual period
NM	nanometer (nm) (10^{-9} meters)	NMR	nuclear magnetic resonance (same as magnetic resonance imaging)
	Negro male		
	neuromuscular	NMRS	nuclear magnetic resonance spectroscopy
	neuronal microdysgenesis		
	nodular melanoma	NMRT (R)	Nuclear Medicine Radiologic Technologist (Registered)
	nonmalignant		
	not measurable		
	not measured	NMS	neonatal morphine solution
	not mentioned		
	nuclear medicine		neuroleptic malignant syndrome
	nurse manager		
N & M	nerves and muscles	NMSC	nonmelanoma skin cancer
	night and morning	NMSE	normalized mean square root
NMB	neuromuscular blockade		
NMBA	neuromuscular blocking agent	NMSIDS	near-miss sudden infant death syndrome
NMC	no malignant cells	NMT	nebulized mist treatment
NMD	Doctor of Naturopathic Medicine		no more than
		NMTB	neuromuscular transmission blockade
	neuromuscular disorders		
	neuronal migration disorders	NMTCB	Nuclear Medicine Technology Certification Board
	Normosol M and 5% Dextrose®		
		NMT(R)	Nuclear Medicine Technologist Registered
NMDA	N-methyl-D-aspartate		
NMDP	National Marrow Donor Pool	NMU	nitrosomethylurea
		NN	narrative notes
NME	new molecular entity		Navajo neuropathy
NMES	neuromuscular electrical stimulation		neonatal
			neural network
NMF	neuromuscular facilitation		normal nursery
NMH	neurally mediated hypotension		nurses' notes
		N/N	negative/negative
NMHH	no medical health history	NNB	normal newborn
NMI	no manifest improvement	NNBC	node-negative breast cancer
	no mental illness		
	no middle initial	NND	neonatal death

	number needed to detain	NOAEL	no observed adverse effect level
NNDSS	National Notifiable Diseases Surveillance System	$N_2O{:}O_2$	nitrous oxide to oxygen ratio
NNE	neonatal necrotizing enterocolitis	NOC	nonorgan-confined Nursing Outcome Classification
NNH	number needed to harm	noc.	night
NNIS	National Nosocomial Infections Surveillance	noct	nocturnal
NNM	Nicolle-Novy-MacNeal (media)	NOD	nonobese diabetic notice of disagreement notify of death
NNL	no new laboratory (test orders)	NOE	naso-orbitoethmoid
NNN	normal newborn nursery	NOED	no observed effect dose
NNO	no new orders	NOEL	no observable effect level
NNP	Neonatal Nurse Practitioner non-nociceptive pain	NOF	National Osteoporosis Foundation (treatment criteria)
N:NPK	grams of nitrogen to non-protein kilocalories	NOFT	nonorganic failure to thrive
NNR	not necessary to return	NOFTT	nonorganic failure to thrive
NNRTI	non-nucleoside reverse transcriptase inhibitor	NOGM	nonoxidative glucose metabolism
NNS	neonatal screen (hematocrit, total bilirubin, and total protein)	NOH	neurogenic orthostatic hypotension
		NOI	nature of illness
	nicotine nasal spray	NOK	next of kin
	non-nutritive sucking	NOL	not on label
	number needed to screen	NOM	nonoperative management nonsuppurative otitis media
NNT	number needed to treat		
NNTB	number needed to treat to benefit	NOMI	nonocclusive mesenteric infarction
NNTB/ NNTH	number needed to treat, benefit-to-harm ratio	NOMS	not on my shift
NNTH	number needed to treat to harm	NO/N_2	nitric oxide; nitrogen
		NONMEM	nonlinear mixed-effects model (modeling)
NNU	net nitrogen utilization		
NNWT	noncontact normothermic wound therapy	non pal	not palpable
NO	nasal oxygen nitric oxide nitroglycerin ointment none obtained nonobese number (no.) nursing office	non-REM	nonrapid eye movement (sleep)
		non rep	do not repeat
		NON VIZ	not visualized
		NOOB	not out of bed
		NOP	not on patient
		NOR	norethynodrel normal nortriptyline
NO_2	nitrogen dioxide		
N_2O	nitrous oxide		
NOAA	National Oceanic and Atmospheric Administration	NOR-EPI	norepinephrine (Levophed)
		norm	normal

NOS	neonatal opium solution (diluted deodorized tincture of opium)	no pain
		not performed
		not pregnant
	new-onset seizures	not present
	nitric oxide synthase	nuclear pharmacist
	no organisms seen	nuclear pharmacy
	not on staff	nursed poorly
	not otherwise specified	nurse practitioner
NOSI	nitric oxide synthase inhibitors	NPA nasal pharyngeal airway
		nasopharyngeal aspirate
NOSIE	Nurse's Observation Scale (Schedule) for Inpatient Evaluation	near point of accommodation
		no previous admission
NOSPECS	categories for classifying eye changes in Graves ophthalmopathy: **n**o signs or symptoms, **o**nly signs, **s**oft tissue involvement with symptoms and signs, **p**roptosis, **e**xtraocular muscle involvement, **c**orneal involvement, and **s**ight loss (visual acuity)	NPAT nonparoxysmal atrial tachycardia
		NPBC node-positive breast cancer
		NPC nasopharyngeal carcinoma
		near-point convergence
		Niemann-Pick disease Type C (sphingomyelin lipidosis)
		nodal premature contractions
		nonpatient contact
NOT	nocturnal oxygen therapy	nonproductive cough
		nonprotein calorie
NOTT	nocturnal oxygen therapy trial	no prenatal care
		no previous complaint(s)
NOU	not on unit	NPCC nonprotein carbohydrate calories
NOV	Novartis	
NOV 70/30	human insulin, regular 30 units/mL with human insulin isophane suspension 70 units/mL (Novolin 70/30)	NPCPAP nasopharyngeal continuous positive airway pressure
		NPD Niemann-Pick disease
		nonprescription drugs
NOV L	human insulin zinc suspension (Novolin L)	no pathological diagnosis
		NPDL nodular poorly differentiated lymphocytic
NOV N	human insulin isophane suspension (Novolin N)	NPDR nonproliferative diabetic retinopathy
NOV R	human insulin regular (Novolin R)	NPE neurogenic pulmonary edema
NP	nasal polyps	neuropsychologic examination
	nasal prongs	no palpable enlargement
	nasopharyngeal	normal pelvic examination
	near point	
	neuropathic pain	
	neurophysin	
	neuropsychiatric	NPEM nocturnal penile erection monitoring
	neutrogenic precautions	
	newly presented	NPF nasopharyngeal fiberscope
	nonpalpable	no predisposing factor

N-PFMSO₄	nebulized preservative-free morphine sulfate (This is a dangerous abbreviation)	NPRM	Notice of Proposed Rulemaking
NPFS	nonpenetrating filtering surgery	NPRS	numerical pain rating scale
NPG	nonpregnant	NPS	National Pharmaceutical Stockpile
	normal-pressure glaucoma		new patient set-up
NPH	isophane insulin (neutral protamine Hagedorn)	NPSA	nonphysician surgical assistant
	no previous history	NPSD	nonpotassium-sparing diuretics
	normal-pressure hydrocephalus	NPSF	National Patient Safety Foundation
NPhx	nasopharynx	NPSG	National Patient Safety Goal
NPI	National Provider Identifier		nocturnal polysomnography
	Neuropsychiatric Inventory	NPSLE	neuropsychiatric systemic lupus erythematosus
	no present illness	NPT	near-patient tests
	Nottingham Prognostic Index		neopyrithiamin hydrochloride
NPIS	Numeric Pain Intensity Scale		nocturnal penile tumescence
NPJT	nonparoxysmal junctional tachycardia		no prior tracings
NPL	insulin lispro protamine suspension		normal pressure and temperature
	neural protamine lispro (insulin)	NPU	net protein utilization
		NPV	negative predictive value
NPLSM	neoplasm		nothing per vagina
NPK	nonprotein kilocalories	NPY	neuropeptide Y
NPM	nothing per mouth	NPZ	neuropsychologic text z
NPN	nonprotein nitrogen	NQECN	nonqueratinizing epidermoid carcinoma
NPNC	no prenatal care		
NPNT	nonpalpable, nontender	NQMI	non-Q wave myocardial infarction
n.p.o.	nothing by mouth		
NPOC	nonpurgeable organic carbon	NQWMI	non-Q wave myocardial infarction
NPOD	Neuropsychiatric Officer of the Day	NR	do not repeat
NPP	nonphysician practitioner		newly reformulated
	normal postpartum		none reported
NPPI	nonpeptidic protease inhibitor		nonreactive
			nonrebreathing
NPPNG	nonpenicillinase-producing *Neisseria gonorrhoeae*		no refills
			no report
			no response
			no return
NPPV	noninvasive positive-pressure ventilation		normal range
			normal reaction
NPR	normal pulse rate		not reached
	nothing per rectum		not reacting
NPRL	normal pupillary reaction to light		not remarkable
			not resolved

	number	NRTs	nitron radical traps
NRAF	nonrheumatic atrial fibrillation	NS	nephrotic syndrome
NRB	Noninstitutional Review Board		neurological signs
			neurosurgery
	nonrebreather (oxygen mask)		nipple stimulation
			nodular sclerosis
NRBC	normal red blood cell		no-show
	nucleated red blood cell		nonsmoker
NRBS	nonrebreathing system		normal saline solution (0.9% sodium chloride solution)
NRC	National Research Council		
	normal retinal correspondence		normospermic
			no sample
	Nuclear Regulatory Commission		not seen
			not significant
NREH	normal renin essential hypertension		nuclear sclerosis
			nursing service
NREM	nonrapid eye movement		nutritive sucking
NREMS	nonrapid eye movement sleep		nylon suture
		NSA	neck-shaft angle
NREMT-P	National Registry of Emergency Medical Technicians–Paramedic level		normal serum albumin (albumin, human)
			no salt added
			no significant abnormalities
NRF	normal renal function		number of signals averaged (radiology)
NRI	nerve root involvement		
	nerve root irritation	NSAA	nonsteroidal antiandrogen
	no recent illnesses	NSABP	National Surgical Adjuvant Breast Project
	norepinephrine reuptake inhibitor		
NRL	natural rubber latex	NSAD	no signs of acute disease
N-RLX	nonrelaxed	NSAIA	nonsteroidal anti-inflammatory agent
NRM	nonrebreathing mask		
	no regular medicines	NSAID	nonsteroidal anti-inflammatory drug
	normal range of motion		
	normal retinal movement	NSAP	nonspecific abdominal pain
NRN	no return necessary		
NRNST	nonreassuring-nonstress test	NSBGP	nonspecific bowel gas pattern
NRO	neurology	NSC	neural stem cells
NROM	normal range of motion		no significant change
NRP	nonreassuring patterns		nonservice-connected
NRPR	nonbreathing pressure relieving	NSCC	nonsmall cell carcinoma
		NSCD	nonservice-connected disability
NRS	Neurobehavioral Rating Scale		
		NSCFPT	no significant change from previous tracing
NRT	neuromuscular reeducation techniques		
		NSCIDRC	National Spinal Cord Injury Data Research Center
	nicotine-replacement therapy		
NRTI	nucleoside reverse transcriptase inhibitor	NSCLC	nonsmall-cell–lung cancer

NSCST	nipple stimulation contraction stress test	NSOP	no soft organs palpable
		NSP	neck and shoulder pain
NSD	nasal septal deviation	NSPs	needle and syringe exchange programs
	nominal standard dose		
	nonstructural deterioration		nonstarch polysaccharides
	normal spontaneous delivery	NSPVT	nonsustained polymorphic ventricular tachycardia
	no significant disease (difference, defect, deviation)	NSR	nasoseptal repair
			nonspecific reaction
			normal sinus rhythm
			not seen regularly
NSDA	nonsteroid dependent asthmatic	NSRP	nerve-sparing radical prostatectomy
NSDU	neonatal stepdown unit	NSS	nephron-sparing surgery
NSE	neuron-specific enolase		neurological signs stable
	normal saline enema (0.9% sodium chloride)		neuropathy symptom score
			normal size and shape
N s E	nausea without emesis		not statistically significant
NSEACS	non-ST-elevation acute coronary syndromes		nutritional support service
NSF	no significant findings		sodium chloride 0.9% (normal saline solution)
NSFTD	normal spontaneous full-term delivery		
		1/2 NSS	sodium chloride 0.45% (1/2 normal saline solution)
NSG	nursing		
NSGCT	nonseminomatous germ-cell tumors		
		NSSC	normal size, shape and consistency (uterus)
NSGCTT	nonseminomatous germ-cell tumor of the testis		
		NSSL	normal size, shape, and location
NSGI	nonspecific genital infection		
		NSSP	normal size, shape, and position
NSGT	nonseminomatous germ-cell tumor		
		NSSTT	nonspecific ST and T-wave
NSHC	no-self-harm contract		
NSHD	nodular sclerosing Hodgkin disease	NSST-TWCs	nonspecific ST-T wave changes
NSI	needlestick injury	NST	nonmyeloablative stem-cell transplant
	negative self-image		
	no signs of infection		Nonsense Syllable Test
	no signs of inflammation		nonstress test
NSICU	neurosurgery intensive care unit		normal sphincter tone
			not sooner than
NSILA	nonsuppressible insulin-like activity		nutritional support team
NSIP	nonspecific interstitial pneumonia	NSTD	nonsexually transmitted disease
NSMMVT	nonsustained monomorphic ventricular tachycardia	NSTEMI	non-ST-segment elevation myocardial infarction
		NSTGCT	nonseminomatous testicular germ cell tumor
NSN	Neo-Synephrine		
	nephrotoxic serum nephritis		
NSO	Neosporin® ointment	NSTI	necrotizing soft-tissue infection
NSOM	near field scanning optical microscope		

NSTT	nonseminomatous testicular tumors	NTIS	National Technical Information Service (U.S. Department of Commerce)
NSU	neurosurgical unit		
	nonspecific urethritis		
NSV	nonspecific vaginitis	NTL	nectar-thick liquid (diet consistency)
NSVD	nonstructural valve deterioration		nortriptyline (Aventyl; Pamelor)
	normal spontaneous vaginal delivery		no time limit
NSVT	nonsustained ventricular tachycardia	NTLE	neocortical temporal-lobe epilepsy
NSX	neurosurgical examination	NTM	nocturnal tumescence monitor
NSY	nursery		nontuberculous mycobacterium
NT	nasotracheal	NTMB	nontuberculous myobacteria
	next time		
	Nordic Track®	NTMI	nontransmural myocardial infarction
	normal temperature		
	normotensive	NTND	not tender, not distended
	nortriptyline	NTP	narcotic treatment program
	not tender		
	not tested		National Toxicology Program
	nourishment taken		
	numbness and tingling		Nitropaste® (nitroglycerin ointment)
	nursing technician		
N&T	nose and throat		nonthrombocytopenic preterm (infant)
	numbness and tingling		
N Tachy	nodal tachycardia		normal temperature and pressure
NT-ANP	N-terminal atrial natriuretic peptide		
			sodium nitroprusside
NTBR	not to be resuscitated	NTPD	nocturnal tidal peritoneal dialysis
NTC	neurotrauma center		
NTCS	no tumor cells seen	NT-proBNP	N-terminal pro-brain natriuretic peptide
NTD	negative to date		
	neural-tube defects	NTS	nasotracheal suction
	nitroblue tetrazolium dye (test)		nicotine transdermal system
NTE	neutral thermal environment		nontyphoidal salmonellae
	not to exceed		nucleus tractus solitarii
NTED	neonatal toxic-shock-syndrome-like exanthematous disease	NTSCI	nontraumatic spinal cord injury
		NTT	nasotracheal tube
NTF	neurotrophic factor		near-total thyroidectomy
	normal throat flora		nonthrombocytopenic term (infant)
NTG	nitroglycerin		
	nontoxic goiter		nontreponemal test
	nontreatment group	NTTP	no tenderness to palpation
	normal tension glaucoma		
NTGO	nitroglycerin ointment	NTU	nephelometric turbidity units
NTI	narrow therapeutic index		
	no treatment indicated	NTX	naltrexone (ReVia)

NTZ	nitazoxanide (Alinia)	NVL	neurovascular laboratory
NTZ Long-acting®	oxymetazoline nasal spray	NVLD	nonverbal learning disability
NU	name unknown	NVM	neovascular membrane
NUD	nonulcer dyspepsia	NVP	nausea and vomiting of pregnancy
NUG	necrotizing ulcerative gingivitis		nevirapine (Viramune)
nullip	nullipara	NVS	neurological vital signs
NUN	nonurea nitrogen		neurovascular status
NV	naked vision	NVSS	normal variant short stature
	nausea and vomiting		
	near vision	NW	naked weight
	negative variation		nasal wash
	neovascularization		normal weight
	neurovascular		not weighed
	new vessel	NWB	nonweight bearing
	next visit	NWBL	nonweight bearing, left
	nonvenereal	NWBR	nonweight bearing, right
	nonveteran	NWC	number of words chosen
	normal value		
	not vaccinated	NWD	neuroleptic withdrawal
	not verified		normal well developed
N&V	nausea and vomiting	NWS	New World screwworm
NVA	near visual acuity		(*Cochliomyia*
NVAF	nonvalvular atrial fibrillation		*hominivorax* [Coquerel])
NVB	Navelbine (vinorelbine tartrate)	NWTS	National Wilms Tumor Study (rating scale)
NVBo	oral vinorelbine		
NVC	neurovascular checks	NWTSG	National Wilms Tumor Study Group
nvCJD	new-variant Creutzfeldt-Jakob disease	Nx	nephrectomy
NVD	nausea, vomiting, and diarrhea	NX211	liposomal lurtotecan
	neck vein distention	NYB	New York Blood Center
	neovascularization of the (optic) disk	NYD	not yet diagnosed
	neurovesicle dysfunction	NYHA	New York Heart Association (classification of heart disease)
	normal vaginal delivery		
	no venereal disease		
	no venous distention	NYST	nystagmus
	nonvalvular disease	NZ	enzyme
NVDC	nausea, vomiting, diarrhea, and constipation		
NVE	native		
	native valve endocarditis		
	neovascularization elsewhere		
NVG	neovascular glaucoma		
	neoviridogrisein		
NVI	neovascularization of the iris		

O

O	eye
	objective findings
	obvious
	occlusal
	often
	open
	oral
	ortho
	other
	oxygen
	pint
	zero
$\bar{o}$	negative
	no
	none
	pint
	without
O+	blood type O positive (O positive is preferred)
O−	blood type O negative (O negative is preferred)
Ⓞ	orally (by mouth)
$_1O_2$	singlet oxygen
O_2	both eyes
	oxygen
O_2^-	superoxide
O_3	ozone
O157	*Escherichia coli* O157
OA	occipital artery
	occipitoatlantal
	occiput anterior
	old age
	on admission
	on arrival
	ophthalmic artery
	oral airway
	oral alimentation
	osteoarthritis
	ovarian ablation
	Overeaters Anonymous
O/A	on or about
O & A	observation and assessment
	odontectomy and alveoloplasty
OAA	Old Age Assistance
OAA/S	Observer's Assessment of Alertness/Sedation

OAB	overactive bladder
OAC	omeprazole, amoxicillin, and clarithromycin
	oral anticoagulant(s)
	overaction
OAD	obstructive airway disease
	occlusive arterial disease
	overall diameter
OAE	otoacoustic emissions
OAF	oral anal fistula
	osteoclast activating factor
OAG	open angle glaucoma
OAP	old age pension
OAR	Ottawa Ankle Rules
OAS	Older Adult Services
	oral allergy syndrome
	organic anxiety syndrome
	outpatient assessment service
	overall survival
	Overt Aggression Scale
OASDHI	Old Age, Survivors, Disability, and Health Insurance
OASI	Old Age and Survivors Insurance
OASIS	Outcomes and Assessment Information Set
OASO	overactive superior oblique
OASR	overactive superior rectus
OASS	Overt Agitation Severity Scale
OAT	ornithine aminotransferase
OATP	organic anion-transporting polypeptide
OATS	osteochondral autograft transfer system
OAV	oculoauriculovertebral (dysplasia)
OAW	oral airway
OB	obese
	obesity
	obstetrics
	occult blood
	osteoblast
OBA	office-based anesthesia
	Office of Biotechnology Activities (NIH)
OB-A	obstetrics-aborted
OB-Del	obstetrics-delivered
OBE	out-of-body experience
OBE-CALP	placebo capsule or tablet

OBF	ocular blood flow	OCC Th	occupational therapy
OBG	obstetrics and gynecology	Occup Rx	occupational therapy
Ob-Gyn	obstetrics and gynecology	OCD	obsessive-compulsive
Obj	objective		disorder
obl	oblique		osteochondritis dissecans
OB marg	obtuse marginal	OCE	outpatient code editor
OB-ND	obstetrics-not delivered	OCG	oral cholecystogram
OBP	office blood pressure	OCI	Obsessive-Compulsive
OBRR	obstetric recovery room		Inventory
OBS	observed	OCL®	oral colonic lavage
	obstetrical service	OCN	obsessive-compulsive
	organic brain syndrome		neurosis
OBT	obtained		Oncology Certified
OBTM	omeprazole, bismuth		Nurse
	subcitrate, tetracycline,	OCNS	Obsessive-Compulsive
	and metronidazole		Neurosis Scale
OBUS	obstetrical ultrasound	O-CNV	occult choroidal
OBW	open bed warmer		neovascularization
OC	observed cases	OCOR	on-call to operating
	obstetrical conjugate		room
	office call	OCP	ocular cicatricial
	on call		pemphigoid
	only child		oral contraceptive pills
	open cholecystectomy		ova, cysts, parasites
	open colectomy	OCR	oculocephalic reflex
	optical chromatography		optical character
	oral care		recognition
	oral contraceptive	OCS	Obsessive-Compulsive
	osteocalcin		Scale
	osteoclast		oral cancer screening
	OxyContin (oxycodone)	11-OCS	11-oxycorticosteroid
O & C	onset and course	OCT	octreotide (Sandostatin)
OCA	oculocutaneous albinism		optical coherence
	open care area		tomograph
	oral contraceptive agent		(tomography)
OCAD	occlusive carotid artery		oral cavity tumors
	disease		ornithine carbamyl
OCB	obstructive chronic		transferase
	bronchitis		oxytocin challenge test
OCBZ	oxcarbazepine(Trileptal)	OCU	observation care unit
OCC	occasionally	OCVM	occult cerebrovascular
	occlusal		malformations
	old chart called	OCX	oral cancer examination
OCCC	open chest cardiac	OD	Doctor of Optometry
	compression		Officer-of-the-Day
	ovarian clear cell		oligodendroglial
	carcinoma		once daily (this is a
occl	occlusion		dangerous abbreviation
OCCM	open chest cardiac		as it is read as right
	massage		eye; use "once daily")
OCC PR	open chest		on duty
	cardiopulmonary		optic disk
	resuscitation		oral-duodenal

	outdoor	ODTS	organic dust toxic
	outside diameter		syndrome
	ovarian dysgerminoma	OE	on examination
	overdose		orthopedic examination
	right eye		otitis externa
Δ OD 450	deviation of optical density at 450	O-E	standard observed minus expected
ODA	occipitodextra anterior	O&E	observation and
	once-daily aminoglycoside		examination
	osmotic driving agent	OEC	outer ear canal
ODAC	Oncologic Drugs Advisory Committee (of the US Food and Drug Administration)	OEI	opioid escalation index
		O_2EI	oxygen extraction index
		OEL	occupational exposure level
	on-demand analgesia computer	OENT	oral endotracheal tube
ODAT	one day at a time	OEP	Office of Emergency Preparedness
ODC	oral disease control		oil of evening primrose (evening primrose oil)
	ornithine decarboxylase		
	outpatient diagnostic center	OEPA	vincristine (Oncovin), etoposide, prednisone, and doxorubicin (Adriamycin)
ODCH	ordinary diseases of childhood		
ODD	oculodentodigital (dysplasia)	OER	oxygen extraction ratios
		O_2ER	oxygen extraction ratio
	opposition defiance disorder	OERR	order entry/results-reports (Veterans Administration's physician computer order entry system)
OD'd	overdosed		
ODed	overdosed		
ODM	occlusion dose monitor		
	ophthalmodynamometry	OET	oral esophageal tube
ODMP	on-going data management plan	OETT	oral endotracheal tube
		OF	occipital-frontal
ODN	optokinetic nystagmus		optic fundi
ODP	occipitodextra posterior		osteitis fibrosa
	offspring of diabetic parents		outlet forceps (delivery)
OD/P	right eye patched	OFC	occipital-frontal circumference
ODQ	on direct questioning		orbitofacial cleft
ODS	Office of Drug Safety (FDA)	OFF	shoes off during weighing
	organized delivery system	OFI	other febrile illness
	osmotic demyelination syndrome	OFLOX	ofloxacin (Floxin)
		OFLX	ofloxacin (Floxin)
ODSS	Office of Disability Support Services	OFM	open-face mask
			oral focal mucinosis
ODSU	oncology day stay unit	OFNE	oxygenated fluorocarbon nutrient emulsion
	One-Day Surgery Unit		
ODT	occipitodextra transerve	OFPF	optic fundi and peripheral fields
	optical Doppler tomography	OFR	oxygen-free radicals
	orally disintegrating tablet	OFTT	organic failure to thrive
		OG	Obstetrics-Gynecology

	orogastric (feeding)	OHRR	open-heart recovery room
	outcome goal (long-term goal)	OHS	obesity hypoventilation syndrome
OGC	oculogyric crisis		occupational health service
OGCT	ovarian germ cell tumor		ocular histoplasmosis syndrome
OGD	oesophagogastro-duodenoscopy (United Kingdom and other countries)		ocular hypoperfusion syndrome
	Office of Generic Drugs (of the Food and Drug Administration)		open-heart surgery
		OHSS	ovarian hyperstimulation syndrome
OGT	orogastric tube	OHT	ocular hypertension
OGTT	oral glucose tolerance test		overhead trapeze
OH	occupational history	OHTN	ocular hypertension
	ocular history	OHTx	orthotopic heart transplantation
	ocular hypertension		
	on hand	OI	opportunistic infection
	open-heart		osteogenesis imperfecta
	oral hygiene		otitis interna
	orthostatic hypotension	OIF	oil-immersion field
	outside hospital	OIG	Office of the Inspector General
17-OH	17-hydroxycorticosteroids		
OHA	oral hypoglycemic agents	OIH	orthoiodohippurate
OHC	outer hair cell (in cochlea)	OIHA	orthoiodohippuric acid
		OI&I	occupational injury and illness
OH Cbl	hydroxycobalamine		
17-OHCS	17-hydroxycorticosteroids	OIM	optical immunoassay
OHD	hydroxy vitamin D	OINT	ointment
	organic heart disease	OIR	oxygen-induced retinopathy
$25(OH)D_3$	25-hydroxy vitamin D (calcifediol, Calderol)		
		OIRDA	occipital intermittent rhythmical delta activity
OHF	old healed fracture		
	Omsk hemorrhagic fever	OIS	ocular ischemic syndrome
	overhead frame		optical intrinsic signal (imaging)
OHFA	hydroxy fatty acid		
OHFT	overhead frame and trapeze		optimum information size
		OIs	opportunistic infections
OHG	oral hypoglycemic	OIT	ovarian immature teratoma
OHI	oral hygiene instructions		
OHIAA	hydroxyindolacetic acid	OIU	optical internal urethrotomy
OHL	oral hairy leukoplakia		
7-OHMTX	7-hydroxymethotrexate	OJ	orange juice (this is a dangerous abbreviation as it is read as OS, left eye)
OHNS	Otolaryngology, Head, and Neck Surgery (Dept.)		
			orthoplast jacket
OHP	obese hypertensive patient	OK	all right
			approved
	oxygen under hyperbaric pressure		correct
		OKAN	optokinetic after nystagmus
17 OHP	17-hydroxyprogesterone		
OHRP	open-heart rehabilitation program	OKC	odontogenic keratocyst

O

	open kinetic chain	OM$_2$	second obtuse marginal (branch)
OKN	optokinetic nystagmus		
OKT	Ortho Kung T-cell, designation for a series of antigens	OMA	older maternal age
		OMAC	otitis media, acute, catarrhal
OL	left eye	OMAS	Olerud-Molander Ankle Score
	open label (study)		
OLA	occiput left anterior occipitolaevoanterior		otitis media, acute, suppurating
OLAP	online analytical processing	OMB	obtuse marginal branch
		OMB$_1$	first obtuse marginal branch
OLB	open-liver biopsy		
	open-lung biopsy	OMB$_2$	second obtuse marginal branch
OLBPQ	Oswestry Low Back Pain Questionnaire	OMC	open mitral commissuortomy
OLC	ouabain-like compound		
OLD	obstructive lung disease		ostiomeatal complex
		OMCA	otitis media, catarrhalis, acute
OLE	olive leaf extract		
OLF	ouabain-like factor	OMCC	otitis media, catarrhalis, chronic
OLM	ocular larva migrans		
	ophthalmic laser microendoscope	OMD	organic mental disorder
		OME	Office of Medical Examiner
OLNM	occult lymph node metastases		
			otitis media with effusion
OLP	abnormal lipoprotein	7-OMEN	menogaril
OLR	optic labyrinthine righting	OMFS	oral and maxillofacial surgery
	otology, laryngology, and rhinology		
		OMG	ocular myasthenia gravis
OLS	ordinary least squares	OMI	old myocardial infarct
	ouabain-like substance	OMIEI	oral medication induced esophageal injury
OLT	occipitolaevoposterior		
	orthotopic liver transplantation	OMP	oculomotor (third nerve) palsy
OLTP	online transaction processing		open mediastinal biopsy
		OMPA	otitis media, purulent, acute
OLTx	orthotopic liver transplantation		
		OMPC	otitis media, purulent, chronic
OLV	one-lung ventilation	OMR	operative mortality rate
OLZ	olanzapine (Zyprexa)	OMS	oral morphine sulfate
OM	every morning (this is a dangerous abbreviation)		organic mental syndrome
			organic mood syndrome
	obtuse marginal	OMSA	otitis media secretory (or suppurative) acute
	ocular melanoma		
	oral motor	OMSC	otitis media secretory (or suppurative) chronic
	oral mucositis		
	organomegaly	OMT	oral mucosal transudate
	osteomalacia		Osteopathic manipulative technique (treatment)
	osteomyelitis		
	otitis media	OMVC	open mitral valve commissurotomy
O$_2$M	oxygen mask		
OM$_1$	first obtuse marginal (branch)		

OMVD	optimized microvessel density (analysis)	OOH	out of hospital
		OOH&NS	ophthalmology, otorhinolaryngology, and head and neck surgery
OMVI	operating motor vehicle intoxicated		
ON	every night (this is a dangerous abbreviation)		
		OOI	out of isolette
	optic nerve	OOL	onset of labor
	optic neurophathy	OOLR	ophthalmology, otology, laryngology, and rhinology
	oronasal		
	Ortho-Novum®		
	overnight	OOM	onset of menarche
ONC	over-the-needle catheter vincristine (Oncovin)	OOP	out of pelvis
			out of plaster
OND	Office of New Drugs (FDA)		out on pass
		OOPS	out of program status
	ondansetron (Zofran)	OOR	out of room
	other neurologic disorder(s)	OORW	out of radiant warmer
		OOS	out of sequence
ONH	optic nerve head		out of specification (deviation from standard)
	optic nerve hypoplasia		
ONM	ocular neuromyotonia		
ON RR	overnight recovery room		out of splint
			out of stock
ONS	Office for National Statistics (United Kingdom)	OOT	out of town
		OOW	out of wedlock
			out of work
ONSD	optic nerve sheath decompression	OP	oblique presentation
			occiput posterior
ONSF	optic nerve sheath fenestration		open
			operation
ONTD	open neural tube defect(s)		organophosphorous
ONTR	orders not to resuscitate		oropharynx
OO	ophthalmic ointment		oscillatory potentials
	oral order		osteoporosis
	other		outpatient
	out of		overpressure
o/o	on account of	O&P	ova and parasites (stool examination)
O&O	off and on		
OOB	out of bed	OPA	oral pharyngeal airway
OOBL	out of bilirubin light		
OOBBRP	out of bed with bathroom privileges		outpatient anesthesia
		OPAC	opacity (opacification)
OOC	onset of contractions	OPAT	outpatient parenteral antibiotic therapy
	out of cast		
	out of control	OPB	outpatient basis
OO Con	out of control	OPC	operable pancreatic carcinoma
OOD	outer orbital diameter		
OO-EMG	electromyographic recording of the orbicularis oculi muscles		oropharyngeal candidiasis
			outpatient care
			outpatient catheterization
			outpatient clinic
OOF	out of facility	OPCA	olivopontocerebellar atrophy

O

263

OPCAB	off-pump coronary artery bypass (grafting)	OPPS	Outpatient Prospective Payment System
op cit	in the work cited	OPQRST	onset, provocation, quality, radiation, severity, and time (an EMT mnemonic used in initial patient questioning)
OPCS-4	Classification of Surgical Operations and Procedures (4th revision)		
OPD	oropharyngeal dysphagia		
	Orphan Products Development (office of)	OPRDU	outpatient renal dialysis unit
	outpatient department	OPS	Objective Pain Scores
O'p'-DDD	mitotane (Lysodren)		operations
OPDRA	Office of Postmarketing Drug Risk Assessment (FDA) (name changed to Office of Drug Safety [ODS])		Orpington prognostic scale
			orthogonal polarization spectral (imaging)
			outpatient surgery
OPDUR	on-line prospective drug utilization review		overnight polysomnography
OPE	oral peripheral examination	OPSI	overwhelming postsplenectomy infection
	outpatient evaluation		
OPEN	vincristine (Oncovin), prednisone, etoposide, and mitoxantrone (Novantrone)	OPSU	oblique partial sit-up
			outpatient surgical unit
		O PSY	open psychiatry
		OPT	optimum
OPERA	outpatient endometrial resection/ablation		outpatient treatment
		OPT c CA	Ohio pediatric tent with compressed air
OPG	ocular plethysmography		
	osteoprotegerin	OPT c O$_2$	Ohio pediatric tent with oxygen
OPIDP	organophosphate-induced delayed polyneuropathy		
		OPTN	Organ Procurement and Transplantation Network
OPL	oral premalignant lesion		
	other party liability		
OPLC	optimum performance liquid chromatography	OPT-NSC	outpatient treatment, nonservice-connected
OPLL	ossification of posterior latitudinal ligament	OPT-SC	outpatient treatment, service-connected
OPM	occult primary malignancy	OPV	oral polio vaccine
			outpatient visit
	oral and pharyngeal mucositis	OR	odds ratio
			oil retention
OPMD	oculopharyngeal muscular dystrophy		open reduction
			operating room
OPN	osteopontin		Orthodox
OPO	organ procurement organizations		own recognizance
		ORA	occiput right anterior
	overnight pulse oximetry	ORC	outpatient rehabilitation centers
OPOC	oral pharynx, oral cavity		
OPP	opposite	ORCH	orchiectomy
OPPG	oculopneumoplethysmography	ORD	orderly
		OREF	open reduction, external fixation
OPPOS	opposition		

ORF	open reading frame		Osgood-Schlatter (disease)
OR&F	open reduction and fixation		osmium
			osteosarcoma
ORIF	open reduction internal fixation		overall survival
		OSA	obstructive sleep apnea
ORL	oblique retinacular ligament		off-site anesthesia
			osteosarcoma
	otorhinolaryngology (otology, rhinology and laryngology)	OSA/HS	obstructive sleep apnea/ hypopnea syndrome
		OSAS	obstructive sleep apnea syndrome
ORMF	open reduction metallic fixation		
		OSC	oral self-care
ORN	operating room nurse osteoradionecrosis	OSCAR	On-line Survey Certification and Reporting
OROS	ostomotic release oral system		
		OSCC	oral squamous cell carcinoma
ORP	occiput right posterior		
ORR	overall response rate	OSCE	Objective Structured Clinical Examination
ORS	oculorespiratory syndrome		
	olfactory reference syndrome	OSD	Osgood-Schlatter disease
			overseas duty
	oral rehydration salts		overside drainage
ORSA	oxacillin-resistant *Staphylococcus aureus*	OSE	ovarian surface epithelium
		OSESC	opening-snap ejection systolic click
ORT	oestrogen (estrogen)- replacement therapy (United Kingdom and elsewhere)		
		OSFT	outstretched fingertips
		OSG	osteosonogram (osteosonogrammetry)
	operating room technician	OSH	outside hospital
	oral rehydration therapy	OSHA	Occupational Safety & Health Administration
	Registered Occupational Therapist		
		OSM S	osmolarity serum
		OSM U	osmolarity urine
OR XI	oriented to time	OSN	off-service note
OR X2	oriented to time and place	OSP	outside pass
		OS/P	left eye patched
OR X3	oriented to time, place, and person	OSS	osseous
			over-shoulder strap
OR X4	oriented to time, place, person, and objects (watch, pen, book)	OSSI	orthognathic surgery simulating instrument
		OST	occipitosubtemporal
OS	left eye		optimal sampling theory
	mouth (this is a dangerous abbreviation as it is read as left eye)		osteogenic sarcoma
		OT	occiput transverse
			occupational therapy
	occipitosacral		old tuberculin
	oligospermic		on-treatment
	opening snap		oral transmucosal
	ophthalmic solution (this is a dangerous abbreviation as it is read as left eye)		orotracheal
			outlier threshold
			oxytocin (Pitocin)
		O/T	oral temperature
	oral surgery	OTA	open to air

OTC	occult tumor cell	OVLT	organum vasculosum of lamina terminalis
	ornithine transcarbamoylase	OVR	Office of Vocational Rehabilitation
	Orthopedic Technician, Certified	OVS	obstructive voiding symptoms (syndrome)
	over-the-counter (sold without prescription)	OW	once weekly (this is a dangerous abbreviation)
OTCD	ornithine-transcarbamylase deficiency		open wound
			oral warts
OTD	optimal therapeutic dose		outer wall
	organ tolerance dose		out of wedlock
	out-the-door		ova weight
OTE	(McMaster) Overall Treatment Evaluation	O/W	oil in water
			otherwise
OTFC	oral transmucosal fentanyl citrate (Fentanyl Oralet; Actiq)	OWL	out of wedlock
		OWNK	out of wedlock, not keeping (baby)
OTH	other	OWR	Osler-Weber-Rendu (disease)
OTHS	occupational therapy home service	OWT	zero work tolerance
OTIS	Organization of Teratology Information Services	OX	oximeter
		O×1	oriented to time
		O×2	oriented to time and place
OTJ	on-the-job (injury; training)	O×3	oriented to time, place, and person
OTO	one-time only	O×4	oriented to time, place, person, and objects (watch, pen, book)
	otolaryngology		
	otology		
OTPT	oral triphasic tablets (contraceptive)	OXA	oxacillinase
			oxaliplatin (Eloxatin)
OTR	Occupational Therapist, Registered	OXC	oxcarbazepine (Trileptal)
		Oxi	oximeter (oximetry)
OTRL	Occupational Therapist, Registered Licensed	Ox-LDL	oxidized low-density lipoprotein
OT/RT	occupational therapy/ recreational therapy	OXPHOS	oxidative phosphorylation
		OxPt	oxaliplatin (Eloxatin)
OTS	orotracheal suction	OXM	pulse oximeter
OTT	oral transit time	OXT	oxytocin (Pitocin)
	orotracheal tube	Oxy-5®	benzoyl peroxide
OTW	off-the-wall	OxyIR®	oxycodone immediate release capsules
OU	each eye		
OUES	oxygen uptake efficiency slope	OXZ	oxazepam (Serax)
		OZ	optical zone
OULQ	outer upper left quadrant		ounce
OU/P	both eyes patched		
OURQ	outer upper right quadrant		
OUS	obstetric ultrasound		
OV	office visit		
	ovary		
	ovum		
OVAL	ovalocytes		
OVF	Octopus® visual field		

P

P	para
	peripheral
	phosphorus
	pint
	plan
	Plasmodium
	poor
	protein
	Protestant
	pulse
	pupil
P	statistical probability value
$\bar{p}$	after
/P	partial lower denture
P/	partial upper denture
P1	pilocarpine 1% ophthalmic solution
P_2	pulmonic second heart sound
P20	Ocusert® P20
^{32}p	radioactive phosphorus
P40	Ocusert® P40
P53	tumor suppressive gene
PA	panic attack
	paranoid
	peanut allergy
	periapical (x-ray)
	pernicious anemia
	phenol alcohol
	physical activity
	Physician Assistant
	pineapple
	platelet aggregometry
	posterior-anterior (posteroanterior) (x-ray)
	premature adrenarche
	presents again
	primary aldosteronism
	professional association (similar to a corporation)
	Pseudomonas aeruginosa
	psychiatric aide
	psychoanalysis
	pulmonary artery
Pa	pascal

P&A	percussion and auscultation
	phenol and alcohol
	position and alignment
$P_2 > A_2$	pulmonic second heart sound greater than aortic second heart sound
PAAA	para-anastomotic aneurysm of the aorta
PAAD	persistently and acutely disabled
PAB	premature atrial beat
	pulmonary artery banding
PABA	aminobenzoic acid (para-aminobenzoic acid)
PABD	preoperative autologous blood donation
PAC	cisplatin (Platinol), doxorubicin (Adriamycin), and cylcophosphamide
	phenacemide
	Physical Assessment Center
	Physician Assistant, Certified
	picture archiving communication (system)
	Port-a-cath®
	premature atrial contraction
	prophylactic anticonvulsants
	pulmonary artery catheter
PA-C	Physician Assistant, Certified
PACATH	pulmonary artery catheter
PACE	population-adjusted clinical epidemiology
PACG	primary angle-closure glaucoma
PACH	pipers to after coming head
PACI	partial anterior cerebral infarct
$PACO_2$	partial pressure (tension) of carbon dioxide, alveolar
$PaCO_2$	partial pressure (tension) of carbon dioxide, artery

PACS	picture archiving and communications systems	PAGA	premature appropriate for gestational age
PACT	prism and alternate cover test	PAGE	polyacrylamide gel electrophoresis
	Program of Assertive Community Treatment	PAH	para-aminohippurate partial abdominal hysterectomy
PAC-V	cisplatin (Platinol), doxorubicin (Adriamycin), and cyclophosphamide		phenylalanine hydroxylase polycyclic aromatic hydrocarbons polynuclear aromatic hydrocarbon
PACU	postanesthesia care unit		predicted adult height
PAD	pelvic adhesive disease peripheral artery disease persistently and acutely disabled pharmacologic atrial defibrillator physician-assisted death preliminary anatomic diagnosis preoperative autologous donation primary affective disorder		primary adrenal hyperplasia pulmonary arterial hypertension
		PAHO	Pan American Health Organization
		PAI	penetrating abdominal injury plasminogen activator inhibitor platelet accumulation index
PADCAB	perfusion-assisted direct coronary artery bypass	PAIDS	pediatric acquired immunodeficiency syndrome
PADP	pulmonary arterial diastolic pressure pulmonary artery diastolic pressure	PAIgG	platelet-associated immunoglobulin G
PADS	Post Anesthesia Discharge Scoring System	PAIR	Puncture, Aspiration, Injection, Reaspiration (technique)
PAE	percutaneous angiographic embolization postanoxic encephalopathy postantibiotic effect pre-admission evaluation progressive assistive exercise	PAIVMs	passive accessory intervertebral movements
		PAIVS	pulmonary atresia with intact ventricular septum
		PAK	pancreas and kidney
PAEDP	pulmonary artery and end-diastole pressure	PAL	physical activity levels posterior axillary line posteroanterior and lateral
PAEE	physical activity energy expenditure	PALA	N-phosphoacetate-L-aspartate
PAF	paroxysmal atrial fibrillation platelet-activating factor population attributable fraction	Pa Line	pulmonary artery line
		PALN	para-aortic lymph node
		PALP	palpation
		PALS	pediatric advanced life support periarterial lymphatic sheath
PA&F	percussion, auscultation, and fremitus		
PAFE	postantifungal effect		

P

PAM	partial allosteric modulators	PaO₂	arterial oxygen pressure (tension)
	potential acuity meter	PAOD	peripheral arterial occlusive disease
	primary acquired melanosis	PAOP	pulmonary artery occlusion pressure
	primary amebic meningoencephalitis	PAP	passive-aggressive personality
	protein A mimetic		patient assistance program
2-PAM	pralidoxime (Protopam)		peroxidase-anti-peroxidase
PAMP	pulmonary arterial (artery) mean pressure		pokeweed antiviral protein
			positive airway pressure
PAN	pancreas		primary atypical pneumonia
	pancreatic		prostatic acid phosphatase
	pancuronium (Pavulon)		pulmonary alveolar proteinosis
	panoral x-ray examination		
	periodic alternating nystagmus		pulmonary artery pressure
	polyacrylonitrile (filter)	PAPS	primary antiphospholipid syndrome
	polyarteritis nodosa		
	polyomavirus-associated nephropathy	Pap smear	Papanicolaou smear
pANCA	perinuclear antineutrophil cytoplasmic antibody	PA/PS	pulmonary atresia/ pulmonary stenosis
PANDAS	pediatric autoimmune neuropsychiatric disorders associated with streptococcal infections	PAPVC	partial anomalous pulmonary venous connection
		PAPVR	partial anomalous pulmonary venous return
PANENDO	panendoscopy		
PANESS	physical and neurological examination for soft signs	PAQLQ	Pediatric Asthma Quality of Life Questionnaire
		PAR	parafin
PanIN-1	pancreatic intraepithelial neoplasm (low grade); there is a 1A and 1B		parainfluenza (paramyxovirus) vaccine
			parallel
PanIN-2	pancreatic intraepithelial neoplasm (moderate grade)		perennial allergic rhinitis
			platelet aggregate ratio
PanIN-3	pancreatic intraepithelial neoplasm (high grade)		population attributable risks
PANP	pelvic autonomic nerve preservation		possible allergic reaction
			postanesthetic recovery
PANSS	Positive and Negative Syndrome Scale		procedures, alternatives, and risks
PANSS-EC	Positive and Negative Symptoms of Schizophrenia-Excited Component		pulmonary arteriolar resistance
		PARA	number of pregnancies producing viable offspring
PAO	peak acid output		paraplegic
	peripheral arterial occlusion		parathyroid
PAO₂	alveolar oxygen pressure (tension)	PARA 1	having borne one child
		Paraflu	Parainfluenza

PARC	perennial allergic rhinoconjunctivitis		patient
			percent acceleration time
PAROM	passive assistance range of motion		peripheral arterial tone
			platelet aggregation test
PARR	plasma aldosterone/renin activity ratio		preadmission testing
			pregnancy at term
	postanesthesia recovery room	PATH	Physicians at Teaching Hospitals (Medicare Audit)
PARS	postanesthesia recovery score		pituitary adrenotropic hormone
PARU	postanesthetic recovery unit		pathology
PAS	aminosalicylic acid (para-aminosalicylic acid)	PATP	preadmission testing program
	periodic acid-Schiff (reagent)	PATS	payment at time of service
		PAV	Pavulon (pancuronium bromide)
	peripheral anterior synechia		pre-admission visit (hospice care initial home visit)
	physician-assisted suicide		
	pneumatic antiembolic stocking	PAVe	procarbazine, melphalan (Alkeran), and vinblastine (Velban)
	postanesthesia score		
	premature auricular systole	PAVF	pulmonary arteriovenous fistula
	Professional Activities Study	PAVM	pulmonary arteriovenous malformation
	pulmonary artery stenosis		
	pulsatile antiembolism system (stockings)	PAVNRT	paroxysmal atrial ventricular nodal re-entrant tachycardia
PA-S	Physician Assistant, Student	PAWP	pulmonary artery wedge pressure
PASA	aminosalicylic acid (para-aminosalicylic acid)	PAX	periapical x-ray
PA/S/D	pulmonary artery systolic/diastolic	PB	barometric pressure
			British Pharmacopeia
PASE	Physical Activity Scale for the Elderly		parafin bath
			phenylbutyrate
Pas Ex	passive exercise		piggyback
PASG	pneumatic antishock garment		powder board
			power building
PASI	Psoriasis Area and Severity Index		premature beat
			Presbyterian
PASK	peripheral anterior stromal keratopathy		protein-bound
			Prussian blue
PASP	pulmonary artery systolic pressure		pudendal block
			pyridostigmine bromide (Mestinon)
PASS	Pain Anxiety Symptoms Scale	Pb	lead
PAT	paroxysmal atrial tachycardia		phenobarbital
		p/b	postburn
	passive alloimmune thrombocytopenia	P&B	pain and burning
	patella		Papanicolaou and breast (examinations)

	phenobarbital and belladonna
PBA	percutaneous bladder aspiration
PBAC	Pharmaceutical Benefits Advisory Committee
PBAL	protected bronchoalveolar lavage
PbB	whole blood lead
PBC	point of basal convergence
	prebed care
	primary biliary cirrhosis
PBD	percutaneous biliary drainage
	postburn day
	proliferative breast disease
PBDs	psychotic and behavioral disturbances
PBE	partial breech extraction
	population bioequivalence
	power building exercise
PBF	peripheral blood film
	placental blood flow
	pulmonary blood flow
PBFS	penile blood flow study
PBG	porphobilinogen
	pressure breathing for G protection
	pupillary block glaucoma
PBI	protein-bound iodine
PBK	pseudophakic bullous keratopathy
PBL	peripheral blood lymphocyte
	primary breast lymphoma
	primary brain lymphoma
	problem-based learning
PBLC	premature birth live child
PBM	pharmacy benefit management (manager)
PBMA	polybutylmethacrylate
PBMC	peripheral blood mononuclear cell
PBMNC	peripheral blood mononuclear cell
PBN	polymyxin B sulfate, bacitracin, and neomycin
PB:ND	problem: nursing diagnosis
PBNS	percutaneous bladder neck stabilization

PBO	placebo
PBP	penicillin-binding protein
	phantom breast pain
	protein-bound polysaccharide
PBPC	peripheral blood progenitor cell
PBPCT	peripheral blood progenitor cell transplantation
PBPI	penile-brachial pulse index
PBPs	penicillin-binding proteins
PBS	phosphate-buffered saline
	prune-belly syndrome
PBSC	peripheral blood stem cells
PBT	primary brain tumor
PBT_4	protein-bound thyroxine
$PbtO_2$	brain tissue partial pressure of oxygen
PBV	percutaneous balloon valvuloplasty
PBZ	phenoxybenzamine (Dibenzyline)
	phenylbutazone
	pyribenzamine
ΦBZ	phenylbutazone
PC	after meals (*p.c.* preferred)
	cisplatin (Platinol AQ) and cyclophosphamide
	packed cells
	paclitaxel; carboplatin
	palliative care
	pancreatic carcinoma
	pathologic consultation
	photocoagulation
	placebo-controlled (study)
	platelet concentrate
	Pneumocystis carinii
	poor condition
	politically correct
	popliteal cyst
	posterior canals (vestibular)
	posterior chamber
	prednicarbate
	premature contractions
	present complaint
	productive cough
	professional corporation
	psychiatric counselor
	pubococcygeus (muscle)

P

p.c.	after meals	PCCI	penetrating craniocerebral injuries
PCA	passive cutaneous anaphylaxis	PCCM	primary care case management
	patient care assistant (aide)	PCCU	postcoronary care unit
	patient-controlled analgesia	PCD	pacer-cardioverter-defibrillator
	penicillamine (Cuprimine)		paroxysmal cerebral dysrhythmia
	porous coated anatomic (joint replacement)		plasma cell dyscrasias
	postcardiac arrest		postmortem cesarean delivery
	postciliary artery		primary ciliary dyskinesia
	postconceptional age		programmed cell death
	posterior cerebral artery	PCDAI	Pediatric Crohn Disease Activity Index
	posterior communicating artery	PCE	physical capacities evaluation
	procainamide		potentially compensable event
	procoagulation activity		
	prostate cancer		pseudophakic corneal edema
PCa	prostate cancer	PCE®	erythromycin particles in tablets
PCAC	Physical Care Assessment Center	PCEA	patient-controlled epidural analgesia
P-CAC	preparative continuous annular chromatography	PCEAO	postcarotid endarterectomy airway obstruction
PCAD	posterior circulation arterial dissection	PCEC	purified chick embryo cell (culture)
PCASSO	patient-centered access to secure systems online	PCECV	purified chick embryo cell vaccine
PCB	pancuronium bromide	PCF	pharyngeal conjunctival fever
	para cervical block		
	placebo	PCFL	primary cutaneous follicular lymphoma
	postcoital bleeding		
	prepared childbirth	PCFT	platelet complement fixation test
	procarbazine (Matulane)		
	Pseudomonas cepacia bacteremia	PCG	phonocardiogram
PCBH	personal care boarding home		plasma cell granuloma
			primary congenital glaucoma
PCBMN	palmar cutaneous branch of the median nerve		pubococcygeus (muscle)
PCBs	polychlorinated biphenyls	PCGG	percutaneous coagulation of gasserian ganglion
PCBUN	palmar cutaneous branch of the ulnar nerve	PCGLV	poorly contractile globular left ventricle
PCC	patient care coordinator	PCG/Ts	Primary Care Groups and Trusts
	petrous carotid canal		
	pheochromocytoma	PCH	paroxysmal cold hemoglobinuria
	pneumatosis cystoides coli		
	poison control center		
	precipitated calcium carbonate		
	progressive cardiac care		
PCCC	pediatric critical care center		

	periocular capillary hemangioma
	personal care home
PCHI	permanent childhood hearing impairment
PCHL	permanent childhood hearing loss
PC&HS	after meals and at bedtime
PCI	percutaneous coronary intervention
	pneumatosis cystoides intestinalis
	prophylactic cranial irradiation
PCINA	patient-controlled intranasal analgesia
PCIOL	posterior chamber intraocular lens
PC-IRV	pressure-controlled inverse-ratio ventilation
PCKD	polycystic kidney disease
PCL	pacing cycle length
	plasma cell leukemia
	posterior chamber lens
	posterior cruciate ligament
	proximal collateral ligament
PCLD	polycystic liver disease
PCLI	plasma cell labeling index
PCLN	psychiatric consultation liaison nurse
PCLR	paid claims loss ratio
PCLS	precision-cut lung slices
PCM	pharmaceutical case management
	primary cutaneous melanoma
	protein-calorie malnutrition
	pubococcygeal muscle
PC-MRI	phase-contrast magnetic resonance imaging
PCMX	chloroxylenol
PCN	penicillin
	percutaneous nephrostomy
	primary care nursing
PCNA	proliferating cell nuclear antigen
PCNL	percutaneous nephrostolithotomy
PCNs	posterior cervical nodes
PCNSL	primary central nervous system lymphoma

PCNT	percutaneous nephrostomy tube
PCO	patient complains of
	polycystic ovary
	posterior capsular opacification
PCO₂	partial pressure (tension) of carbon dioxide, artery
PCOD	polycystic ovarian disease
PCOE	prescriber (physician) computer order entry
P COMM A	posterior communicating artery
PCOS	polycystic ovary syndrome
PCP	Palliative Care Program
	patient care plan
	phencyclidine (phenylcyclohexyl piperidine)
	Pneumocystis carinii pneumonia
	primary care person
	primary care physician
	primary care provider
	prochlorperazine (Compazine)
	pulmonary capillary pressure
PCR	patient care report
	percutaneous coronary revascularization
	polymerase chain reaction
	protein catabolic rate
PCr	plasma creatinine
PCRA	pure red-cell aplasia
PCR/PSA	polymerase chain reaction analysis of prostate-specific antigen
PCS	patient care system
	patient-controlled sedation
	personal care service
	photon correlation spectroscopy
	physical component summary
	portable cervical spine
	portacaval shunt
	postconcussion syndrome
P c/s	primary cesarean section
PC-SPES	an herbal refined powder preparation of eight medicinal plants

P

PCT	parasite-clearance time		prism diopter
	percent		probing depth (dental)
	poker chip tool (for rating pain)		progressive disease
			pupillary distance
	porphyria cutanea tarda	P/D	packs per day (cigarettes)
	postcoital test	2PD	two point discriminatory test
	posterior chest tube		
	Primary Care Trust	^{103}Pd	palladium 103
	primary chemotherapy	PDA	parenteral drug abuser
	progesterone challenge test		patent ductus arteriosus
PCTA	percutaneous transluminal angioplasty		pathological demand avoidance (syndrome)
			personal digital assistant
PCU	palliative care unit		poorly differentiated adenocarcinoma
	primary care unit		
	progressive care unit		posterior descending (coronary) artery
	protective care unit		
PCV	packed cell volume		property damage accident
	polycythemia vera	PDAD	photodiode array detector
	pressure-controlled ventilation	PDAF	platelet-derived angiogenesis factor
	procarbazine, lomustine (CCNU [Cee Nu]), and vincristine	PDAP	peritoneal dialysis-associated peritonitis
		PDB	preperitoneal distention balloon
PCV 7	pneumococcal 7-valent conjugate vaccine (Prevnar)	PDC	patient denies complaints
			poorly differentiated carcinoma
PCV 23	pneumococcal vaccine polyvalent (Pneumovax 23; Pnu-Imune 23)		private diagnostic clinic
			property damage collision (crash)
PCVC	percutaneous central venous catheter		pyruvate dehydogenase complex
PCWP	pulmonary capillary wedge pressure	PD&C	postural drainage and clapping
PCX	paracervical		
PCXR	portable chest radiograph	PDCA	Plan-Do-Check-Act (process improvement)
PCZ	procarbazine (Matulane)	PDD	cisplatin (Platinol AQ)
	prochlorperazine (Compazine)		Parkinson disease cases with dementia
PD	interpupillary distance		pervasive developmental disorder
	Paget disease		
	pancreaticoduodenectomy		premenstrual dysphoric disorder
	panic disorder		
	Parkinson disease		primary degenerative dementia
	percutaneous drain		
	peritoneal dialysis	PDDNOS	pervasive developmental disorder, not otherwise specified
	personality disorder		
	pharmacodynamics		
	pocket depth (dental)	PDDs	pervasive developmental disorders
	poorly differentiated		
	postural drainage	PDE	paroxysmal dyspnea on exertion
	pressure dressing		

	pulsed Doppler echocardiography	PDQ-39	Parkinson Disease Questionnaire
PDE 5	phosphodiesterase type 5	PDQ-R	Personality Diagnostic Questionnaire-Revised
PDEGF	platelet-derived epidermal growth factor	PDR	patients' dining room
PDF	Portable Document Format		*Physicians' Desk Reference*
PDFC	premature dead female child		point of decreasing response
PDGF	platelet-derived growth factor		postdelivery room
PDGXT	predischarge graded exercise test		proliferative diabetic retinopathy
PDH	past dental history		prospective drug review
	pyruvate dehydrogenase	PDRcVH	proliferative diabetic retinopathy with vitreous hemorrhage
PDI	Pain Disability Index		
	phasic detrusor instability		
	psychomotor developmental index	PDRP	proliferative diabetic retinopathy
PDIGC	patient dismissed in good condition	PDS	pain dysfunction syndrome
PDL	periodontal ligament		persistent developmental stuttering
	poorly differentiated lymphocytic		polydioxanone suture
	postures of daily living		power Doppler sonography
	preferred drug list		
	progressively diffused leukoencephalopathy		Progressive Deterioration Scale
	pulsed-dye laser	PDSA	Plan, Do, Study, and Act
PDL-D	poorly differentiated lymphocytic-diffuse	PDSS	Postpartum Depression Screening Scale
PDL-N	poorly differentiated lymphocytic-nodular	PDT	percutaneous dilatational tracheostomy
PDMC	premature dead male child		photodynamic therapy
PDN	Paget disease of the nipple		postdisaster trauma
	painful diabetic neuropathy	PDTC	pyrrolidine dithiocarbamate
	prednisone	PDU	pulsed Doppler ultrasonography
	private duty nurse	PDUFA	Prescription Drug User Fee Act (1992)
	prosthetic disk nucleus	PDUR	postdialysis urea rebound
PDNE	poorly differentiated neuroendocrine (carcinoma)		prospective drug utilization review
PDOX	pegylated doxorubicin	PDW	platelet distribution width
PDP	pachydermoperiostosis	PDWHF	platelet-derived wound healing factors
	peak diastolic pressure		
PD & P	postural drainage and percussion	PDWI	proton-density-weighted image(s)
PDPH	postdural puncture headache	PDX	pyridoxine (vitamin B_6)
		PDx	principal diagnosis
PDQ	pretty damn quick (at once)	pDXA	peripheral dual energy x-ray absorptiometry

P

PE	cisplatin (Platinol AQ) and etoposide	PED	paroxysmal exertion-induced dyskinesia
	pedal edema		pediatrics
	pelvic examination		pigment epithelial detachments
	pharyngoesophageal		
	phenytoin equivalent (150 mg of fosphenytoin sodium is equivalent to 100 mg of phenytoin sodium)	PEDD	proton-electron dipole-dipole
		PEDI	pediatric evaluation of disability inventory
		PEDI-DEG	pediatric deglycerolized red blood cells
	physical education (gym)		
	physical examination	Peds	pediatrics
	physical exercise	PEE	punctate epithelial erosion
	plasma exchange	PEEP	positive end-expiratory pressure
	pleural effusion		
	pneumatic equalization	PEF	cisplatin (Platinol AQ), epirubicin, and fluorouracil
	polyethylene		
	preeclampsia		
	premature ejaculation		peak expiratory flow
	pressure equalization	PEFR	peak expiratory flow rate
	pulmonary edema		
	pulmonary embolism	PEFSR	partial expiratory flow static recoil curve
P_1E_1®	epinephrine 1%, pilocarpine 1% ophthalmic solution	PEG	pegylated
			percutaneous endoscopic gastrostomy
P&E	prep and enema		pneumoencephalogram
PE24	Preemie Enfamil 24		polyethylene glycol
PEA	pelvic examination under anesthesia	PEG-ELS	polyethylene glycol and iso-osmolar electrolyte solution
	pre-emptive analgesia		
	pulseless electrical activity		
PEARL	physiologic endometrial ablation/resection loop	PEGG	Parent Education and Guidance Group
	pupils equal accommodation, reactive to light	PEG-J	percutaneous endoscopic gastrojejunostomy
		PEG-JET	percutaneous endoscopic gastrostomy with jejunal extension tube
	pupils equal and reactive to light		
PEARLA	pupils equal and react to light and accommodation	PEG-SOD	polyethylene glycol-conjugated superoxide dismutase (pegorgotein)
PEB	cisplatin, etoposide, and bleomycin	PEI	cisplatin (Platinol AQ), etoposide, and ifosfamide
PEC	pectoralis		
	pulmonary ejection click		percutaneous ethanol injection
PECCE	planned extracapsular cataract extraction		phosphate excretion index
PECHO	prostatic echogram		physical efficiency index
PECHR	peripheral exudative choroidal hemorrhagic retinopathy		polyethylenimine
		PEIT	percutaneous ethanol injection therapy
$PECO_2$	mixed expired carbon dioxide tension	PEJ	percutaneous endoscopic jejunostomy

P

276

PEK	punctate epithelial keratopathy	PERC	perceptual percutaneous
PEL	permissible exposure limits	PERF	perfect perforation
	primary effusion lymphomas	Peri Care	perineum care
PELD	percutaneous endoscopic lumbar diskectomy	PERIO	periodontal disease periodontitis
PELOD	pediatric logistic organ dysfunction (score)	peri-pads PERL	perineal pads pupils equal, reactive to light
PELV	pelvimetry	PERLA	pupils equally reactive to
PEM	prescription event monitoring		light and accommodation
	protein-energy malnutrition	per os	by mouth (this is a
PEMA	phenylethylmalonamide		dangerous abbreviation
PEMS	physical, emotional, mental, and safety		as it is read as left eye)
	post-exercise muscle soreness	PERR	pattern evoked retinal response
PEN	pancreatic endocrine neoplasm	PERRL	pupils equal, round, and reactive to light
	parenteral and enteral nutrition	PERRLA	pupils equal, round, reactive to light and
	Pharmacy Equivalent Name	PERR-LADC	accommodation pupils equal, round,
PENS	percutaneous electrical nerve stimulation		reactive to light and accommodation directly
	percutaneous epidural nerve stimulator	PERRRLA	and consensually pupils equal, round,
PEO	progressive external ophthalmoplegia		regular, react to light and accommodation
PEP	patient education program	PERS	personal emergency response systems
	pharmacologic erection program	PERT	pancreatic enzyme replacement therapy
	positive expiratory pressure		program evaluation and review technique
	postexposure prophylaxis	PERV	porcine endogenous
	preejection period		retroviruses
	protein electrophoresis	PER$_w$	pertussis, whole-cell
PEP/ET	pre-ejection period/ ejection time	PES	antigens, vaccine polyethersulfone
PEPI	preejection period index		preexcitation syndrome
PEPP	payment error prevention program		programmed electrical stimulation
PER	by		pseudoexfoliation
	pediatric emergency room		syndrome
	pertussis (whooping cough) vaccine,	PESA	percutaneous epididymal sperm aspiration
	antigens not otherwise unspecified	peSPL	peak equivalent sound pressure level
	protein efficiency ratio	PET	poor exercise tolerance
PER$_a$	pertussis, acellular antigen(s), vaccine		positron-emission tomography

P

	preeclamptic toxemia	PFGE	pulsed field gel
	pressure equalizing tubes		electrophoresis
	problem elicitation	PfHRP-2	*Plasmodium falciparum*
	technique		histidine-rich protein 2
PETN	pentaerythritol tetranitrate	PFHx	positive family history
PEX	plasma exchange	PFI	pill-free intervals
	pseudoexfoliation		progression-free interval
	(glaucoma)	PFJ	patellofemoral joint
PEx	physical examination	PFJS	patellofemoral joint
PEX# 3	plasma exchange number		syndrome
	three	PFL	cisplatin (Platinol AQ),
PF	patellofemoral		fluorouracil, and
	peak flow		leucovorin
	peripheral fields	PFL+IFN	cisplatin (Platinol AQ),
	plantar flexion		fluorouracil, leucovorin,
	Pontiac fever		and interferon alfa 2b
	power factor	PFM	peak flow meter
	preservative free		porcelain fused to metal
	prostatic fluid		primary fibromyalgia
	pulmonary fibrosis	PFME	pelvic floor muscle
	push fluids		exercise
Pf	*Plasmodium falciparum*	PFO	patent foramen ovale
PF3	platelet factor 3	PFP	progression free
PF4	platelet factor 4		probability
16PF	The Sixteen Personality		proinsulin fusion protein
	Factors test	PFPC	Pall filtered packed cells
PFA	foscarnet	PFPS	patellofemoral pain
	(phosphonoformatic		syndrome
	acid) (Foscavir)	PFR	parotid flow rate
	patellofemoral arthritis		peak flow rate
	platelet function analysis	PFRC	plasma-free red cells
	psychological first aid	PFROM	pain-free range of motion
	pure free acid	PFS	patellar femoral syndrome
PFB	potential for breakdown		patient financial services
	pseudofolliculitis barbae		prefilled syringe
PFC	patient-focused care		preservative-free solution
	perfluorochemical		(system)
	permanent flexure		primary fibromyalgia
	contracture		syndrome
	persistent fetal circulation		progression-free survival
	prolonged febrile		pulmonary function
	convulsions		studies (study)
P̄ FEEDS	after feedings	PFSH	past, family, and social
PFFD	proximal femoral focal		history (histories)
	deficiency (defect)	PFT	parafascicular thalamotomy
PFFFP	Pall filtered fresh frozen		pulmonary function test
	plasma	PFTC	primary fallopian tube
PFG	patellofemoral grind		carcinoma
	percutaneous fluoroscopic	PFU	plaque-forming unit
	gastrostomy	PFW	pHisoHex® face wash
	proximal femur	PFWB	Pall filtered whole blood
	geometry		Psychological General
	pulsed-field gradient		Well-Being (index)

P

PFWT	pain-free walking time		primary gastric lymphoma
PG	paged in hospital	PGM	paternal grandmother
	paregoric		phosphoglucomutase
	performance goal (short-term goal)	PGP	paternal grandparent
	phosphatidylglycerol	Pgp	P-glycoprotein
	picogram (pg) (10^{-12} gram)	PGR	pulse-generated runoff
		PgR	progesterone receptor
	placental grade (biophysical profile)	P-graph	penile plethysmograph
	polygalacturonate	PGS	Persian Gulf syndrome
	practice guidelines	PGT	play-group therapy
	pregnant	P±GTC	partial seizures with or without generalized tonic-clonic seizures
	prostaglandin		
	pyoderma gangrenosum		
PGA	prostaglandin A	pGTD	persistent gestational trophoblastic disease
	prothrombin time, **g**amma-glutamyl transpeptidase activity, and serum **a**polipoprotein AI concentration	PG-TXL	poly (L-glutamic acid)-paclitaxel
		PGU	postgonococcal urethritis
		PGW	person gametocyte week
		PGY-1	postgraduate year one (first year resident)
PGBD	polyglucosan body disease	pH	hydrogen ion concentration
PGCH	postinfantile giant cell hepatitis	PH	past history
			personal history
PGCR	pharyngoglottal closure reflex		pinhole
			poor health
PGCs	primordial germ cells		pubic hair
PGD	preimplantation genetic diagnosis		public health
			pulmonary hypertension
PGE	partial generalized epilepsy	P&H	physical and history
		Ph[1]	Philadelphia chromosome
	posterior gastroenterostomy	PHA	arterial pH
			passive hemagglutinating
	proximal gastric exclusion		paternal history of alcoholism
PGE₁	alprostadil (prostaglandin E₁)		peripheral hyperalimentation
PGE₂	dinoprostone (prostaglandin E₂)		phenylalanine
PGF	paternal grandfather		phytohemagglutinin antigen
PGF₂∝	dinoprost (prostaglandin F₂∝)		postoperative holding area
PGGF	paternal great-grandfather		
PGGM	paternal great-grandmother	PHACO	phacoemulsification
		PHACO OD	phacoemulsification of the right eye
PGH	pituitary growth hormones	PHACO OS	phacoemulsification of the left eye
PGI	potassium, glucose, and insulin	PHAL	peripheral hyperalimentation
PGI₂	epoprostenol (Prostacyclin)	PHAR	pharmacist
			pharmacy
PGL	persistent generalized lymphadenopathy		pharynx

P

Pharm	Pharmacy
PharmD	Doctor of Pharmacy
PHb	pyridoxylated hemoglobin
PHC	permissive hypercapnia
	posthospital care
	primary health care
	primary hepatocellular carcinoma
PHCA	profound hypothermic cardiac arrest
PHD	paroxysmal hypnogenic dyskinesia
	Public Health Department
PhD	Doctor of Philosophy
PHE	periodic health examination
PHEN-FEN	phentermine and fenfluramine
PHEO	pheochromocytoma
PHEP	progressive home exercise program
PHF	paired helical filament
PHG	portal hypertensive gastropathy
PHH	paraesophageal hiatus hernia
	posthemorrhagic hydrocephalus
PHHI	persistent hyperinsulinemic hypoglycemia of infancy
PHI	patient health information
	phosphohexose isomerase
	prehospital index
	protected health information
PHIS	posthead injury syndrome
PHL	permanent hearing loss
	Philadelphia (chromosome)
PHLIS	Public Health Laboratory Information System
PHLS	Public Health Laboratory Service (United Kingdom)
PHM	partial hydatidiform mole
	preventative health maintenance
PHMB	polyhexamethylene biguanide
PHMD	polyhexamethylene (Baquacil, a pool cleaner)

PHN	postherpetic neuralgia
	public health nurse
	Puritan® heated nebulizer
PHNC	public health nurse coordinator
PHNI	pinhole no improvement
PHO	Physician/Hospital Organization
PHOB	phobic anxiety
PHP	pooled human plasma
	postheparin plasma
	prepaid health plan
	pseudohypoparathyroidism
	pyridoxalated hemoglobin polyoxyethylene conjugate
PHPPO	Public Health Practice Program Office
PHPT	primary hyperparathyroidism
PHPV	persistent hyperplastic primary vitreous
PHR	peak heart rate
	personal health record
PhRMA	Pharmaceutical Research and Manufacturers of America
PHS	partial hospitalization program
	US Public Health Service
PHT	phenytoin (Dilantin)
	portal hypertension
	posterior hyaloidal traction
	postmenopausal hormone therapy
	primary hyperthyroidism
	pulmonary hypertension
PHTC	pulmonary hypertensive crises
PHV	peak height velocity
	pediatric health visit
PHVA	pinhole visual acuity
pHVA	plasma homovanillic acid
PHVD	posthemorrhagic ventricular dilatation
PHx	past history
Phx	pharynx
PHY	physician
PhyO	physician's orders
PI	package insert
	pallidal index

pancreatic insufficiency

Pearl Index

performance improvement

peripheral iridectomy

persistent illness

physically impaired

poison ivy

postincident

postinjury

premature infant

present illness

principal investigator

protease inhibitor

pulmonary infarction

pulmonic insufficiency

PI-3   parainfluenza 3 virus

P & I   probe and irrigation

PIA   personal injury
    accident

polysaccharide
    intercellular adhesine

PIAT   Peabody Individual
    Achievement Test

PIB   partial ileal bypass

professional information
    brochure

PIBD   paucity of interlobular
    bile ducts

PIBF   progesterone-induced
    blocking factor

PIC   penicillin-inhibitor
    combinations

peripherally inserted
    catheter

personal injury collision
    (crash)

polysaccharide-iron
    complex

postintercourse

PICA   Porch Index of
    Communicative Ability

posterior inferior
    cerebellar artery

posterior inferior
    communicating artery

PICC   peripherally inserted
    central catheter

PICHI   pulse-inversion contrast
    harmonic imaging

PICT   pancreatic islet cell
    transplantation

PICU   pediatric intensive care
    unit

psychiatric intensive care
    unit

PICVA   percutaneous *in situ*
    coronary venous
    arterialization

PICVC   peripherally inserted
    central venous catheter

PID   pelvic inflammatory
    disease

primary
    immunodeficiency

prolapsed intervertebral
    disk

proportional-integral-
    derivative (controller)

PIE   pulmonary infiltration
    with eosinophilia

pulmonary interstitial
    emphysema

PIEE   pulsed irrigation for
    enhanced evacuation

PIF   peak inspiratory flow

PIFG   poor intrauterine fetal
    growth

PIG   pertussis immune
    globulin

PIGI   pregnancy-induced
    glucose intolerance

PIGN   postinfectious
    glomerulonephritis

PIH   pregnancy-induced
    hypertension

preventricular
    intraventricular
    hemorrhage

prolactin-inhibiting
    hormone

PIIID   peripheral indwelling
    intermediate infusion
    device

PIIIP   aminoterminal type three
    procollagen propeptide

PIIS   posterior inferior iliac
    spine

PIL   patient information
    leaflet

purpose in life

PILO   pilocarpine

PIM   Program Integrity Manual

pulse-inversion mode
    (ultrasound)

PIMIA   potentiometric ionophore
    mediated immunoassay

P

PIMS	programmable implantable medication system	
PIN	pain in the neck (no place for such a term in a written document)	
	personal identification number	
	posterior interosseous nerve	
	prostatic intraepithelial neoplasia	
	provider identification number	
PIND	progressive intellectual and neurological deterioration	
PINS	persons in need of supervision	
PIO	pemoline (Cylert)	
PIO_2	partial pressure of inspired oxygen	
PIOK	poikilocytosis	
PIP	peak inspiratory pressure	
	postictal psychosis	
	postinfusion phlebitis	
	proximal interphalangeal (joint)	
	pulmonary immaturity of prematurity	
	pulmonary insufficiency of the premature	
PIPB	performance index phonetic balance	
PI-PB	performance intensity-phonemically balanced	
PIPIDA	N-para-isopropyl-acetanilide-iminodiacetic acid	
PIPJ	proximal interphalangeal joint	
PIPP	Premature Infant Pain Profile	
PIP/TZ	piperacillin-tazobactam (Zosyn)	
PIQ	Performance Intelligence Quotient (part of Wechsler tests)	
PIR	pirarubicin	
PIS	pregnancy interruption service	
PISA	phase invariant signature algorithm	

proximal isovelocity surface area

PIT	patellar inhibition test
	peak isometric torque
	Pitocin (oxytocin)
	Pitressin (vasopressin) (this is a dangerous abbreviation as it can be taken for Pitocin)
	pituitary
	pulsed-inotrope therapy
PITP	pseudo-idiopathic thrombocytopenic purpura
PITR	plasma iron turnover rate
PIV	peripheral intravenous
PIV-3	parainfluenza virus type 3
PIVD	protruded intervertebral disk
PIVH	periventricular-intraventricular hemorrhage
PIVKA	proteins induced in vitamin K absence
PIWT	partially impacted wisdom teeth
PIXI	Peripheral Instantaneous X-ray Imaging (dual-energy x-ray absorptiometry system)
PJ	procelin jacket (crown)
PJB	premature junctional beat
PJC	premature junctional contractions
PJI	prosthetic joint infection
PJRT	permanent form of junctional reciprocating tachycardia
PJS	peritoneojugular shunt
	Peutz-Jeghers syndrome
PJT	paroxysmal junctional tachycardia
PJVT	paroxysmal junctional-ventricular tachycardia
PK	penetrating keratoplasty
	pharmacokinetics
	plasma potassium
	pyruvate kinase
PKB	prone knee bend
PKC	protein kinase C
PKD	paroxysmal kinesigenic dyskinesia
	polycystic kidney disease

PKDL	post-kala-azar dermal leishmaniasis	PLC	peripheral lymphocyte count
PKI	public key infrastructure		pityriasis lichenoides chronica
PKND	paroxysmal nonkinesigenic dyskinesia	PLCH	pulmonary Langerhans cell histiocytosis
PKP	penetrating keratoplasty	PLD	partial lower denture
PK/PD	pharmacokinetic/ pharmacodynamic		pegylated liposomal doxorubicin
PKR	phased knee rehabilitation		percutaneous laser diskectomy
PK Test	Prausnitz-Küstner transfer test	PLDD	percutaneous laser disk decompression
PKU	phenylketonuria	PLE	polymorphic light eruption
pk yrs	pack-years (smoking one pack of cigarettes a day for one year is termed 1 pack-year of smoking, thus 2 packs a day for 20 years would be 40 pack-years)		protein-losing enteropathy
		PLED	periodic lateralizing epileptiform discharge
		PLEVA	pityriasis lichenoides et varioliformis acuta
PL	light perception	PLF	prior level of function
	palmaris longus	PLFC	premature living female child
	peroneus longus		
	pharyngolaryngectomy	PLG	plague (*Yersinia pestis*) (*la Peste*) vaccine
	place		
	placebo	PlGF	placental growth factor
	plantar	PLH	paroxysmal localized hyperhidrosis
	plethoric (infant color)		
	transpulmonary pressure	PLIF	posterior lumbar interbody fusion
PLA	placebo		
	Plasma-Lyte A	PLIL	partial laryngectomy with imbrication laryngoplasty
	polylactic acid		
	posterolateral (coronary) artery	PLL	posterior longitudinal ligament
	potentially lethal arrhythmia		prolymphocytic leukemia
		PLLA	poly-l-lactic acid (Sculptra)
	Product License Application	PLM	partial lateral meniscectomy
	pulpolinguoaxial		
PLAD	proximal left anterior descending (artery)		periodic leg movement
			Plasma-Lyte M
Plan B®	levonorgestrel (a progestogen emergency contraceptive)		polarized-light microscope
			precise lesion measuring (device)
PLAP	placental alkaline phosphatase		product-line manager
PLAT C	platelet concentration	PLMC	premature living male child
PLAT P	platelet pheresis		
PLAX	parasternal long axis	PLMD	periodic limb movement disorder
PLB	phospholamban		
	placebo	PLMS	periodic limb movements during sleep
	posterolateral branch		
PLBO	placebo		

PLN	pelvic lymph node		physical medicine
	popliteal lymph node		pneumomediastinum
PLND	pelvic lymph node		poliomyelitis
	dissection		polymyositis
PLO	pluronic lecithin		poor metabolizers
	organogels		postmenopausal
PLOF	previous level of		postmortem
	functioning		presents mainly
PLOSA	physiologic low stress		pretibial myxedema
	angioplasty		primary motivation
PLP	partial		prostatic massage
	laryngopharyngectomy		pulpomesial
	phantom limb pain	Pm	*Plasmodium malariae*
	protolipid protein	PM$_{10}$	particulate matter less
PLPH	postlumbar puncture		than 10 micrometers
	headache		diameter
PLR	pupillary light reflex	PMA	positive mental attitude
PLRT	postlumpectomy		premarket approval
	radiotherapy		(application) (for
PLS	Papillon-Lefèvre		medical devices)
	syndrome		premenstrual asthma
	phantom limb syndrome		primary meningococcal
	plastic surgery		arthritis
	point locator stimulator		Prinzmetal angina
	Preschool Language Scale		progress myoclonic ataxia
	primary lateral sclerosis	PMAA	Premarket Approval
PLs	premalignant lesions		Application (medical
PLSD	protected least significant		devices)
	difference (statistical	PMB	polymorphonuclear
	test)		basophil (leukocytes)
PLSO	posterior leafspring		polymyxin B
	orthosis		postmenopausal bleeding
PLST	progressively lowered	PMC	premature mitral closure
	stress threshold		pseudomembranous colitis
PLSURG	plastic surgery	PMCP	para-monochlorophenol
PLT	platelet		perinatal mortality
PLT EST	platelet estimate		counseling program
PLTF	plaintiff	PMCT	perinatal mortality
PLTS	platelets		counseling team
PLUG	plug the lung until it		postmortem computed
	grows		tomography
PLV	posterior left ventricular	PMD	perceptual motor
PLX	plexus		development
PLYO	plyometric		primary myocardial
PLZF	promyelocytic leukemia		disease
	zinc finger		primidone (Mysoline)
PM	afternoon		private medical doctor
	evening		progressive muscular
	pacemaker		dystrophy
	papillary muscles	PMDD	premenstrual dysphoric
	paraspinal mapping		disorder
	particulate matter	pMDI	pressurized metered-dose
	petit mal		inhaler

PM/DM	polymyositis and dermatomyositis	PMO	postmenopausal osteoporosis
PME	pelvic muscle exercise	pmol	picomole
	phosphomonoester(s)	PMP	pain management program
	polymorphonuclear esosinophil (leukocytes)		previous menstrual period
	postmenopausal estrogen		psychotropic medication plan
	progressive myoclonus epilepsy	PMPA	tenofovir (Viread)
PMEALS	after meals	PMPM	per member, per month
PMEC	pseudomembranous enterocolitis	PMPO	postmenopausal palpable ovary
PMF	peptide mass fingerprinting	PMPY	per member, per year
	progressive massive fibrosis	PMR	pacemaker rhythm
	pupils mid-position, fixed		percutaneous revascularization
PMH	past medical history		polymorphic reticulosis
PMHx	past medical history		polymyalgia rheumatica
PMI	Pain Management Index		premedication regimen
	past medical illness		prior medical record
	patient medication instructions		progressive muscle relaxation
	plea of mental incompetence		proportional mortality ratios
	point of maximal impulse	PM&R	physical medicine and rehabilitation
	posterior myocardial infarction	PMRT	postmastectomy radiation
PMID	PubMed Unique Identifier (National Library of Medicine)	PMS	performance measurement system
			periodic movements of sleep
PML	polymorphonuclear leukocytes		poor miserable soul
	posterior mitral leaflet		postmarketing surveillance
	premature labor		postmenopausal syndrome
	progressive multifocal leukoencephalopathy		premenstrual syndrome
	promyelocytic leukemia		pulse, motor, and sensory
PMLCL	primary mediastinal large-cell lymphoma	PMSF	phenylmethylsulfonyl fluoride
PMMA	polymethyl methacrylate	PMT	pacemaker-mediated tachycardia
PMMF	pectoralis major myocutaneous flap		point of maximum tenderness
PMN	polymodal nociceptors		premenstrual tension
	polymorphonuclear leukocyte	PMTS	premenstrual tension syndrome
	Premarket Notification (medical devices)	PMV	percutaneous mitral (balloon) valvuloplasty
PMNL	polymorphonuclear leukocyte		prolapse of mitral valve
		PMW	pacemaker wires
PMNN	polymorphonuclear neutrophil	PMZ	postmenopausal zest
		PN	parenteral nutrition
PMNS	postmalarial neurological syndrome		peanut (when testing for an allergy)

P

percussion note
percutaneous nephrosonogram
percutaneous nucleotomy
periarteritis nodosa
peripheral neuropathy
pneumonia
polyarteritis nodosa
poorly nourished
positional nystagmus
postnasal
postnatal
practical nurse
premie nipple
primary nurse
progress note
pyelonephritis

P & N pins and needles
psychiatry and neurology

PN₂ partial pressure of nitrogen

PNA Pediatric Nurse Associate
pneumonia
polynitroxyl albumin

PNa plasma sodium

PNAB percutaneous needle aspiration biopsy

PNAC parenteral nutrition associated cholestasis

PNAR perennial nonallergic rhinitis

PNAS prudent no added salt

PNB percutaneous needle biopsy
popliteal nerve block
premature newborn
premature nodal beat
prostate needle biopsy

PNC penicillin
peripheral nerve conduction
postnecrotic cirrhosis
premature nodal contraction
prenatal care
prenatal course
Psychiatric Nurse Clinician

PNCV7 pneumococcal 7-valent conjugate vaccine (Prevnar)

PND paroxysmal nocturnal dyspnea
pelvic node dissection

postnasal drip
pregnancy, not delivered

PNDS Perioperative Nursing Data Set
postnasal drip syndrome

PNE peripheral neuroepithelioma
primary nocturnal enuresis

PNET primitive neuroectodermal tumors

PNET-MB primitive neuroectodermal tumors-medulloblastoma

PNEUMO pneumothorax

PNF primary nonfunction
proprioceptive neuromuscular fasciculation (reaction)

PNFA progressive nonfluent aphasia

PNH paroxysmal nocturnal hemoglobinuria
polynitroxyl-hemoglobin

PNI peripheral nerve injury
Prognostic Nutrition Index

PNKD paroxysmal nonkinesigenic dyskinesia

PNL percutaneous nephrolithotomy

PNMG persistent neonatal myasthenia gravis

PNMT phenylethanolamine-N-methyltransferase

PNNP Perinatal Nurse Practitioner

PNP peak negative pressure
Pediatric Nurse Practitioner
progressive nuclear palsy
purine nucleoside phosphorylase

PNR physician's nutritional recommendation

PNRB partial non-rebreather (oxygen mask)

PNS partial nonprogressing stroke
peripheral nerve stimulator
peripheral nervous system
practical nursing student

PNSP penicillin-nonsusceptible *Streptococcus pneumoniae*

PNT	percutaneous nephrostomy tube	POB	phenoxybenzamine (Dibenzyline)
	percutaneous neuromodulatory therapy		place of birth
		POBC	primary operable breast cancer
pnthx	pneumothorax	POC	plans of care
PNTML	pudendal-nerve terminal motor latency		point-of-care
			position of comfort
PNU	pneumococcal (*Streptococcus pneumoniae*) vaccine, not otherwise specified		postoperative care
			product of conception
		POCD	postoperative cognitive dysfunction
	protein nitrogen units	POCT	point-of-care testing (test)
PNUcn-7	pneumococcal (*Streptococcus pneumoniae*) conjugate vaccine, 7-valent vaccine (Prevnar)		point-of-care therapy
		POD	pacing on demand
			place of death
			Podiatry
			polycystic ovarian disease
PNUps23	pneumococcal (*Streptococcus pneumoniae*) polysaccharide, 23-valent vaccine (Pneumovax-23; Pnu-Imune-23)	POD 1	postoperative day one
		PODx	preoperative diagnosis
		POE	patient-oriented evidence
			point (portal, port) of entry
			position of ease
			prone on elbows
			provider order entry
PNV	postoperative nausea and vomiting	POEM	Patient-Oriented Evidence That Matters
	prenatal vitamins	POEMS	plasma cell dyscrasia with polyneuropathy, organomegaly, endocrinopathy, monoclonal protein (M-protein), and skin changes
Pnx	pneumonectomy
	pneumothorax
PO	by mouth
	phone order
	polonium
	postoperative
Po	*Plasmodium ovale*	POEx	postoperative exercise
	punctal occlusion	POF	physician's order form
P&O	parasites and ova		position of function
	prosthetics and orthotics		premature ovarian failure
PO_2	partial pressure (tension) of oxygen, artery	P of I	proof of illness
		POG	Pediatric Oncology Group
PO_4	phosphate		Penthrane,® oxygen, and gas (nitrous oxide)
POA	pancreatic oncofetal antigen		products of gestation
	power of attorney	POGO	percentage of glottic opening
	present on arrival	POH	perillyl alcohol
	primary optic atrophy		personal oral hygiene
POACH	prednisone, vincristine (Oncovin), doxorubicin (Adriamycin), cyclophosphamide, and cytarabine		presumed ocular histoplasmosis
			progressive osseous heteroplasia
			prone on hands
POAG	primary open-angle glaucoma	POHA	preoperative holding area

POHI	physically or otherwise health impaired		persistent organic pollutants
POHS	by mouth, at bedtime		plaster of paris
	presumed ocular histoplasmosis syndrome		popiliteal
			posterior oral pharynx
		POp	postoperative
POI	Personal Orientation Inventory	POPC	Pediatric Overall Performance Category (scale)
	postoperative ileus		
	postoperative instructions	poplit	popliteal
POIB	place outpatient in inpatient bed	POPs	persistent organic pollutants
POIK	poikilocytosis		progesterone-only pills
POL	physician's office laboratory	POR	physician of record
			problem-oriented record
	poliovirus vaccine, not otherwise specified	PORP	partial ossicular replacement prosthesis
	premature onset of labor	PORR	postoperative recovery room
POLS	postoperative length of stay	PORT	perioperative respiratory therapy
POLY	polychromic erythrocytes		portable
	polymorphonuclear leukocyte		postoperative radiotherapy
POLY-CHR	polychromatophilia		postoperative respiratory therapy
POM	pain on motion		
	polyoximethylene	POS	parosteal osteosarcoma
	prescription-only medication		physician's order sheet
			point-of-service
POMA	Performance-Oriented Mobility Assessment		positive
POMC	pro-opiomelanocortin	POSHPATE	problem, onset, associated symptoms, previous history, precipitating factors, alleviating/ aggravation factors, timing, an etiology (prompts for taking history and chief complaint)
POMP	prednisone, vincristine (Oncovin), methotrexate, and mercaptopurine (Purinthol)		
POMR	problem-oriented medical record		
POMS	Profile of Mood States	poss	possible
POMS-FI	Fatigue-Inertia Subscale of the Profile of Mood States	post	posterior
			postmortem examination (autopsy)
PON	postoperative note	PostC	posterior chamber
PONI	postoperative narcotic infusion	PostCap	posterior capsule
		Post-M	urine specimen after prostate massage
PONV	postoperative nausea and vomiting	post op	postoperative
POOH	postoperative open heart (surgery)	Post Sag D	posterior sagittal diameter
		post tib	posterial tibial
POOL	premature onset of labor	PostVD	posterior vitreous detachment
POP	pain on palpation		
	persistent occipitoposterior	POSYC	Pain Observation Scale for Young Children

POT	peak occupancy time		postpartum amenorrhea
	plans of treatment		primary progressive
	potassium		aphasia
	potential	PP&A	palpation, percussion, and
	primary orthostatic tremor		auscultation
POTS	postural tachycardia	PPAR$_g$	peroxisome-proliferator-
	syndrome		activated receptor
POU	placenta, ovaries, and		gamma
	uterus	PPARs	peroxisome proliferator-
POV	privately owned vehicle		activated receptors
POW	Powassan (virus)	PPAS	postpolio atrophy
	prisoner of war		syndrome
POWSBP	pulse oximetry waveform	PPB	parts per billion
	systolic blood pressure		pleuropulmonary blastoma
POX	pulse oximeter (reading)		positive pressure breathing
PP	near point of		prostate puncture biopsy
	accommodation	PPBE	postpartum breast
	pancreatic pseudocyst		engorgment
	paradoxical pulse	PPBS	postprandial blood sugar
	partial upper and lower	PPBTL	postpartum bilateral tubal
	dentures		ligation
	pedal pulse	PPC	plaster of paris cast
	per protocol		positive product control
	periodontal pockets		primary peritoneal
	peripheral pulses		carcinoma
	pin prick		progressive patient care
	pink puffer (emphysema)	PPCD	posterior polymorphous
	Planned Parenthood		corneal dystrophy
	plasmapheresis	PPCF	plasma prothrombin
	plaster of paris		conversion factor
	poor person	PPD	packs per day
	posterior pituitary		permanent partial
	postpartum		disability (rating)
	postprandial		pinch-point density
	presenting part		(histologic)
	private patient		posterior polymorphous
	prophylactics		dystrophy
	protoporphyria		postpartum day
	proximal phalanx		postpartum depression
	pulse pressure		probing pocket depth
	push pills		(dental)
P-P	probability-probability		purified protein derivative
	(plots)		(of tuberculin)
P&P	pins and plaster		pylorus-sparing
	policy and procedure		pancreaticoduodenectomy
PIIIP	aminoterminal type three	P & PD	percussion & postural
	protocollegan		drainage
	propeptide	PPD-B	purified protein
PPIX	protoporphyrin nine		derivative, Battey
PPA	palpation, percussion, and	PPDR	preproliferative diabetic
	auscultation		retinopathy
	phenylpropanolamine	PPD-S	purified protein
	phenylpyruvic acid		derivative, standard

P

PPE	palmar-plantar erythro-dysesthesia (syndrome)	PPL	pars plana lensectomy
		Ppl	pleural pressure
	personal protective equipment	PPLO	pleuropneumonia-like organisms
	professional performance evaluation	PPLOV	painless progressive loss of vision
	pruritic papular eruption	PPM	parts per million
PPES	palmar-plantar erythrodysesthesia syndrome		permanent pacemaker
			persistent pupillary membrane
	pedal pulses equal and strong		physician practice management
PPF	pellagra preventive factor	PPMA	postpoliomyelitis muscular atrophy
	plasma protein fraction	PPMS	psychophysiologic musculoskeletal (reaction)
PPG	photoplethysmography		
	portal pressure gradients		
	postprandial glucose		
	pylorus-preserving gastrectomy	PPMs	potentially pathogenic microorganisms
PPGI	psychophysiologic gastrointestinal (reaction)	PPN	peripheral parenteral nutrition
PPGSS	papular-purpuric "glove and socks" syndrome	PPNAD	primary pigmented nodular adrenocortical disease
PPH	postpartum hemorrhage	PPNG	penicillinase-producing *Neisseria gonorrhoeae*
	primary postpartum hemorrhage	PPO	permanent punctal occlusion
	primary pulmonary hypertension		preferred provider organization
PPHN	persistent pulmonary hypertension of the newborn		pump-prime only
		PPOB	postpartum obstetrics
PPHTN	portopulmonary hypertension	PPP	patient prepped and positioned
PPHx	previous psychiatric history		pearly penile papules
			pedal pulse present
PPIX	protoporphyrin nine		peripheral pulses palpable (present)
PPI	patient package insert		platelet-poor plasma
	permanent pacemaker insertion		postpartum psychosis
	prepulse inhibition		preferred practice patterns
	Present Pain Intensity		proportional pulse pressure (SBP minus DBP)/SBP
	proton-pump inhibitor		
	Psychopathic Personality Inventory		
PPIA	parental presence during induction of anesthesia		protamine paracoagulation phenomenon
PPIVMs	passive physiological intervertebral movements	PPPBL	peripheral pulses palpable both legs
PPJ	pure pancreatic juice	PPPD	pylorus-preserving pancreatoduodenectomy
PPK	population pharmacokinetics	PPPG	postprandial plasma glucose

PPPM	Parents' Postoperative Pain Measure	PPVT	Peabody Picture Vocabulary Test
	per patient, per month	PPW	plantar puncture wound
PPPY	per patient, per year		premature P-wave
PPQ	Postoperative Pain Questionnaire	PPY	packs per year (cigarettes)
PPR	patient progress record	PQ	pronator quadratus
PPr	periodontal prophylactics	pQCT	peripheral quantitative computed tomography
PPRC	Physician Payment Review Commission	PQOCN	Psychiatric Questionnaire Obsessive-Compulsive Neurosis
pPROM	premature rupture of the membranes before 37 weeks gestation	PQRI	Product Quality Research Initiative
PPS	pentosan polysulfate (Elmiron)	PR	far point of accommodation
	peripheral pulmonary stenosis		pack removal
	per protocol set		partial remission
	postpartum sterilization		partial response
	post-pericardiotomy syndrome		patient relations
	postperfusion syndrome		perennial rhinitis
	postpoliomyelitis syndrome		per rectum
			pityriasis rosea
	postpump syndrome		premature
	prospective payment system		profile
			progressive resistance
	pulses per second		prolonged remission
PPSS	peripheral protein sparing solution		prone
			Protestant
PPT	parts-per-trillion		Puerto Rican
	person, place, and time		pulmonic regurgitation
	Physical Performance Test	P=R	pulse rate
	posterior pelvic tilt	P=R	pupils equal in size and reaction
PPTg	pedunculopontine tegmental nucleus	P & R	pelvic and rectal
PPTL	postpartum tubal ligation		pulse and respiration
PPTR	pulsed photothermal radiometry	PR-2	Bennett pressure ventilator
PPU	perforated peptic ulcer	PRA	panel reactive antibodies (organ transplants)
PPV	pars plana vitrectomy		percent reactive antibody
	patent processus vaginalum		plasma renin activity
	percutaneous polymethylmethacrylate vertebroplasty	PRAFO	pressure relief ankle-foot orthosis
	phakomatosis pigmentovascularis	PRAMS	Pregnancy Risk Assessment Monitoring System
	pneumococcal polysaccharide vaccine	PRAT	platelet radioactive antiglobulin test
	positive predictive value	PRBC	packed red blood cells
	positive-pressure ventilation	PRC	packed red cells
			peer review committee

PRCA	pure red cell aplasia	passive range of motion
PrCa	prostate cancer	phosphoribomutase
PRD	polycystic renal disease	photoreceptor membrane
PRE	passive resistance exercises	prematurely ruptured membrane
	progressive resistive exercise	primidone (Mysoline)
		PRMF — preretinal macular fibrosis
	proton relaxation enhancement	PRM-SDX — pyrimethamine; sulfadoxine (Fansidar)
Pred	prednisone	*p.r.n.* — as occasion requires
PREG	Pregestimil® (infant formula)	PRNS — phrenic repetitive nerve stimulation
Pre-M	urine specimen before prostate massage	PRO — Professional Review Organization
PREMIE	premature infant	proline
pre-op	before surgery	pronation
prep	prepare for surgery	protein
	preposition	prothrombin
PRERLA	pupils round, equal, react to light and accommodation	prob — probable
		PROCTO — procotoscopic proctology
prev	prevent previous	PROG — prognathism prognosis program progressive
PRFD	percutaneous radio-frequency denervation	
PRFNB	percutaneous radio-frequency facet nerve block	PROM — passive range of motion premature rupture of membranes
PRG	phleborheogram	ProMACE — prednisone, methotrexate, calcium leucovorin, doxorubicin (Adriamycin), cyclophosphamide, and etoposide
PRH	past relevant history postocclusive reactive hyperemia preretinal hemorrhage	
PRI	Pain Rating Index Patient Review Instrument	PROMM — passive range of motion machine
prim	primary	
PRIMIP	primipara (1st pregnancy)	Promy — promyelocyte
PR interval	part of the electrocardiographic cycle from onset of atrial depolarization on onset of ventricular depolarization	PRO MYELO — promyelocytes
		PRON — pronation
		PROS — prostate prosthesis
PRISM	Pediatric Risk of Mortality Score	PROT REL — protrusive relationship
PRIT®	pretargeted radioimmunotherapy	prov — provisional
		PROVIMI — proteins, vitamins, and minerals
PRK	photorefractive keratectomy	PROX — proximal
PRL	prolactin	PRP — panretinal photocoagulation patient recovery plan penicllinase-resistant penicillin
PRLA	pupils react to light and accommodation	
PRM	partial rebreathing mask	

	penicillin-resistant pneumococci	PRZF	pyrazofurin
	pityriasis rubra pilaris	PS	paradoxic sleep
	platelet rich plasma		paranoid schizophrenia
	polyribose ribitol phosphate		pathologic stage
			patient's serum
	poor progression of R wave in precordial leads		performance status
			peripheral smear
			physical status
	progressive rubella panencephalitis		plastic surgery (surgeon)
			polysulfone (filter)
PrP	prion protein		posterior synechiae
PRP-D	*Haemophilus influenzae,* type b diphtheria conjugate vaccine		posterior synechiotomy
			pressure sore
			pressure support
			protective services
PRPP	5-phosphoribosyl-1-pyrophosphate		Proteus syndrome
			pulmonary stenosis
PRP-T	polysaccharide tetanus conjugate vaccine		pyloric stenosis
			pyrimethamine; sulfadoxine (Fansidar)
PRRE	pupils round, regular, and equal		serum from pregnant women
PRRERLA	pupils round, regular, equal; react to light and accommodation	P/S	polyunsaturated to saturated fatty acids ratio
PRRs	proportional reporting ratios	P & S	pain and suffering
			paracentesis and suction
PRS	photon radiosurgery system		permanent and stationary
	postradiation sarcoma	PS I	healthy patient with localized pathological process
	prolonged respiratory support		
PRSL	potential renal solute load	PS II	a patient with mild to moderate systemic disease
PRSP	penicillinase-resistant synthetic penicillins		
		PS III	a patient with severe systemic disease limiting activity but not incapacitating
	penicillin-resistant *Streptococcus pneumoniae*		
PRSs	positive rolandic spikes		
PRST	Blood Pressure, Heart Rate, Sweating, and Tears (scale to assess analgesic needs)	PS IV	a patient with incapacitating systemic disease
		PS V	moribund patient not expected to live
PRT	pelvic radiation therapy		(These are American Society of Anesthesiologists' physical status patient classifications. Emergency operations are designated by "E" after the classification.)
	protamine response test		
PRTCA	percutaneous rotational transluminal coronary angioplasty		
PRTH-C	prothrombin time control		
PRV	polycythemia rubra vera		
PRVEP	pattern reversal visual evoked potentials		
PRW	past relevant work		
	polymerized ragweed	PSA	polysubstance abuse
PRX	panoramic facial x-ray		power spectral analysis

P

	product selection allowed	PSE	portal systemic encephalopathy
	prostate-specific antigen		pseudoephedrine
	Pseudomonas aeruginosa	PSF	posterior spinal fusion
PsA	psoriatic arthritis	PSG	peak systolic gradient
PSAB	pretreatment prostate-specific antigen		polysomnogram
			portosystemic gradient
PSAD	prostate-specific antigen density	PSGN	poststreptococcal glomerulonephritis
PSADT	prostate-specific antigen doubling time	PSH	past surgical history
			postspinal headache
PSAG	*Pseudomonas aeruginosa*	PSHx	past surgical history
PSAV	prostate-specific antigen velocity	PSI	passenger space intrusion (motor vehicle accident)
PSBO	partial small bowel obstruction		Physiologic Stability Index
PSC	Pediatric Symptom Checklist		pounds per square inch
			prostate seed implant
	percutaneous suprapubic cystostomy		punctate subepithelial infiltrate
	posterior semicircular canal	PSIC	pediatric surgical intensive care
	posterior subcapsular cataract	PSIG	pounds per square inch gauge
	primary sclerosing cholangitis	PSIS	posterior superior iliac spine
	pronation spring control	PSM	patient self-management
			presystolic murmur
	pubosacrococcygeal (diameter)	PSMA	personal self-maintenance activities
PSCA	prostate stem cell antigen		progressive spinal muscular atrophy
PSCC	posterior subcapsular cataract		prostate-specific membrane antigen
PSC Cat	posterior subcapsular cataract	PSMF	protein-sparing modified fasting (Blackburn diet)
PSCH	peripheral stem cell harvest	PSM-R	Optimism-Pessimism Scale, revised
PSCP	papillary serous carcinoma of the peritoneum	PSMS	Physical Self Maintenance Scale
	posterior subcapsular precipitates	PSNP	progressive supranuclear palsy
PSCT	peripheral stem cell transplant	PSO	pelvic stabilization orthosis
PSCU	pediatric special care unit		physician supplemental order
PSD	partial sleep deprivation		Polysporin ointment
	pilonidal sinus disease		proximal subungual onychomycosis
	poststroke depression		
	power spectral density	pSO$_2$	arterial oxygen saturation
	psychosomatic disease	PSOC	Puget Sound Oncology Consortium
PSDA	Patient Self-Determination Act		
PSDS	palmar surface desensitization	P/sore	pressure sore

P

PTB	patellar tendon bearing		pharmacy to dose
	prior to birth		pharyngotracheal duct
	pulmonary tuberculosis		preterm delivery
PTBA	percutaneous transluminal		prior to delivery
	balloon angioplasty	PTDM	post-transplant diabetes
PTBD	percutaneous transhepatic		mellitus
	biliary drain	PTDP	permanent transvenous
	(drainage)		demand pacemaker
PTBD-EF	percutaneous transhepatic	PTE	pretibial edema
	biliary drainage—		proximal tibial epiphysis
	enteric feeding		pulmonary
PTBS	post-traumatic brain		thromboembolectomy
	syndrome		pulmonary
PTB-	patellar tendon		thromboembolism
SC-SP	bearing-supracondylar-	PTE-4®	trace metal elements
	suprapatellar		injection (there is also a
PTC	patient to call		#5 and #6)
	percutaneous transhepatic	PTED	pulmonary
	cholangiography		thromboembolic disease
	Pharmacy and	PTER	percutaneous transluminal
	Therapeutics		endomyocardial
	Committee		revascularization
	plasma thromboplastin	PTF	patient transfer form
	components		Patient Treatment File
	post-tetanic count		pentoxifylline (Trental)
	premature tricuspid		post-tetanic facilitation
	closure	PTFE	polytetrafluoroethylene
	prior to conception	PTG	parathyroid gland
	pseudotumor cerebri		photoplethysmogram
PT-C	prothrombin time control	PTGBD	percutaneous transhepatic
PTCA	percutaneous transluminal		gallbladder drainage
	coronary angioplasty	PTH	parathyroid hormone
PTCDLF	pregnancy, term,		post-transfusion hepatitis
	complicated delivered,		prior to hospitalization
	living female	PTHC	percutaneous transhepatic
PTCDLM	pregnancy, term,		cholangiography
	complicated delivered,	PTHrP	parathyroid hormone-
	living male		related protein
PTCL	peripheral T-cell	PTHS	post-traumatic
	lymphoma		hyperirritability
PTCR	percutaneous transluminal		syndrome
	coronary recanalization	PTI	pressure-time integral
PTCRA	percutaneous transluminal		prior to induction
	coronary rotational	PTJV	percutaneous transtracheal
	atherectomy		jet ventilation
PTD	percutaneous	PTK	pancreas-after-kidney
	transpedicular		(transplantation)
	diskectomy		phototherapeutic
	period to discharge		keratectomy
	permanent and total	PTL	preterm labor
	disability		pudding-thick liquid (diet
	persistent trophoblastic		consistency)
	disease		Sodium Pentothal

PTLD	post-transplantation lymphoproliferative disorder (disease)	PTT	partial thromboplastin time
			pharyngeal transit time
PTLR	percutaneous transmyocardial laser revascularization		platelet transfusion therapy
			posterior tibial tendon
PTM	patient monitored		protein truncation testing
	posterior trabecular meshwork		pulse transit time
		PTT-C	partial thromboplastin time control
PTMC	percutaneous transvenous mitral commissurotomy	PTTG	pituitary tumor transforming gene
PTMDF	pupils, tension, media, disk, and fundus	PTTW	patient tolerated traction well
PTMR	percutaneous transmyocardial revascularization	PTU	pain treatment unit
			pregnancy, term, uncomplicated
PT-NANB	post-transfusion non-A, non-B (hepatitis C)		propylthiouracil
PTNB	preterm newborn	PTUCA	percutaneous transluminal ultrasonic coronary angioplasty
pTNM	postsurgical resection-pathologic staging of cancer	PTUDLF	pregnancy, term, uncomplicated delivered, living female
PTNS	percutaneous tibial nerve stimulation	PTUDLM	pregnancy, term, uncomplicated delivered, living male
PTO	part-time occlusion (eye patch)	PTV	patient-triggered ventilation
	please turn over		posterior tibial vein
	proximal tubal obstruction	PTWTKG	patient's weight in kilograms
PTP	phonation threshold pressure	PTX	paclitaxel (Taxol)
	posterior tibial pulse		parathyroidectomy
	post-transfusion purpura		pelvic traction
PTPM	post-traumatic progressive myelopathy		pentoxifylline (Trental)
			phototherapy
PTPN	peripheral (vein) total parenteral nutrition		pneumothorax
P-to-P	point-to-point	PTZ	pentylenetetrazol
PTR	paratesticular rhabdomyosarcoma		phenothiazine
	patella tendon reflex	PU	pelvic-ureteric
	patient to return		pelviureteral
	prothrombin time ratio		peptic ulcer
PT-R	prothrombin time ratio		pregnancy urine
PTRA	percutaneous transluminal renal angioplasty	P & U	Pharmacia & Upjohn Company
PTR-MS	proton transfer reaction mass spectrometry	PUA	pelvic (examination) under anesthesia
PTS	patellar tendon suspension	PUB	pubic
	Pediatric Trauma Score	PUBS	percutaneous umbilical blood sampling
	permanent threshold shift		
	prior to surgery	PUC	pediatric urine collector
PTSD	post-traumatic stress disorder		

P

PUD	partial upper denture		popliteal vein
	peptic ulcer disease		portal vein
	percutaneous ureteral dilatation		postvoiding
			prenatal vitamins
PUE	pyrexia of unknown etiology		projectile vomiting
			pulmonary vein
PUF	pure ultrafiltration	Pv	*Plasmodium vivax*
PUFA	polyunsaturated fatty acids	P & V	peak and valley (this is a dangerous abbreviation, use peak and trough)
PUFFA	polyunsaturated free fatty acids		pyloroplasty and vagotomy
PUJ	pelviureteral junction		
pul.	pulmonary	PVA	polyethylene vinyl acetate
PULP	pulpotomy		polyvinyl alcohol
Pulse A	pulse apical		Prinzmetal variant angina
PULSE OX	pulse oximetry	PVAD	prolonged venous access devices
Pulse R	pulse radial	PVAM	potential visual acuity meter
PULSES	(physical profile) physical condition, upper limb functions, lower limb functions, sensory components, excretory functions, and support factors	PVAR	pulmonary vein atrial reversal
		PVB	cisplatin, (Platinol AQ) vinblastine, and bleomycin
PUN	plasma urea nitrogen		paravertebral block
PUND	pregnancy, uterine, not delivered		porcelain veneer bridge
			premature ventricular beat
PUNL	percutaneous ultrasonic nephrolithotripsy	PVC	paclitaxel, vinblastine, and cisplatin
PUO	pyrexia of unknown origin		polyethylene vacuum cup
PUP	percutaneous ultrasonic pyelolithotomy		polyvinyl chloride
			porcelain veneer crown
	previously untreated patient		postvoiding cystogram
PU/PL	partial upper and lower dentures		premature ventricular contraction
			pulmonary venous congestion
PUPPP	pruritic urticarial papules and plaque of pregnancy	Pv_{CO_2}	partial pressure (tension) of carbon dioxide, vein
PUS	percutaneous ureteral stent	PVD	patient very disturbed
	preoperative ultrasound		peripheral vascular disease
PUU	Puumala hantavirus		posterior vitreous detachment
PUV	posterior urethral valves		premature ventricular depolarization
PUVA	psoralen-ultraviolet-light (treatment)		
		PVDA	prednisone, vincristine, daunorubicin, and asparaginase
PUW	pick-up walker		
PV	papillomavirus	PVDF	polyvinylidene difluoride
	Parvovirus	PVE	perivenous encephalomyelitis
	per vagina		
	plasma volume		premature ventricular extrasystole
	polio vaccine		
	polycythemia vera		

P

298

	prosthetic value endocarditis		Photoselective Vaporization of the Prostate (procedure)
P vera	polycythemia vera		polyvinylpyrrolidone
PVF	peripheral visual field		posteroventral pallidotomy
PVFS	postviral fatigue syndrome	P-VP-B	cisplatin (Platinol AQ), etoposide (VP-16), and bleomycin
PVGM	perifoveolar vitreoglial membrane		
PVH	periventricular hemorrhage	PVR	peripheral vascular resistance
	periventricular hyperintensity		perspective volume rendering
	pulmonary vascular hypertension		postvoiding residual
PVI	pelvic venous incompetence		proliferative vitreoretinopathy
	peripheral vascular insufficiency		pulmonary valve replacement
	portal-vein infusion		pulmonary vascular resistance
	protracted venous infusion		pulse-volume recording
	pulmonary valve insufficiency	PVRI	pulmonary vascular resistance index
PVK	penicillin V potassium		
PVL	Panton-Valentine leukocidin	PVS	percussion, vibration and suction
	peripheral vascular laboratory		peripheral vascular surgery
	periventricular leukomalacia		peritoneovenous shunt
PVM	paraverteabral muscle		persistent vegetative state
	proteins, vitamins, and minerals		Plummer-Vinson syndrome
PVMS	paravertebral muscle spasms		pulmonic valve stenosis
PVN	peripheral venous nutrition	PVT	paroxysmal ventricular tachycardia
PVNS	pigmented villonodular synovitis		physical volume test
PVO	peripheral vascular occlusion		portal vein thrombosis
			previous trouble
	portal vein occlusion		private
	pulmonary venous occlusion		proximal vein thrombosis
PVo	pulmonary valve opening	PVTT	tumor thrombus in the portal vein
Pvo₂	partial pressure (tension) of oxygen, vein	PVV	persistent varicose veins
	peripheral vascular occlusive disease	PW	pacing wires
			patient waiting
PVOD	pulmonary vascular obstructive disease		plantar wart
			posterior wall
PVP	cisplatin (Platinol AQ) and etoposide (VePesid)		pulse width
			puncture wound
	penicillin V potassium	P&W	pressures and waves
	peripheral venous pressure	PWA	persons with AIDS
			P-wave axis
		PWACR	Prader-Willi/Angelman critical region

P

P wave	part of the electrocardio-graphic cycle representing atrial depolarization	PXF	pseudoexfoliation
		PXL	paclitaxel (Taxol)
		PXS	dental prophylaxis (cleaning)
PWB	partial weight bearing	PY	pack-years (see pk yrs)
	Positive Well-being (scale)	PYE	person-years of exposure
	psychological well-being	PYHx	packs per year history
PWBL	partial weight bearing, left	PYLL	potential years of life lost
PWBR	partial weight bearing, right	PYP	pyrophosphate
		PYP®	technetium Tc 99m pyrophosphate kit
PWC	personal watercraft	PZ	peripheral zone
	physical working capacity	PZA	pyrazinamide
	powered wheelchair		pyrazoloacridine (a drug class of sedative/hypnotics)
PWCA	personal watercraft accident		
PWD	patients with diabetes	PZD	partial zona drilling
	person(s) with a disability		partial zonal dissection
	powder	PZI	protamine zinc insulin
PWE	people with epilepsy	PZR	posterior zygomatic root
PWI	pediatric walk-in clinic		
	perfusion-weighted (magnetic resonance) imaging		
	posterior wall infarct		
PWLV	posterior wall of left ventricle		
PWM	pokeweed mitogens		
PWMI	posterior wall myocardial infarction		
PWO	persistent withdrawal occlusion		
PWP	pulmonary wedge pressure		
PWS	plagiocephaly without synostosis		
	port-wine stain		
	Prader-Willi syndrome		
PWT	pad weight test(s)		
	posterior wall thickness		
	primary writing tremor		
PWTd	posterior wall thickness at end-diastole		
PWV	polistes wasp venom		
	pulse-wave velocity		
Px	physical exam		
	pneumothorax		
	prognosis		
	prophylaxis		
PXAT	paroxysmal atrial tachycardia		
PXE	pseudoxanthoma elasticum		

Q

Q every
   quadriceps
QA quality assurance
QAC before every meal (this is a
     dangerous abbreviation)
QALE quality-adjusted life
      expectancy
QALYs quality-adjusted life
       years
QAM every morning (this is a
     dangerous abbreviation
     because the Q can be
     read as a 9)
QAPI quality assessment and
      performance
      improvement
QAS quality-adjusted survival
QATTP quality-adjusted time to
       progression
QB blood flow
QC quad cane
    quality checks
    quality control
    quick catheter
QCA quantitative coronary
     angiography
Q Chinese cucumber
compound
QCSW Qualified Clinical Social
      Worker
QCT quantitative computed
     tomography
QD dialysate flow
    every day (this is a
    dangerous abbreviation
    as it is read as four
    times daily-QID; use
    "once daily")
    quinupristin and
    dalfopristin (Synercid)
QDAM once daily in the
      morning (this is a
      dangerous abbreviation)
QDAY every day
QDNs quantum dot nanocrystals
QDPM once daily in the evening
      (This is a dangerous
      abbreviation)

QDS United Kingdom
     abbreviation for four
     times a day
QE quinidine effect
QED every even day (this is a
     dangerous abbreviation
     as it will be read as
     four times daily-QID)
     quick and early diagnosis
QEE quadriceps extension
     exercise
QEMG quantitative
      electromyography
QF quadriceps femoris
    (muscle)
QFB Qu'mico Farmacéutico
     Bi-logo (Chemist
     Pharmacist Biologist;
     Pharmacist in Mexico)
QF-PCR quantitative fluorescence
        polymerase chain
        reaction
QFV Q fever (*Coxiella burnetii*)
     vaccine
QGS quantitative gate SPECT
     (single photon
     emission computed
     tomography)
q4h every four hours
q.h. every hour
qhs once daily at bedtime,
     each day (this is a
     dangerous abbreviation
     as it is read as every
     hour-QHR or four times
     daily-QID)
QIAD Quantitative Inventory of
      Alcohol Disorders
q.i.d. four times daily
QIDM four times daily with
      meals and at bedtime
QIG quantitative
     immunoglobulins
QIMT quantitative intima media
      thickness
QIO Quality Improvement
     Organization
QIW four times a week (this is
     a dangerous
     abbreviation)
QJ quadriceps jerk
QKD Korotkoff sounds
interval

Q

QL	quality of life	QRC	qualitative radiocardiography
QLI	Quality of Life Index		
QLS	quality of life score	QRDR	quinolone resistance-determining region(s)
QM	every morning (this is a dangerous abbreviation as it will not be understood)		
		QRE	quality-related event
		QRNG	quinolone-resistant *N. gonorrhoeae*
Qmax	maximal flow rate	QRS	part of electrocardiographic wave representing ventricular depolarization
QMB	qualified Medicare beneficiary		
QMI	Q-wave myocardial infarction		
		QS	every shift
QMRP	qualified mental retardation professional		quadriceps set
			quadrilateral socket
QMT	quantitative muscle testing		Quality Services (Department)
q.n.	every night (this is a dangerous abbreviation as it is read as every hour)		sufficient quantity
		qs ad	a sufficient quantity to make
q.n.s.	quantity not sufficient	QS&L	quarters, subsistence, and laundry
qod	every other day (this is a dangerous abbreviation as it is read as every day or four times a day-QID)		
		Qs/Qt	intrapulmonary shunt fraction
		QSP	physiological shunt fraction
qoh	every other hour (this is a dangerous abbreviation as it is read as every day or four times a day-QID)	QT	the time between the beginning of the QRS complex and the end of the T-wave
		qt	quart
qohs	every other day at bedtime (this is a dangerous abbreviation as it is read as every hour-QHR or four times daily-QID)	QTB	quadriceps tendon bearing
		QTC	quantitative tip cultures
		QTc	the QTc interval is the length of time it takes the electrical system in the heart to repolarize, adjusted for heart rate (normal 350-440 milliseconds)
QOL	quality of life		
QOLIE-31	quality of life in epilepsy		
QOM	quality of motion		
QON	every other night (this is a dangerous abbreviation)	QTL	quantitative trait locus
		QTP	quetiapine fumarate (Seroquel)
QPCR	quantitative polymerase chain reaction		
		Q-TWiST	quality-adjusted time without symptoms (of disease) and toxicity
qpm	every evening (this is a dangerous abbreviation)		
QPOS	Quality Point of Service	QTY	quantity
QP/QS	ratio of pulmonary blood to systemic blood flow	QUAD	quadrant
			quadriceps
			quadriplegic
qqh	every four hours (United Kingdom)	QU	quiet
qqs	every four hours (United Kingdom)	QUART	quadrantectomy, axillary dissection, and radiotherapy
QR	quiet room		

QUEST	Quality of Upper Extremity Skills Test
QuMA	quantitative microsatellite analysis
QUS	quantitative (bone) ultrasound
QW	every week (this is a dangerous abbreviation)
q4w	every 4 weeks (this is a dangerous abbreviation)
QWB	Quality of Well-Being (scale)
QWE	every weekend (this is a dangerous abbreviation)
QWK	once a week (this is a dangerous abbreviation)
Q4wk	every four weeks (this is a dangerous abbreviation)
QWMI	Q-wave myocardial infarction

R	radial
	rate
	ratio
	reacting
	rectal
	rectum
	regular
	regular insulin
	resistant
	respiration
	reticulocyte
	retinoscopy
	rifampicin [part of tuberculosis regimen, see RHZ(E/S)/HR]
	right (this a dangerous abbreviation; spell out "right" to avoid surgical errors)
	Ritalin (methylphenidate) as in vitamin R
	roentgen
	rub
^{r}	recombinant
®	registered trademark
	right (this is a dangerous abbreviation; spell out "right" to avoid surgical errors)
−R	Rinne test, negative
+R	Rinne test, positive
RA	radial artery
	radiographic absorptiometry
	rales
	readmission
	renal artery
	repeat action
	retinoic acid
	rheumatoid arthritis
	right arm
	right atrium
	right auricle
	room air
	rotational atherectomy
RAA	renin-angiotensin-aldosterone
	right atrial abnormality

	right atrial appendage
RAAS	renin-angiotensin-aldosterone system
RAB	rabies vaccine, not otherwise specified
	rice (rice cereal), applesauce, and banana (diet)
RAB$_{DEV}$	rabies vaccine, duck embryo culture
RAB$_{FRhL-2}$	rabies vaccine, diploid fetal-rhesus-lung-2 cell line
RABG	room air blood gas
RAB$_{HDCV}$	rabies vaccine, human diploid cell culture
RABig	rabies immune globulin
RAB$_{PCEC}$	rabies vaccine, purified chick embryo cell culture
RAC	Recombinant DNA Advisory Committee
	right antecubital
	right atrial catheter
RACCO	right anterior caudocranial oblique
RACT	recalcified whole-blood activated clotting time
RACZ	a procedure of dissolving lumbar scar tissue (epidurolysis)
RAD	ionizing radiation unit
	radical
	radiology
	rapid antigen detection
	reactive airway disease
	reactive attachment disorder
	right axis deviation
RADCA	right anterior descending coronary artery
RADE	reactive airway disease exacerbation
RADISH	rheumatoid arthritis diffuse idiopathic skeletal hyperostosis
RADS	ionizing radiation units
	rapid assay delivery systems
	reactive airway disease syndrome
RADT	rapid antigen detection testing
RAE	right atrial enlargement

RAEB	refractory anemia, erythroblastic
RAEB-T	refractory anemia with excess blasts in transition
RAF	rapid atrial fibrillation
RAFF	rectus abdominis free flap
RAFT	Rehabilitative Addicted Family Treatment
RAG	room air gas
RAH	right atrial hypertrophy
RAHB	right anterior hemiblock
rAHF	antihemophilic factor (recombinant)
RAI	radioactive iodine
	Resident Assessment Instrument
RAID	radioimmunodetection
RAIT	radioimmunotherapy
RAIU	radioactive iodine uptake
RALT	routine admission laboratory tests
RAM	radioactive material
	rapid alternating movements
	rectus abdominis myocutaneous
RAN	resident's admission notes
R$_2$AN	second year resident's admission notes
RANTES	regulated upon activation, normal T cell expressed and secreted
RAO	right anterior oblique
rAOM	recurrent acute otitis media
RAP	renal artery pseudoaneurysm
	request for advance payment
	right abdominal pain
	right atrial pressure
RAPA	radial artery pseudoaneurysm
RAQ	right anterior quadrant
RAP	recurrent abdominal pain
	Resident Assessment Protocol
RAPD	random amplified polymorphic DNA
	relative afferent pupillary defect
RAPs	Resident Assessment Protocols

RAR	right arm, reclining	RBILD	respiratory bronchiolitis-associated interstitial lung disease
RARs	retinoic acid receptors		
RAS	recurrent aphthous stomatitis		
	renal artery stenosis	RBL	Roche Biomedical Laboratory
	renin-angiotensin system	RBON	retrobulbar optic neuritis
	reticular activating system	RBOW	rupture bag of water
	right arm, sitting	RBP	retinol-binding protein
RASE	rapid-acquisition spin echo	RBRVS	Medicare resource-based relative-value scale
RAST	radioallergosorbent test	RBS	random blood sugar
RAT	right anterior thigh		redback spider
RA test	test for rheumatoid factor	RBT	rational behavior therapy
RATG	rabbit antithymocyte globulin	RBV	right brachial vein
		RBVO	right brachial vein occlusion
RATx	radiation therapy		
RAU	recurrent aphthous ulcers	RC	race
RAVLT	Rey Auditory Verbal Learning Test		radiocarpal (joint)
			Red Cross
R(AW)	airway resistance		report called
RB	relieved by		retention catheter
	retinoblastoma		retrograde cystogram
	retrobulbar		retruded contact (position)
	right breast		right coronary
	right buttock		Roman Catholic
R & B	right and below		root canal
RBA	right basilar artery		rotator cuff
	right brachial artery	R/C	reclining chair
	risks, benefits, and alternatives (discussion with patient)	R & C	reasonable and customary
		RCA	radiographic contrast agent
			radionuclide cerebral angiogram
RBB	right breast biopsy		right carotid artery
RBBB	right bundle branch block		right coronary artery
RBBX	right breast biopsy examination		rolling circle amplification
			root cause analysis
RBC	ranitidine bismuth citrate	RC/AL	residential care, assisted living
	red blood cell (count)		
RBCD	right border cardiac dullness	RCBF	regional cerebral blood flow
RBCM	red blood cell mass	RCC	rape crisis center
RBC s/f	red blood cells spun filtration		resectable colon cancer
			renal cell carcinoma
RBCV	red blood cell volume		Roman Catholic Church
RBD	REM (rapid eye movement sleep) behavior disorder	RCCA	right common carotid artery
		RCCT	randomized controlled clinical trial
	right border of dullness		
RbDe	residue-based diagram editor	RCD	relative cardiac dullness
		RCE	right carotid endarterectomy
RBE	relative biologic effectiveness		
		RCF	Reiter complement fixation
RBF	renal blood flow		
RBG	random blood glucose	RCF®	enteral nutrition product

R

RCFA	right common femoral angioplasty right common femoral artery	RCT	randomized clinical trial Registered Care Technologist root canal therapy Rorschach Content Test rotator cuff tear
RCFE	residential care facility for the elderly		
RCH	residential care home	RCU	respiratory care unit
RCHF	right-sided congestive heart failure	RCV	red cell volume right colic vein
R-CHOP	rituximab (Rituxan), cyclophosphamide, doxorubicin (hydroxydaunorubicin), vincristine (Oncovin), and prednisone	RCX	ramus circumflexus
		RD	radial deviation Raynaud disease reaction of degeneration reading disability reflex decay Registered Dietitian renal disease respiratory disease respiratory distress restricted duty retinal detachment Reye disease rhabdomyosarcoma right deltoid ruptured disk
RCIN	radiographic-contrast-media-induced nephropathy		
RCIP	rape crisis intervention program		
RCL	radial collateral ligament range of comfortable loudness		
RCM	radiographic contrast media restricted cardiomyopathy retinal capillary microaneurysm right costal margin		
		RDA	recommended daily allowance Registered Dental Assistant representational difference analysis
RCN	radiocontrast-agent-induced nephrotoxicity		
RCO	revoked court order		
RCOG	Royal College of Obstetricians and Gynaecologists	RDB	randomized double-blind (trial)
RCOT	revoked court-ordered treatment	RDCS	Registered Diagnostic Cardiac Sonographer
RCP	respiratory care plan retrograde cerebral perfusion Royal College of Physicians	RDD	renal dose dopamine
		RDE	remote data entry respiratory disturbance events
		RDEA	right deviation of electrical axis
RCPM	raven-colored progressive matrices	RDG	right dorsogluteal
RCPT	Registered Cardio-pulmonary Technician	RDH	Registered Dental Hygienist
		RDI	respiratory disturbance (distress) index
RCR	replication-competent retrovirus (assay) rotator cuff repair	RDIH	right direct inguinal hernia
RCS	repeat cesarean section reticulum cell sarcoma Royal College of Surgeons	RDLBBB	rate-dependent left bundle branch block
		RDM	right deltoid muscle

RDMS	Registered Diagnostic Medical Sonographer	REC	gingival recession
			rear-end collision
RDMs	reactive drug metabolites		recommend
RDOD	retinal detachment, right eye		record
			recovery
RDOS	retinal detachment, left eye		recreation
RDP	random donor platelets		recur
	right dorsoposterior	RECA	right external carotid artery
RDPE	reticular degeneration of the pigment epithelium	RECT	rectum
RDS	research diagnostic criteria	REDA	Registered Eating Disorders Associate
	respiratory distress syndrome	REDs	reproductive endocrine diseases
RDT	rapid diagnostic test	RED SUBS	reducing substances
	regular dialysis (hemodialysis) treatment	REE	resting energy expenditure
		RE-ED	re-education
RDTD	referral, diagnosis, treatment, and discharge	R-EEG	resting electroencephalogram
RDU	recreational drug use	REEGT	Registered Electroencephalogram Technologist
RDVT	recurrent deep vein thrombosis	REF	referred
RDW	red (cell) distribution width		refused
			renal erythropoietic factor
RE	concerning	ref→	refer to
	Rasmussen encephalitis	REG	radioencephalogram
	rectal examination		regression analysis
	reflux esophagitis	Reg block	regional block anesthesia
	regarding	regurg	regurgitation
	regional enteritis	rehab	rehabilitation
	reticuloendothelial	REL	relative
	retinol equivalents		religion
	right ear (this is a dangerous abbreviation as it can be read as right eye)	RELE	resistive exercise, lower extremities
		REM	rapid eye movement
	right eye (this a dangerous abbreviation as it can be read as right ear)		recent event memory
			remarried
			remission
	rowing ergometer		roentgen equivalent unit
^{186}Re	rhenium 186	REMS	rapid eye movement sleep
R & E	rest and exercise	REO	respiratory and enteric orphan (viruses)
	round and equal	REP	rapid electrophoresis
R ↑ E	right upper extremity		repair
R ↓ E	right lower extremity		repeat
RE✓	recheck		report
READM	readmission	REP CK	rapid electrophoresis creatine kinase
REAL	Revised European American Lymphoma (classification)	REPL	recurrent early pregnancy loss
REALM	Rapid Estimation of Adult Literacy in Medicine	repol	repolarization
		REPS	repetitions

R

REPT	Registered Evoked Potential Technologist	RFB	retained foreign body
RER	renal excretion rate		radial flow chromatography
RER+	replication error positive		residual functional capacity
RES	recurrent erosion syndrome	RFC	reduced folate carrier
	resection	RFCA	radiofrequency catheter ablation
	resident		
	reticuloendothelial system	RFD	residue-free diet
RESC	resuscitation	RFDT	Reach in Four Directions Test
RESP	respirations		
	respiratory	RFE	return flow enema
REST	restoration	RFFF	radial forearm free flap (reconstruction of pharyngeal defect)
	restriction of environmental stimulation therapy		
		RFFIT	rapid fluorescent focus inhibition test
RET	retention		
	reticulocyte	rFVIII FS	antihemophilic factor (recombinant), formulated with sucrose (Kogenate)
	retina		
	retired		
	return		
	right esotropia	RFg	visual fields by Goldmann-type perimeter
ret detach	retinal detachment		
retic	reticulocyte		
RETRO	retrograde	rFGF-2	recombinant fibroblast growth factor-2
RETRX	retractions		
REUE	resistive exercise, upper extremities	RFID	radio frequency identification
REV	reverse	RFIPC	Rating Form of IBD (inflammatory bowel disease) Patient Concerns
	review		
	revolutions		
RF	radiofrequency		
	reduction fixation	RFL	radionuclide functional lymphoscintigraphy
	refill; refilled (prescriptions)		
			right frontolateral
	renal failure	RFLF	retained fetal lung fluid
	respiratory failure	RFLP	restriction fragment length polymorphism (patterns)
	restricted fluids		
	rheumatic fever		
	rheumatoid factor	RFM	rifampin (Rifadin)
	ring finger	RFP	Renal function panel (see page 392)
	right foot		
	risk factor		request for payment
	radiofrequency		request for proposal
R/F	retroflexed		right frontoposterior
R&F	radiographic and fluoroscopic	RFS	rapid frozen section
			refeeding syndrome
RF6	rejection-free survival at 6 months		relapse-free survival
		RFT	respiratory function test
RFA	radiofrequency ablation		right frontotransverse
	right femoral artery		routine fever therapy
	right forearm	RFTA	radiofrequency thermal ablation
	right frontoanterior		

RFTC	radiofrequency thermocoagulation	relative hepatic dullness
		rheumatic heart disease
RFUT	radioactive fibrinogen uptake	right-hand dominant
rh-DNase		dornase alfa (Pulmozyme)
RFV	reason for visit	RHF	rheumatic fever vaccine
	right femoral vein		right heart failure
RFVTR	radiofrequency volumetric tissue reduction	RHG	right-hand grip
r-hGH(m)		mammalian-cell–derived recombinant human growth hormone (Serostim)
RG	regurgitated (infant feeding)		
	right (upper outer) gluteus		
		RHH	right homonymous hemianopsia
R/G	red/green		
RGA	right gastroepiploic artery	RHIA	Registered Health Information Administrator
RGM	rapidly growing *Mycobacteria*		
		RHINO	rhinoplasty
	recurrent glioblastoma multiforme	RHIT	Registered Health Information Technician
	right gluteus medius		
RGO	reciprocating gait orthosis	RHL	right hemisphere lesions
			right heptic lobe
RGP	rigid gas-permeable (contact lens)	rhm	roentgens per hour at one meter
Rh	Rhesus factor in blood	RHO	right heel off
RH	radical hysterectomy	Rho(D)	immune globulin to an Rh-negative woman
	reduced haloperidol		
	relative humidity	RhoGAM®	Rh$_O$ (D) immune globulin
	rest home	RHP	resting head pressure
	retinal hemorrhage	rhPDGF	recombinant human platelet-derived growth factor
	right hand		
	right hemisphere		
	right hyperphoria		
	room humidifier	RHR	resting heart rate
Rh+	Rhesus positive	RHS	right-hand side
Rh−	Rhesus negative	RHT	regional hyperthermia
RHA	rheumatoid arthritis (therapeutic) vaccine		right hypertropia
		rHuEPO	recombinant human erythropoietin
	right hepatic artery		
rHA	recombinant human albumin	Rhupus	coexistence of rheumatoid arthritis and systemic lupus erythematosus
rhAPC	recombinant human activated protein C		
		RHV	right hepatic vein
RHB	raise head of bed	RHW	radiant heat warmer
	right heart border	RHZ(E/S)/ HR	a tuberculosis treatment regimen consisting of rifampicin, isoniazid, pyrazinamide, ethambutol, streptomycin, isoniazid, and rifampicin (also see 2EHRZ/6HE)
RH/BSO	radial hysterectomy and bilateral salpingo-oophorectomy		
RHC	respiration has ceased		
	right heart catheterization		
	right hemicolectomy		
	routine health care	RI	ramus intermedius (coronary artery)
	rural health clinic		
RHD	radial head dislocation		

R

309

refractive index
regular insulin
relapse incidence
renal insufficiency
respiratory illness
retroillumination
rooming in

RIA radioimmunoassay
reversible ischemic attack

RIAT radioimmune antiglobulin test

RIBA recombinant immunoblot assay

RIBC residual infiltrating breast cancer

RIC reduced intensity conditioning
right iliac crest
right internal carotid (artery)

RICA right internal carotid artery

RICE rest, ice, compression, and elevation

RICM right intercostal margin

RICS right intercostal space

RICU respiratory intensive care unit

RID radial immunodiffusion
ruptured intervertebral disk

RIDL Release of Insects with a Dominant Lethal (mutations)

RIE radiation induced emesis
reactive ion etching
rocket immunoelectrophoresis

RIF rifampin
right iliac fossa
right index finger
rigid internal fixation

RIG rabies immune globulin

RIGS radioimmunoguided surgery

RIH right inguinal hernia

RIHP renal interstitial hydrostatic pressure

RIJ right internal jugular

RIMA reversible inhibitor of monoamine oxidase-type A

right internal mammary anastamosis
right internal mammary artery

RIN radiocontrast-induced nephropathy

RIND reversible ischemic neurologic defect

RINV radiation-induced nausea and vomiting

RIO right inferior oblique (muscle)

RIOJ recurrent intrahepatic obstructive jaundice

R-IOL remove intraocular lens

RIP radioimmunoprecipitin test
rapid infusion pump
respiratory inductance plethysmograph
rhythmic inhibitory pattern

RIPA ristocetin-induced platelet agglutination

RIR right inferior rectus

RIS responding to internal stimuli
risperidone (Risperdal)

RISA radioactive iodinated serum albumin

RIST radioimmunosorbent test

RIT radioimmunotherapy
ritonavir (Norvir)
Rorschach Inkblot Test

RITA right internal thoracic artery

RIVD ruptured intervertebral disk

RIX radiation-induced xerostomia

RJ radial jerk (reflex)
right jugular

RK radial keratotomy
right kidney

RKS renal kidney stone

RKT Registered Kinesiotherapist

RL right lateral
right leg
right lower
right lung
Ringer lactate
rotation left

R → L	right to left		right lower extremity
RLA	right lower arm	RM	radical mastectomy
RLB	right lateral bending		repetitions maximum
	right lateral border		respiratory movement
RLBCD	right lower border of cardiac dullness		risk manager (management)
RLC	residual lung capacity		risk model
RLD	reference listed drug		room
	related living donor	R&M	routine and microscopic
	remaining life expectancy	1-RM	single repetition maximum lift
	right lateral decubitus		
	ruptured lumbar disk	RMA	reduction in metabolic activity
RLDP	right lateral decubital position		Registered Medical Assistant
RLE	right lower extremity		right mentoanterior
RLF	retrolental fibroplasia		Rivermead motor assessment
	right lateral femoral		
RLFP	Remaining Lifetime Fracture Probability	RMB	right main bronchus
RLG	right lateral gaze	RMBPC	Revise Memory and Behavior Problems Checklist
RLGS	restriction landmark genomic scanning		
RLH	reactive lymphoid hyperplasia	RMCA	right main coronary artery right middle cerebral artery
RLL	right liver lobe	RMCAT	right middle cerebral artery thrombosis
	right lower lid		
	right lower lobe	RMCL	right midclavicular line
RLN	recurrent laryngeal nerve	RMD	recommended maintenance dose
	regional lymph node(s)		
RLND	regional lymph node dissection		rippling muscle disease
		RME	reasonable maximum exposure
RLQ	right lower quadrant		
RLQD	right lower quadrant defect		resting metabolic expenditure
RLR	right lateral rectus		right mediolateral episiotomy
RLRTD	recurrent lower respiratory tract disease		
		RMEE	right middle ear exploration
RLS	resonance light scattering	rMET	recombinant methioninase
	restless legs syndrome	RMF	right middle finger
	Ringer lactate solution	RMI	Rivermead Mobility Index
	stammerer who has difficulty in enunciating R, L, and S	RMK #1	remark number 1
		RML	right mediolateral
			right middle lobe
RLSB	right lower scapular border	RMLE	right mediolateral episiotomy
	right lower sternal border	RMMA	rhythmic masticatory muscle activity
RLT	right lateral thigh		
RLTCS	repeat low transverse cesarean section	RMO	responsible medical officer
RLUs	relative light units		
RLWD	routine laboratory work done	rMOG	recombinant myelin oligodendrocyte glycoprotein
RLX	raloxifene (Evista)		

R

RMP	right mentoposterior	RNF	regular nursing floor
	risk management program	RNFA	registered nurse first assistant
RMR	resting metabolic rate	RNFL	retinal nerve fiber layer
	right medial rectus	RNFLT	retinal nerve fiber layer thickness
	root mean square residue	RNI	reactive nitrogen intermediates
RMRM	right modified radical mastectomy		rubella nonimmune
RMS	red-man syndrome	RNLP	Registered Nurse, license pending
	Rehabilitation Medicine Service	RNP	Registered Nurse Practitioner
	repetitive motion syndrome		restorative nursing program
	rhabdomyosarcoma		ribonucleoprotein
	Rocky Mountain spotted fever vaccine	RNS	recurrent nephrotic syndrome
	root-mean-square		replacement normal saline (0.9% sodium chloride)
RMS®	rectal morphine sulfate (suppository)	RNST	reactive nonstress test
RMSB	right middle sternal border	RNUD	recurrent nonulcer dyspepsia
RMSE	root-mean-square error	RO	reality orientation
RMSF	Rocky Mountain spotted fever		relative odds
RMT	Registered Music Therapist		report of
			reverse osmosis
	right mentotransverse		routine order(s)
RMV	respiratory minute volume		Russian Orthodox
RN	Registered Nurse	R/O	rule out
	right nostril (nare)	ROA	radiographic osteoarthritis
Rn	radon		right occiput anterior
R/N	renew	ROAC	repeated oral doses of activated charcoal
RNA	radionuclide angiography	ROAD	reversible obstructive airway disease
	Restorative Nursing Assistant	ROBE	routine operative breast endoscopy
	ribonucleic acid		
	routine nursing assistance	ROC	receiver operating characteristic
RNC	Registered Nurse, Certified		record of contact
RNCD	Registered Nurse, Chemical Dependency		resident on call
RNCNA	Registered Nurse Certified in Nursing Administration		residual organic carbon
		ROCF	Rey-Osterrieth complex figure
RNCNAA	Registered Nurse Certified in Nursing Administration Advanced	ROD	rapid opioid detoxification
		RODA	rapid opiate detoxification under anesthesia
RNCS	Registered Nurse Certified Specialist	ROE	report of event
RND	radical neck dissection		right otitis externa
RNEF	resting (radio-) nuclide ejection fraction	ROF	review of outside films
		ROG	rogletimide

ROH	rubbing alcohol	ROUL	rouleaux (rouleau)
ROI	region of interest (radiology)	ROW	rest of (the) week
		RP	radial pulse
	release of information		radical prostatectomy
ROIDS	hemorrhoids		radiopharmaceutical
ROIH	right oblique inguinal hernia		Raynaud phenomenon
			responsible party
ROJM	range of joint motion		resting position
ROL	right occipitolateral		restorative proctocolectomy
ROLC	roentgenologically occult lung cancer		retinitis pigmentosa
ROM	range of motion		retrograde pyelogram
	rifampicin 600 mg, ofloxacin 400 mg, and minocycline 100 mg		retropubic prostatectomy
			root plane
		RPA	radial photon absorptiometry
	right otitis media		recursive partitioning analysis
	rupture of membranes		
Romb	Romberg		Registered Physician's Assistant
ROMCP	range of motion complete and painfree		repolarization alternans
ROMI	rule out myocardial infarction		restenosis postangioplasty
ROMSA	right otitis media, suppurative, acute		ribonuclease protection assay
			right pulmonary artery
ROMSC	right otitis media, suppurative, chronic	RPAC	Registered Physician's Assistant Certified
ROMWNL	range of motion within normal limits	RPC	root planing and curettage
RON	radiation optic neuropathy		
RONTD	risk of neural tube defect	RPCDBM	randomized, placebo-controlled, double-blind, multinational (study)
ROP	retinopathy of prematurity		
	right occiput posterior		
ROPS	roll-over protection structures	RPCF	Reiter protein complement fixation
ROR	the French acronym for measles-mumps-rubella vaccine	RPD	removable partial denture
		RPE	rating of perceived exertion
	reporting odds ratio		retinal pigment epithelium
R or L	right or left	RPED	retinal pigment epithelium detachment
ROS	review of systems		
	rod outer segments	RPEP	rabies postexposure prophylaxis
	rule out sepsis		
ROSA	rank-order stability analysis		right pre-ejection period
		RPF	relaxed pelvic floor
ROSC	restoration of spontaneous circulation		renal plasma flow
			retroperitoneal fibrosis
ROSS	review of signs and symptoms	RPFT	Registered Pulmonary Function Technologist
ROT	remedial occupational therapy	RPG	retrograde percutaneous gastrostomy
	right occipital transverse rotator		retrograde pyelogram
ROU	recurrent oral ulcer		

R

RPGN	rapidly progressive glomerulonephritis	
RPH	retroperitoneal hemorrhage	
RPh	Registered Pharmacist	
RPHA	reverse passive hemagglutination	
RPI	resting pressure index	
	reticulocyte production index	
RPICA	right posterior internal carotid artery	
RPICCE	round pupil intracapsular cataract extraction	
RPL	retroperitoneal lymphadenectomy	
RPLC	reversed-phase liquid chromatography	
RPLND	retroperitoneal lymph node dissection	
RPLS	reversible posterior leukoencephalopathy syndrome	
RPN	renal papillary necrosis	
	resident's progress notes	
R₂PN	second year resident's progress notes	
RPO	right posterior oblique	
RPP	radical perineal prostatectomy	
	rate-pressure product	
	retropubic prostatectomy	
RPPS	retropatellar pain syndrome	
RPR	rapid plasma reagin (test for syphilis)	
	Reiter protein reagin	
RPS	rhabdoid predisposition syndrome	
RPSGT	Registered Polysomnography Technician	
RPT	Registered Physical Therapist	
RPTA	Registered Physical Therapist Assistant	
RPU	retropubic urethropexy	
RPV	right portal vein	
	right pulmonary vein	
RQ	respiratory quotient	
RQLQ	Respiratory Quality of Life Questionnaire	
RR	recovery room	

	regular rate
	regular respirations
	relative risk
	respiratory rate
	response rate
	retinal reflex
	rotation right
R/R	rales-rhonchi
R&R	rate and rhythm
	recent and remote
	recession and resection
	resect and recess (muscle surgery)
	rest and recuperation
	remove and replace
RRA	radioreceptor assay
	Registered Record Administrator (for newer title, see RHIA)
	right radial artery
	right renal artery
RRAM	rapid rhythmic alternating movements
RRC	cohort relative risk
RRCT, no(m)	regular rate, clear tones, no murmurs
RRD	removable rigid dressing
	rhegmatogenous retinal detachment
RRE	round, regular, and equal (pupils)
RRED®	Rapid Rare Event Detection
RREF	resting radionuclide ejection fraction
RRI	renal resistive index
RR-IOL	remove and replace intraocular lens
RRM	reduced renal mass
	right radial mastectomy
	risk-reducing mastectomy
RRMS	relapsing-remitting multiple sclerosis
RRNA	Resident Registered Nurse Anesthetist
rRNA	ribosomal ribonucleic acid
RRND	right radical neck dissection
RROM	resistive range of motion
R rot	right rotation
RRP	radical retropubic prostatectomy

R

RRR	recovery room routine	RSBQ	Rett Syndrome Behavior Questionnaire
	regular rhythm and rate		
	relative risk reduction	RSC	right subclavian (artery) (vein)
RRRN	round, regular, and react normally	RScA	right scapuloanterior
RRRsM	regular rate and rhythm without murmur	RSCL	Rotterdam Symptom Check List
RRSO	risk-reducing salpingo-oophorectomy	RScP	right scapuloposterior
		RSCS	respiratory system compliance score
RRT	Registered Respiratory Therapist	rscu-PA	recombinant, single-chain, urokinase-type plasminogen activator
RRU	rapid reintegration unit		
RRVO	repair relaxed vaginal outlet		
		RSD	reflex sympathetic dystrophy
RRVS	recovery room vital signs		relative standard deviation
RRV-TV	rhesus rotavirus tetravalent (vaccine)	RSDS	reflex-sympathetic dystrophy syndrome
RRW	rales, rhonchi or wheezes	RSE	rattlesnake envenomation
RS	Raynaud syndrome		reactive subdural effusion
	rectal swab		refractory status epilepticus
	recurrent seizures		
	Reed-Sternberg (cell)		right sternal edge
	Reiter syndrome	RSI	rapid sequence intubation
	remote sensing		repetitive strain (stress) injury
	reschedule		
	restart	R-SICU	respiratory-surgical intensive care unit
	Rett syndrome		
	Reye syndrome	RSL	renal solute load
	rhythm strip	RSLR	reverse straight leg raise
	right side	RSM	remote study monitoring
	Ringer solution	RSNI	round spermatid nuclear injection
	rumination syndrome		
R/S	reschedule	RSO	right salpingooophorectomy
	rest stress		
	rupture spontaneous		right superior oblique
R & S	restraint and seclusion	rS02	regional oxygen saturation
R/S I	resuscitation status one (full resuscitative effort)	RSOC	regular source of care
		RSOP	right superior oblique palsy
R/S II	resuscitation status two (no code, therapeutic measures only)	RSP	rapid straight pacing
			respirable suspended particles
R/S III	resuscitation status three (no code, comfort measures only)		restriction site polymophism
			right sacroposterior
RSA	right sacrum anterior	RSR	regular sinus rhythm
	right subclavian artery		relative survival rate
RSAPE	remitting seronegative arthritis with pitting edema		right superior rectus
		RSRI	renal:systemic renin index
RSB	right sternal border	RSS	reduced space symbologies
RSBI	rapid shallow breathing index		

	representative sample	RTFS	return to flying status
	sectioned	RTH	right total hip
	Russell-Silver syndrome		(arthroplasty)
RSSE	Russian spring-summer	RTI	respiratory tract infection
	encephalitis		reverse transcriptase
RST	rapid simple tests		inhibitor
	rapid Streptococcal test	RTK	rhabdoid tumor of the
	right sacrum transverse		kidney
RSTs	Rodney Smith tubes		right total knee
RSV	respiratory syncytial virus		(arthroplasty)
	right subclavian vein	RTL	reactive to light
RSVC	right superior vena cava		right temporal lobectomy
RSV$_{IGIV}$	respiratory syncytial virus	RTLF	respiratory-tract lining
	immune globulin,		fluids
	intravenous	RTM	regression to the mean
RSV$_{mab}$	respiratory syncytial virus		routine medical care
	monoclonal antibody,	RTMD	right mid-deltoid
	intramuscular	rTMS	repetitive transcranial
	(palivizumab; Synagis)		magnetic stimulation
RSVP	rapid serial visual	RTN	renal tubular necrosis
	presentation	RTNM	retreatment staging of
RSW	right-sided weakness		cancer
RT	radiation therapy	RTO	return to office
	Radiologic Technologist	RTOG	Radiation Therapy
	recreational therapy		Oncology Group
	rectal temperature	RTP	renal transplant patient
	renal transplant		return to pharmacy
	repetition time		return-to-play
	resistance training	rtPA	alteplase (recombinant
	Respiratory Therapist		tissue-type plasminogen
	reverse transcriptase		activator) (Activase)
	right	RT-PCR	reverse transcription
	right thigh		polymerase chain
	room temperature		reaction
R/t	related to	RTR	renal transplant
RTA	ready to administer		recipient(s)
	renal tubular acidosis		return to room
	road traffic accident	RT (R)	Radiologic Technologist
t-RA	tretinoin (*trans*-retinoic		(Registered)
	acid)	RTRR	return to recovery room
RTAE	right atrial enlargement	RTS	radial tunnel syndrome
RTAH	right anterior hemiblock		raised toilet seat
RTAT	right anterior thigh		real-time scan
RTB	return to baseline		Resolve Through Sharing
RTC	Readiness to Change		return to school
	(questionnaire)		return to sender
	return to clinic		Revised Trauma Score
	round the clock		Rothmund-Thomson
RTCA	ribavirin		syndrome
RTER	return to emergency room		Rubinstein-Taybi
rt.↑ext.	right upper extremity		syndrome
RTF	ready-to-feed	RTT	Respiratory Therapy
	return to flow		Technician

RT$_3$U	resin triiodothyronine uptake		residual volume
			respiratory volume
RTUS	realtime ultrasound		retinal vasculitis
RTV	ritonavir (Norvir)		return visit
	rotavirus vaccine, not otherwise specified		right ventricle
			rubella vaccine
RTV$_{rr}$	rotavirus vaccine, rhesus reassortant	RVA	rabies vaccine, adsorbed
			right ventricular apex
RTW	return to ward		right vertebral artery
	return to work	RVAD	right ventricular assist device
	Richard Turner Warwick (urethroplasty)		
		RVCD	right ventricular conduction deficit
RTWD	return to work determination	RVD	relative vertebral density
			renal vascular disease
RTX	resiniferatoxin	RVDP	right ventricular diastolic pressure
RTx	radiation therapy		
	renal transplantation	RVE	right ventricular enlargement
RU	residual urine		
	resin uptake	RVEDP	right ventricular end-diastolic pressure
	retrograde ureterogram		
	right upper	RVEDV	right ventricular end-diastolic volume
	routine urinalysis		
RU 486	mifepristone (Mifeprex)	RVEF	right ventricular ejection fraction
RUA	right upper arm		
	routine urine analysis	RVET	right ventricular ejection time
RUB	rubella virus vaccine		
RUE	right upper extremity	RVF	Rift Valley fever
RUG	resource utilization group		right ventricular function
			right visual field
	retrograde urethrogram	RVG	radionuclide ventriculography
RUI	recurring urinary infections		
			Radio VisioGraphy
RUL	right upper lid		right ventrogluteal
	right upper lobe	RVH	renovascular hypertension
RUOQ	right upper outer quadrant		right ventricular hypertrophy
rupt.	ruptured		
RUQ	right upper quadrant	RVHT	renovascular hypertension
RUQD	right upper quadrant defect	RVI	right ventricle infarction
		RVIDd	right ventricle internal dimension diastole
RURTI	recurrent upper respiratory tract infection		
		RVL	right vastus lateralis
RUSB	right upper scapular border	RVO	relaxed vaginal outlet
			retinal vein occlusion
	right upper sternal border		right ventricular outflow
RUT	rapid urease test		right ventricular overactivity
RUTF	ready-to-use therapeutic food		
		RVOT	right ventricular outflow tract
RUTI	recurring urinary tract infections	RVOTH	right ventricular outflow tract hypertrophy
RUV	residual urine volume		
RUX	right upper extremity	RVP	right ventricular pressure
RV	rectovaginal	RVR	rapid ventricular response

R

			S
	renal vascular resistance		
	right ventricular rhythm		
RVSP	right ventricular systolic pressure		
RVSW	right ventricular stroke work	S	sacral
RVSWI	right ventricular stroke work index		second (s)
			sensitive
RVT	recurrent ventricular tachycardia		serum
			single
	renal vein thrombosis		sister
RV/TLC	residual volume to total lung capacity ratio		son
			South (as in the location 2S would be second floor, South wing)
RVU	relative-value units		
RVV	rubella vaccine virus		
RVVC	recurrent vulvovaginal candidiasis		sponge
			Staphylococcus
RVVT	Russell viper venom time		streptomycin [part of tuberculosis regimen as in RHZ(E/S)/HR]
RW	radiant warmer		
	ragweed		
	red welt		subjective findings
	rolling walker		suicide
R/W	return to work		suction
RWM	regional wall motion		sulfur
RWMA	regional wall motion abnormalities		supervision
			surgery
RWP	ragweed pollen		susceptible
RWS	ragweed sensitivity	/S/	signature
RWT	relative wall thickness	$\bar{s}$	without (this is a dangerous abbreviation)
Rx	drug		
	medication	S'	shoulder
	pharmacy	S_1	first heart sound
	prescription	$S^{-1}...S^{-4}$	suicide risk classifications
	radiotherapy	S_2	second heart sound
	take	S_3	third heart sound (ventricular filling gallop)
	therapy		
	treatment		
RXN	reaction	S_4	fourth heart sound (atrial gallop)
RXRs	retinoid X receptors		
RXT	radiation therapy	$S_1...S_5$	sacral vertebra or nerves 1 through 5
	right exotropia		
RYGBP	Roux-en-Y gastric bypass (surgery)	SI..SIV	symbols for the first to fourth heart sounds
		SA	sacroanterior
			salicylic acid
			semen analysis
			Sexoholics Anonymous
			sinoatrial
			sleep apnea
			slow acetylator
			Spanish American
			spinal anesthesia
			Staphylococcus aureus

R

	subarachnoid		subacromial
	substance abuse		decompression
	suicide alert		subacute dialysis
	suicide attempt		sugar and acetone
	surface area		determination
	surgical assistant		superior axis deviation
	sustained action	SADBE	squaric acid dibutyl
Sa	Saturday		ester
S/A	same as	SADD	Students Against Drunk
	sugar and acetone		Driving
S&A	sugar and acetone	SADL	simulated activities of
SAA	same as above		daily living
	serum amyloid A	SADR	suspected adverse drug
	Stokes-Adams attacks		reaction
	synthetic amino acids	SADS	Schedule for Affective
SAAG	serum-ascites albumin		Disorders and
	gradient		Schizophrenia
SAANDs	selective apoptotic		sudden arrhythmic death
	antineoplastic drugs		syndrome
SAARDs	slow-acting antirheumatic	SADs	severe autoimmune
	drugs		diseases
SAB	serum albumin	SADS-C	Schedule for Affective
	sinoatrial block		Disorders And
	Spanish-American Black		Schizophrenia –
	spontaneous abortion		Change Version
	Staphylococcus aureus	SAE	serious adverse event
	bacteremia		short above elbow (cast)
	subarachnoid bleed	SAEG	signal averaging
	subarachnoid block		electrocardiogram
SABA	short-acting beta-agonist	SAEKG	signaled average
SABR	screening auditory		electrocardiogram
	brainstem response	SAESU	Substance Abuse
SABs	side air bags		valuating Screen Unit
SAC	school-age children	SAF	Self-Analysis Form
	segmental antigen		self-articulating femoral
	challenge		Spanish-American female
	serial abdominal closure		subcutaneous abdominal
	serum aminoglycoside		fat
	concentration	SAFHS	sonic accelerated fracture
	short arm cast		healing system
	substance abuse counselor	SAG	sodium antimony
SACC	short arm cylinder cast		gluconate
SACD	subacute combined	Sag D	sagittal diameter
	degeneration	SAGE	serial analysis of gene
SACH	solid ankle, cushioned		expression
	heel	SAH	subarachnoid hemorrhage
SACT	sinoatrial conduction time		systemic arterial
SAD	schizoaffective disorder		hypertension
	seasonal affective disorder	SAHA	suberoylanilide
	Self-Assessment		hydroxamic acid
	Depression (scale)	SAHS	sleep apnea/hypopnea
	social anxiety disorder		(hypersomnolence)
	source-axis distance		syndrome

S

SAI	self-administered injectable Sodium Amytal® interview	sang	sanguinous
		SANS	Schedule (Scale) for the Assessment of Negative Symptoms sympathetic autonomic nervous system
SAL	salicylate salmeterol (Serevent) *Salmonella* sensory acuity level sterility assurance level	SAO	small airway obstruction Southeast Asian ovalocytosis
SAL 12	sequential analysis of 12 chemistry constituents (see page 392)	SaO₂	arterial oxygen percent saturation
		SAP	serum alkaline phosphate serum amyloid P sporadic adenomatous polyps statistical analysis plan
SALK	surgical arthroscopy, left knee		
SAM	methylprednisolone sodium succinate (Solu-Medrol), aminophylline, and metaproterenol (Metaprel) selective antimicrobial modulation self-administered medication short arc motion sleep apnea monitor Spanish-American male systolic anterior motion	SAPD	self-administration of psychotropic drugs
		SAPH	saphenous
		SAPHO	synovitis, acne, pustulosis, hyperostosis, and osteomyelitis (syndrome)
		SAPS	Scale for the Assessment of Positive Symptoms short-arm plaster splint Simplified Acute Physiology Score
SAME	syndrome of arthralgias, myalgias, and edema		
SAMe	*S*-adenosylmethionine (ademetionine)	SAPs	shock-absorbing pylons
SAMHSA	Substance Abuse and Mental Health Services Administration	SAPS II	Simplified Acute Physiology Score version II
		SAQ	saquinavir (Invirase) Sexual Adjustment Questionnaire short-arc quadriceps
SAMPLE	symptoms/signs, allergies, medications, past medical history, last oral intake, and events prior to arrival (an EMT mnemonic used in initial patient questioning)	SAR	seasonal allergic rhinitis Senior Assistant Resident sexual attitudes reassessment structural activity relationships
SAMU	Service d'Aide Médicale Urgente (French prehospital emergency system)	SARA	sexually acquired reactive arthritis SQUID (superconducting quantum interference device) array for reproductive assessment system for anesthetic and respiratory administration analysis
SAN	side-arm nebulizer sinoatrial node slept all night		
SANC	short-arm navicular cast		
SANE	Sexual Assault Nurse Examiner		

SARAN	senior admitting resident's admission note		subacute thyroiditis
SARC	seasonal allergic rhinoconjunctivitis		subcutaneous adipose tissue
		SATC	substance abuse treatment clinic
SARK	surgical arthroscopy, right knee	SATL	surgical Achilles tendon lengthening
S Arrh	sinus arrhythmia		
SARS	severe acute respiratory syndrome	SATP	substance abuse treatment program
SARS-CoV	severe acute respiratory syndrome-associated coronavirus	SATS	refers to oxygen saturation levels
SART	standard acid reflux test	SATU	substance abuse treatment unit
SAS	saline, agent, and saline	SAV	supra-annular valve
	scalenus anticus syndrome	SAVD	spontaneous assisted vaginal delivery
	Sedation-Agitation Scale		
	see assessment sheet	SB	safety belt
	Self-rating Anxiety Scale		sandbag
	short-arm splint		scleral buckling
	Simpson-Angus Scale		seat belt
	sleep apnea syndrome		seen by
	Social Adjustment Scale		Sengstaken-Blakemore (tube)
	Specific Activity Scale		sick boy
	statistical applications software		side bend
	subarachnoid space		side bending
	subaxial subluxation		sinus bradycardia
	sulfasalazine (Azulfidine)		slide board
	synthetic absorbable sutures		small bowel
			spina bifida
SASA	Sex Abuse Survivors Anonymous		sponge bath
			stand-by
SASH	saline, agent, saline, and heparin		Stanford-Binet (test)
			sternal border
SASP	sulfasalazine (salicylazo-sulfapyridine; Azulfidine)		stillbirth
			stillborn
			stone basketing
SASS	Social Adaptation Self-Evaluation Scale	Sb	antimony
		SB+	wearing seat belt
SAST	slide agglutination serotyping	SB−	not wearing seat belt
		SBA	serum bactericidal activity
SAT	methylprednisolone sodium succinate (Solu-Medrol), aminophylline, and terbutaline		standby angioplasty
			standby assistant (assistance)
			Summary Basis of Approval
	saturated	SBAC	small bowel adenocarcinoma
	saturation		
	Saturday	SBB	stereotactic breast biopsy
	self-administered therapy	SBBO	small-bowel bacterial overgrowth
	Senior Apperception Test		
	speech awareness threshold	SBC	sensory binocular cooperation

S

	single base cane		shaken baby syndrome
	standard bicarbonate		short (small) bowel
	strict bed confinement		syndrome
	superficial bladder		sick-building syndrome
	cancer		side-by-side
SBD	sleep-related breathing		small bowel series
	disorder	SBT	serum bactericidal titers
	straight bag drainage		special baby Travesol
SBE	saturated base excess		spontaneous breathing
	self-breast examination		trial
	short below-elbow (cast)	SBTB	sinus breakthrough
	shortness of breath on		beat
	exertion	SBTT	small bowel transit time
	subacute bacterial	SBV	single binocular vision
	endocarditis	SBW	seat belts worn
SBFT	small bowel follow	SBX	symphysis, buttocks, and
	through		xiphoid
SBG	stand-by guard	SC	schizophrenia
SBGM	self blood-glucose		Schwann cell
	monitoring		self-care
SBH	State Board of Health		serum creatinine
SBI	silicone (gel-containing)		service connected
	breast implants		sick call
	systemic bacterial		sickle cell
	infection		small (blood pressure)
SBJ	skin, bones, and joints		cuff
SBK	spinnbarkeit		Snellen chart
SBL	sponge blood loss		spinal cord
sBLA	supplemental Biologic		sport cord
	License Application		sternoclavicular
SB-LM	Stanford-Binet		subclavian
	Intelligence Test-Form		subclavian catheter
	LM		subcutaneous
SBO	small bowel obstruction		succinylcholine
	specified bovine offals		sugar-coated (tablets)
SBOD	scleral buckle, right eye		sulfur colloid
SBOE	surgical blood order		supportive care
	equation		surveillance cultures
SBOH	State Board of Health	s̄c	without correction
SBOM	soybean oil meal		(without glasses)
SBOS	scleral buckle, left eye	S&C	sclerae and conjunctivae
SBP	school breakfast program	SCA	sickle cell anemia
	scleral buckling procedure		spinocerebellar ataxia
	small bowel phytobezoars		subclavian artery
	spontaneous bacterial		subcutaneous abdominal
	peritonitis		(block)
	systolic blood pressure		sudden cardiac arrest
SBQC	small-based quad cane		superior cerebellar artery
SBR	sluggish blood return	SCa	serum calcium
	strict bed rest	ScA	*Scedosporium*
SBRN	sensory branch of the		*apiospermum*
	radial nerve	SCA1	spinocerebellar ataxia
SBS	serum blood sugar		type 1

SCAD	short chain acyl-coenzyme A dehydrogenase	SCDM	soybean-casein digest medium
	spontaneous cervical artery dissection	ScDP	scapulodextra posterior
SCAN	suspected child abuse and neglect	SCE	sister chromatid exchange
SCAP	scapula; scapulae; scapular		soft cooked egg
			specialized columnar epithelium
	stem cell apheresis		spinal cord ependymoma
SCARMD	severe childhood autosomal recessive muscular dystrophy	SCEMIA	self-contained enzymatic membrane immunoassay
SCAT	sheep cell agglutination titer	SCEP	somatosensory cortical evoked potential
	sickle cell anemia test	SCF	special care formula
SCB	strictly confined to bed		stem cell factor
SCBC	small cell bronchogenic carcinoma		supra ciliochoroidal fluid
		SCFA	short-chain fatty acid
SCBE	single-contrast barium enema	SCFE	slipped capital femoral epiphysis
SCBF	spinal cord blood flow	SCFGT	Southern California Figure Ground Test
SCC	short course chemotherapy (for tuberculosis)	SCG	seismocardiography
			serum Chemogram
	sickle cell crisis		sodium cromoglycate
	small cell carcinoma		substitute care giver
	spinal cord compression	SCH	schistosomiasis (*Schistosoma* sp.) vaccine
	squamous cell carcinoma		
SCCA	semi-closed circle absorber		subclinical hypothyroidism
	squamous cell carcinoma antigen	SCh	succinylcholine chloride
		SCHISTO	schistocytes
SCCa	squamous cell carcinoma	SCHIZ	schizocytes
SCCB	small cell cancer of the bladder		schizophrenia
		SCHLP	supracricord hemilaryngopharyngec-tomy
SCCE	squamous cell carcinoma of the esophagus		
SCCHN	squamous cell carcinoma of the head and neck	SCHNC	squamous cell head and neck cancer
SCCI	subcutaneous continuous infusion	SCI	silent cerebral infarct
			specific COX-2 inhibitor
SCCOT	squamous cell carcinoma of the oral tongue		spinal cord injury
			subcoma insulin
SCD	sequential compression device	SCID	severe combined immunodeficiency disorders (disease)
	service connected disability		
	sickle cell disease		structured clinical inter-view for DSM-III-R
	spinal cord disease	SCII	Strong-Campbell Interest Inventory
	subacute combined degeneration		
	sudden cardiac death	SCIP	Screening and Crisis Intervention Program
ScDA	scapulodextra anterior		

S

SCIPP	sacrococcygeal to inferior pubic point	SCPF	stem cell proliferation factor
SCIT	single-chain immunotoxin	S-CPK	serum creatine phosphokinase
SCIU	spinal cord injury unit		
SCIV	subclavian intravenous	SCPP	spinal cord perfusion pressure
SCI-WORA	spinal cord injury without radiographic abnormalities	SCR	special care room (seclusion room)
SCJ	squamocolumnar junction sternoclavicular joint		spondylitic caudal radioculopathy standard care regimen
sCJD	sporadic Creutzfeldt-Jakob disease		stem cell rescue
SCL	skin conductance level symptom checklist	SCr	serum creatinine
		sCR	soluble complement receptor
SCL-90	Symptoms Checklist—90 items	SCRIPT	prescription
ScLA	scapulolaeva anterior	SC/RP	scaling and root planing
SCLAX	subcostal long axis	SC-RNV	subcutaneous radionuclide venography
SCLC	small cell lung cancer		
SCLD	sickle cell lung disease	SCS	spinal cord stimulation
SCLE	subacute cutaneous lupus erythematosis		splatter control shield stem cell support
ScLP	scapulolaeva posterior		suspected catheter sepsis
SCLs	soft contact lenses		
	synthetic combinatorial libraries	SCSAX	subcostal short axis
SCM	scalene muscle	SCSIT	Southern California Sensory Integration Tests
	sensation, circulation, and motion		
	spondylitic caudal myelopathy	SCSVT	Southern California Space Visualization Test
	sternocleidomastoid supraclavicular muscle	SCT	Sertoli cell tumor sex chromatin test
SCMD	senile choroidal macular degeneration		sickle cell trait stem cell transplant
SCMV	serogroup C meningococcal vaccine		sugar-coated tablet
		SCTX	static cervical traction
SCN	severe congenital neutropenia	SCU	self-care unit special care unit
	special care nursery suprachiasmatic nucleus (nuclei)	SCUCP	small cell undifferentiated carcinoma of the prostate
SCNT	somatic-cell nuclear transfer	SCUF	slow continuous ultrafiltration
S/CO	signal-to-cut-off (ratios)	SCUT	schizophrenia, chronic undifferentiated type
SCOB	Schedule-Controlled Operant Behavior	SCV	subclavian vein subcutaneous vaginal (block)
SCOP	scopolamine		
SCOPE	arthroscopy	SCY	scytonemin
SCP	secondary care provider sodium cellulose phosphate standardized care plan	SD	scleroderma senile dementia sensory deficit

severe deficit
septal defect
severely disabled
shallow distance (aquatic therapy)
shoulder disarticulation
single dose
skin dose
sleep deprived
solvent-detergent
somatic dysfunction
spasmodic dysphonia
speech discrimination
spontaneous delivery
stable disease
standard deviation
standard diet
step-down
sterile dressing
straight drainage
streptozocin and doxorubicin
sudden death
surgical drain

S & D seen and discussed
stomach and duodenum

S/D sharp/dull
systolic-diastolic ratio

SDA sacrodextra anterior
same day admission
serotonin/dopamine antagonist
Seventh-Day Adventist
steroid-dependent asthmatic

SDAT senile dementia of Alzheimer type

SDB Sabouraud dextrose broth
self-destructive behavior
sleep disordered breathing

SDBP seated diastolic blood pressure
standing diastolic blood pressure
supine diastolic blood pressure

SDC serum digoxin concentration
serum drug concentration
Sleep Disorders Center
sodium deoxycholate

SD&C suction, dilation, and curettage

SDD selective digestive (tract) decontamination
sterile dry dressing
subantimicrobial dose doxycycline (dental; Periostat)

SDDT selective decontamination of the digestive tract

SDE subdural empyema

SDES symptomatic diffuse esophageal spasm

SDF sexual dysfunction
stromal-cell-derived factor

SDH spinal detrusor hyperreflexia
subdural hematoma

SDHD succinate dehydrogenase complex subunit D

SDI Sandimmune (cyclosporine)
State Disability Insurance

SDII sudden death in infancy

SDL serum digoxin level
serum drug level
speech discrimination loss

SDLE sex-difference in life expectancy
somatic dysfunction lower extremity

SDM soft drusen maculopathy
standard deviation of the mean

S/D/M systolic, diastolic, mean

SDMC safety and data monitoring committee

SD/N signal-difference-to-noise ratio

SDNN standard deviation of normal-to-normal beats

SDO surgical diagnostic oncology

SDP sacrodextra posterior
single donor platelets
solvent-detergent plasma
stomach, duodenum, and pancreas

SDPTG second derivative of photoplethysmogram

SDR selective dorsal rhizotomy
short-duration response

SDS same day surgery

S

	Self-Rating Depression Scale		surrogate end-point biomarker
	Shwachman-Diamond Syndrome	SEC	second
	sodium dodecyl sulfate		secondary
	somatropin deficiency syndrome		secretary
	Speech Discrimination Score		size exclusion chromatography
	standard deviation score		spontaneous echo contrast
	sudden death syndrome		steric exclusion chromatography
	Symptom Distress Scale	SECG	scalp electrocardiogram
SDSO	same day surgery overnight	SECL	seclusion
SDS-PAGE	sodium dodecyl sulfate – polyacrylamide gel electrophoresis	SECPR	standard external cardiopulmonary resuscitation
SDT	sacrodextra transversa	SE-CPT	single-electrode current perception threshold
	speech detection threshold	SED	sedimentation
SDU	step-down unit		skin erythema dose
SDUE	somatic dysfunction upper extremity		socially and emotionally disturbed
SDV	single-dose vial		spondyloepiphyseal dysplasia
SDX/PYR	sulfadoxine; pyrimethamine (Fansidar)	SeDBP	seated diastolic blood pressure
SE	saline enema (0.9% sodium chloride)	SEDDS	self-emulsifying drug-delivery system
	self-examination	SED-NET	severely emotional disturbed - network
	side effect	sed rt	sedimentation rate
	soft exudates	SEER	Surveillance, Epidemiology, and End Results (program)
	special education		
	spin echo		
	staff escort		
	standard error	SEF	spectral edge frequency (anesthesia-depth monitor)
	Starr-Edwards (valve, pacemaker)		
	status epilepticus	SEG	segment
Se	selenium		sonoencephalogram
S/E	suicidal and eloper	segs	segmented neutrophils
S & E	seen and examined	SEH	spinal epidural hematomas
SEA	sheep erythrocyte agglutination (test)		subependymal hemorrhage
	side-entry (venous) access	SEI	subepithelial (comeal) infiltrate
	Southeast Asia		
	Staphylococcal enterotoxin A	SELDI	surface enhanced laser desorption/ionization
	subdural electrode array		
	synaptic electronic activation	SELFVD	sterile elective low forceps vaginal delivery
SEAR	Southeast Asia refugee	SEM	scanning electron microscopy
SEB	Staphylococcus enterotoxin B		semen

S

	slow eye movement		skin end-point titration
	standard error of mean		social environmental therapy
	systolic ejection murmur		systolic ejection time
SEMI	subendocardial myocardial infarction	SEV	sevoflurane (Ultane)
SEN	spray each nostril	SEWHO	shoulder-elbow-wrist-hand orthosis
SENS	sensitivity		
	sensorium	SF	salt-free
SEOC	serous epithelial ovarian carcinoma		saturated fat
			scarlet fever
SEP	multiple sclerosis (French)		seizure frequency
	separate		seminal fluid
	serum electrophoresis		skull fracture
	somatosensory evoked potential		small finger
			soft feces
	syringe exchange program		sound field
			spinal fluid
	systolic ejection period		starch-free
SEPS	subfascial endoscopic perforator surgery		sugar-free
			symptom-free
SEQ	sequela		synovial fluid
SER	scanning equalization radiography	S&F	slip and fall
			soft and flat
	sertraline (Zoloft)	SF-6	sulfahexafluoride
	side effects records	SF 36	36-item short form health survey
	signal enhancement ratio		
SERA-TEK	technetium-99m hexametazime	SFA	saturated fatty acids
			superficial femoral artery
SERF	Severity of Exacerbation and Risk Factors	SFB	single frequency bioimpedance
Serial 7's	a mental status examination (starting with a 100, count backward by 7's)	SFC	spinal fluid count
			subarachnoid fluid collection
		SFD	scaphoid fossa depression
SER-IV	supination external rotation, type 4 fracture		small for dates
		SFE	supercritical fluid extraction
SERM	selective estrogen-receptor modulator		
		SFEMG	single-fiber electromyography
SERO-SANG	serosanguineous		
		SFH	schizophrenia family history
SERP-ACWA	Skin Exposure Reduction Paste Against Chemical Warfare Agents		
		SFJ	saphenofemoral junction
		SFM	scanning force microscopy
SERs	somatosensory evoked responses		
		SFNM	subfoveal neovascular membranes
SES	sick euthyroid syndrome		
	socioeconomic status	SFP	simulated fluorescence process
	standard electrolyte solution		simultaneous foveal perception
SeSBP	seated systolic blood pressure		
			spinal fluid pressure
SET	signal extraction technology	SFPT	standard fixation preference test

S

SFRT	stereotactic fractionated radiotherapy	SGP	Schering-Plough Corporation
SFS	split function studies	SGPT	serum glutamate pyruvate transaminase (same as ALT)
SFT	solitary fibrous tumor		
SFTR	sagittal, frontal, transverse, rotation	SGRQ-A	St. George's Respiratory Questionnaire translated into American English
SFTs	solitary fibrous tumors		
SFUP	surgical follow-up	SGS	second-generation sulfonylurea
SFV	simian foamy viruses superficial femoral vein		subglottic stenosis
SFW	shell fragment wound	sGS	surgical Gleason score
SFWB	social/family well-being	SGTCS	secondarily generalized tonic-clonic seizures
SFWD	symptom-free walking distance		
SG	salivary gland	SH	serum hepatitis
	scrotography		sexual harassment
	serum glucose		short
	side glide		shoulder
	skin graft		shower
	specific gravity		social history
	Swan-Ganz (catheter)		sulfhydryl (group)
S/G	swallow/gag		surgical history
SGA	small for gestational age		systemic hypertension
	subjective global assessment (dietary history and physical examination)	S&H	speech and hearing
			suicidal and homicidal
		S/H	suicidal/homicidal ideation
	substantial gainful activity (employment)	SH2	sarc homology region 2
		SHA	super-heated aerosol
SGAs	second-generation antihistamines second-generation antipsychotics	SHAFT	*s*hopping, *h*ousework, *a*ccounting (bills), *f*ood preparation, and *t*ransportation (driving); (instrumental activities of daily living)
SGB	Swiss gym ball		
SGC	Swan-Ganz catheter		
SGCNB	stereotactic guided core-needle biopsy	SHAL	standard hyperalimentation
SGD	salivary gland dysfunction	SHAS	supravalvular hypertrophic aortic stenosis
	specific granule deficiency		
	specific growth delay		
	speech generating device	S Hb	sickle hemoglobin screen
	straight gravity drainage	SHBG	sex hormone-binding globulin
	sweat gland density		
SGE	significant glandular enlargement	sHBO₂T	systemic hyperbaric oxygen therapy
SGHL	superior glenohumeral ligament	SHC	subsequent hospital care
s̄ gl	without correction (without glasses)	SHEENT	skin, head, eyes, ears, nose, and throat
SGM	serum glucose monitoring	SHG	shigellosis (*Shigella* sp.) vaccine
SGOT	serum glutamic oxalo-acetic transaminase (same as AST)	SHGT	somatic-cell human gene therapy

SHI	Self-Harm Inventory		Standard Industrial Classification
	standard heparin infusion		
Shig	*Shigella*	SICD	sudden infant crib death
SHIV	simian-human immunodeficiency virus	SICOG	Southern Italy Cooperative Oncology Group
SHL	sudden hearing loss		
	supraglottic horizontal laryngectomy	SICT	selective intracoronary thrombolysis
SHMB	severe hypersensitivity to mosquito bites	SICU	surgical intensive care unit
		SID	once daily (used in veterinary medicine)
SHO	Senior House Officer		
SHP	secondary hypertension, pulmonary	SIDA	French and Spanish abbreviation for AIDS
SHR	scapulohumeral rhythm	SIDAM	structured interview for the diagnosis of dementia of Alzheimer type
SHRC	shortened, held, resisted contraction		
SHS	student health service		
SHV	short hepatic vein	SIDAM-A	structured interview for the diagnosis of dementia of the Alzheimer type, multi-infarct dementia, and dementias of other etiology according to ICD-10 and DSM-III-R
	sulfhydryl variant		
SHx	social history		
SI	International System of Units		
	sacroiliac		
	sagittal index		
	sector iridectomy		
	self-inflicted	SIDD	syndrome of isolated diastolic dysfunction
	sensory integration		
	seriously ill	SIDERO	siderocyte
	sexual intercourse	SIDFF	superimposed dorsiflexion of foot
	signal intensity		
	small intestine	SIDS	sudden infant death syndrome
	strict isolation		
	stress incontinence	SIEP	serum immunoelectrophoresis
	stroke index		
	suicidal ideation	*SIG*	let it be marked (appears on prescription before directions for patient)
Si	silicon		
S & I	suction and irrigation		
	support and interpretation		sigmoidoscopy
SIA	small intestinal atresia	Signal 99	patient in cardiac or respiratory distress
SIADH	syndrome of inappropriate antidiuretic hormone secretion		
		SI/HI	suicidal/homicidal ideations
SIAT	supervised intermittent ambulatory treatment	SIJ	sacroiliac joint
		SIJS	sacroiliac joint syndrome
SIB	self-inflating bulb	SIL	seriously ill list
	self-injurious behavior		sister-in-law
SIBC	serum iron-binding capacity		squamous intraepithelial lesion
sibs	siblings	SILFVD	sterile indicated low forceps vaginal delivery
SIC	self-intermittent catherization		
	squamous intraepithelial cells	SILV	simultaneous independent lung ventilation

S

329

SIM	selective ion monitoring	SIVP	slow intravenous push
	Similac®	SIW	self-inflicted wound
	surface-induced	SJC	swollen joint count
	mineralization	SJCRH	St. Jude Children's
SIMCU	surgical intermediate care		Research Hospital
	unit	SJM	St. Jude Medical (heart
Sim c Fe	Similac with iron®		valve prosthesis)
SIMV	synchronized intermittent	S-JRA	systemic juvenile
	mandatory ventilation		rheumatoid arthritis
SIN	salpingitis isthmica	SJS	Schwartz-Jampel
	nodose		syndrome
SIOD	Schimke immuno-osseous		Stevens-Johnson
	dysplasia		syndrome
SIP	Sickness Impact Profile		Swyer-James syndrome
	stroke in progression	S_{jv02}	jugular venous oxygen
	sympathetically		saturation
	independent pain	SK	seborrheic keratosis
SIQ	sick in quarters		senile keratosis
SIQ-JR	Suicidal Ideation		solar keratosis
	Questionnaire-Junior		streptokinase
SIR	standardized incidence	S & K	single and keeping
	rate (ratio)		(baby)
SIRS	systemic inflammatory	SKAO	supracondylar knee-ankle
	response syndrome		orthosis
SIS	sister	SKAs	skills, knowledge, and
	small intestinal submucosa		abilities (ratings)
	Surgical Infection	SKB	SmithKline Beecham
	Stratification (system)	SKC	single knee to chest
SISI	Short Increment	SKINT	skinfold thickness
	Sensitivity Index	SK-SD	streptokinase
SISS	severe invasion		streptodornase
	streptococcal syndrome	SKU	stock keeping unit
SIT	serum inhibitory titers		(related to product
	silicon-intensified target		identification)
	Slossen Intelligence Test	SKY	spectral karyotyping
	specific immunotherapy	SL	scapholunate
	(allergy)		secondary leukemia
	sperm immobilization test		sensation level
	structured interrupted		sentinel lymphadenectomy
	therapy		serious list
	supraspinatus,		shortleg
	infraspinatus, teres		side-lying
	(insertions)		staging laparoscopy
	surgical intensive therapy		slight
SITA	standard infertility		sublingual
	treatment algorithm	S/L	slit lamp (examination)
SIT BAL	sitting balance	SLA	sacrolaeva anterior
SIT TOL	sitting tolerance		sex and love addictions
SIV	simian immunodeficiency		slide latex agglutination
	virus		The Satisfaction with Life
SIVD	subcortical ischemic		Areas
	vascular dementia	SLAA	Sex and Love Addicts
	(disease)		Anonymous

SLAC	scapholunate advanced collapse	SLNM	sentinel lymph node mapping
SLAM	Systemic Lupus Activity Measure	SLNTG	sublingual nitroglycerin
		SLNWBC	short leg nonweight-bearing cast
SLAP	serum leucine amino-peptidase	SLNWC	short leg nonwalking cast
	superior labral anteroposterior (shoulder lesion)	SLO	scanning laser ophthalmoscope
			second-look operation
SLB	short leg brace		shark liver oil
SLBB	single-living baby boy		Smith-Lemli-Opitz (syndrome)
SLBG	single-living baby girl		streptolysin O
SLC	short leg cast	SLOA	short leave of absence
SLCC	short leg cylinder cast	SLOM	serous left otitis media
SLCG	sulfolithocholylglycine	SLP	scanning laser polarimeter
SLCT	Sertoli-Leydig cell tumor		single-limb progression
SLD	specific language disorder		Speech Language Pathologist
	stealth liposomal doxorubicin		speech language pathology
SLE	slit-lamp examination		superficial lamina propria
	St. Louis encephalitis	SLPI	secretory leukocyte protease inhibitor
	systemic lupus erythematosus	SLPMS	short-leg posterior-molded splint
SLEDAI	Systemic Lupus Erythematosus Disease Activity Index	SLR	straight-leg raising
		SLRS	stereotactic linac radiosurgery
SLEX	slit-lamp examination (biomicroscopy)	SLRT	straight-leg raising tenderness
SLFVD	sterile low forceps vaginal delivery		straight-leg raising test
SLGXT	symptom-limited graded exercise test	SLS	second-look sonography
			short leg splint
SLI	specific language impairment		shrinking lungs syndrome
			single leg stance
SLIT	sublingual immunotherapy		single limb support
SLK	superior limbic keratoconjunctivitis	SLT	sacrolaeva transversa
			scanning laser tomography
SLL	second-look laparotomy		single lung transplantation
	small lymphocytic lymphoma		Speech Language Therapist
SLMFVD	sterile low midforceps vaginal delivery		spontaneous labor at term
SLMMS	slightly more marked since		swing light test
SLMP	since last menstrual period	SLT-I	Shiga-like toxin I
		SLTA	severe life-threatening asthma
SLN	sentinel lymph node(s)		standard language test for aphasia
	superior laryngeal nerve		
SLNB	sentinel lymph node biopsy	SLTEC	Shiga-like toxin-producing *Escherichia coli*
SLND	sentinel lymph node detection		

sl. tr.	slight trace
SLUD	salivation, lacrimation, urination, and defecation
SLUDGE	**s**alivation, **l**acrimation, **u**rination, **d**iarrhea, **g**astrointestinal upset, and **e**mesis (signs and symptoms of cholinergic excess)
SLV	since last visit
SLVD	systolic left ventricular dysfunction
SLWB	severely low birth weight
SLWC	short leg walking cast
SM	sadomasochism
	service mark (such as The Pause that Refreshes)
	skim milk
	small
	sports medicine
	Stairmaster®
	streptomycin
	systolic motion
	systolic murmur
^{153}Sm	samarium 153
SMA	smallpox vaccine, not otherwise specified
	smooth muscle antibody
	spinal muscular atrophy
	superior mesenteric artery
SMA-II	spinal muscular atrophy type II
SMA-6	simultaneous multichannel autoanalyzer (page 358)
SMA-7	See page 392
SMA-12	See page 392
SMA-18	See page 392
SMA-23	See page 392
SMAO	superior mesenteric artery occlusion
SMAR	self-medication administration record
SMAS	superficial musculoaponeurotic system (graft; flat)
	superior mesenteric artery syndrome
SMAST	Short Michigan Alcohol-ism Screening Test
SMAvac	smallpox (vaccinia virus) vaccine

SMB	simulated moving bed (chromatography)
SMBG	self-monitoring blood glucose
SMC	skeletal myxoid chondrosarcoma
	special mouth care
SMCA	sorbitol MacConkey agar
SMCD	senile macular chorio-retinal degeneration
SMCs	smooth muscle cells
SMD	senile macular degeneration
	standardized mean difference
SMDA	Safe Medical Defice Act
SME	significant medical event
SMF	streptozocin, mitomycin, and fluorouracil
SMFA	sodium monofluoroacetate
SMFVD	sterile midforceps vaginal delivery
SMG	submandibular gland
SMH	state mental hospital
SMI	sensory motor integration (group)
	serious mental illness
	severely mentally impaired
	service mix index
	small volume infusion
	suggested minimum increment
	sustained maximal inspiration
SMIDS	suppertime mixed insulin and daytime sulfonylureas
SMILE	safety, monitoring, intervention, length of stay and evaluation
	sustained maximal inspiratory lung exercises
SMIT	standard mycological identification techniques
SMMVT	sustained monomorphic ventricular tachycardia
SMN	second malignant neoplasia
SMO	Senior Medical Officer

	site management organization(s)
	slip made out
SMON	subacute myelo-opticoneuropathy
SMORs	standardized mortality odds ratios
SMP	safety management plan
	self-management program
	sympathetic maintained plan
SmPC	Summary of Product Characteristics (European Union)
SMPN	sensorimotor polyneuropathy
SMR	senior medical resident
	skeletal muscle relaxant
	sleeping metabolic rate
	standardized mortality ratio
	submucous resection
SMRR	submucous resection and rhinoplasty
SMS	scalded mouth syndrome
	senior medical student
	Smith-Magenis syndrome
	somatostatin (Zecnil)
	stiff-man syndrome
SMSA	standard metropolitan statistical area
SMT	smooth muscle tumors
	standard medical therapy
	study management team
SMV	stentless mitral valve
	submentovertical
	superior mesenteric vein
SMVT	sustained monomorphic ventricular tachycardia
SMX-TMP	sulfamethoxazole and trimethoprim (SMZ-TMP)
SN	sciatic notch
	sinus node
	staff nurse
	student nurse
	suprasternal notch
	superior nasal
Sn	tin
sN	sentinel lymph node
S/N	signal to noise ratio
SNA	specimen not available
	Student Nursing Assistant
SNa	serum sodium

SNAE	sustained pain-free and no adverse events
SNAP	scheduled nursing activities program
	Score for Neonatal Acute Physiology
	sensory nerve action potential
	Swanson, Nolan, and Pelham (rating scale)
SNAP-PE	Score for Neonatal Acute Physiology-Perinatal Extension
SNaRI	serotonin noradrenergic reuptake inhibitor
SNASA	Salford Needs Assessment Schedule for Adolescents
SNAT	suspected nonaccidental trauma
SNB	scalene node biopsy
	sentinel (lymph) node biopsy
SNC	skilled nursing care
SNc	substantia nigra compacta
SNCV	sensory nerve conduction velocity
SND	selective neck dissection
	single needle device
	sinus node dysfunction
SNDA	Supplemental New Drug Application
SNE	subacute necrotizing encephalomyelopathy
SNEP	student nurse extern program
SnET2	tin ethyl etiopurpurin
SNF	Simon nitinol filter
	skilled nursing facility
SnF$_2$	stannous fluoride
SNF/MR	skilled nursing facility for the mentally retarded
SNGFR	single nephron glomerular filtration rate
SNGP	supranuclear gaze palsy
SNHL	sensorineural hearing loss
SNIP	silver nitrate immunoperoxidase
	strict no information in paper
SNK	Student-Newman-Keuls (test)

S

SNM	sentinel (lymph) node mapping	SNUB	super neurotransmitter uptake blocker
	serotoninergic neuroenteric modulators	SNV	Sin Nombre virus
			skilled nursing visit
	student nurse midwife		spleen necrosis virus
SnMp	tin-mesoporphyrin	SO	second opinion
SNOMED	Systematized Nomenclature of Medicine		sex offender
			shoulder orthosis
			significant other
SNOMED CT	Systemized Nomenclature of Medicine, Clinical Terms		special observation
			sphincter of Oddi
			standing orders
			suboccipital
SNOMED RT	Systemized Nomenclature of Medicine, Reference Terminology		suggestive of
			superior oblique
			supraoptic
			supraorbital
SNOOP	Systematic Nursing Observation of Psychopathology		sutures out
			sympathetic ophthalmia
		S/O	suggestive of
SNOs	S-nitrosothiols	S-O	salpingo-oophorectomy
SNP	simple neonatal procedure	S&O	salpingo-oophorectomy
	single nucleotide polymorphism	SO_2	sulfur dioxide
		SO_3	sulfite
	sodium nitroprusside (Nipride)	SO_4	sulfate
		SOA	serum opsonic activity
SNP-LP	single nucleotide polymorphisms – linkage disequilibrium		shortness of air
			spinal opioid analgesia
			supraorbital artery
SNPs	single nucleotide polymorphisms		swelling of ankles
		SOAA	signed out against advice
SNR	signal-to-noise ratio (radiology)	SOAM	sutures out in the morning
		SOAMA	signed out against medical advice
SNr	substantia nigra reticularis		
SNRB	selective nerve root block	SOAP	subjective, objective, assessment, and plans
SNRI	selective noradrenergic reuptake inhibitor	SOAPIE	subjective, objective, assessment, plan, implementation, (intervention), and evaluation
	serotonin norepinephrine reuptake inhibitor		
SNRT	sinus node recovery time		
SNS	sterile normal saline (0.9% sodium chloride, sterile)	SOB	see order book
			shortness of breath (this abbreviation has caused problems)
	Strategic National Stockpile		side of bed
	sympathetic nervous system	SOBE	short of breath on exertion
SNSA	sympathetic nervous system activity	SOBOE	short of breath on exertion
SNT	sinuses, nose, and throat	SOC	see old chart
	suppan nail technique		socialization
SNU	skilled nursing unit		stages of change

	standard of care	SOP	standard operating procedure
	start of care		
	state of consciousness	SOPM	sutures out in afternoon (or evening)
	system organ class		
S & OC	signed and on chart (e.g. permit)	SOR	sign own release strength of recommendation
SOD	sinovenous occlusive disease	SORA	stable on room air
	sphincter of Oddi dysfunction	SOS	if there is need may be repeated once if urgently required (Latin: *si opus sit*) self-obtained smear suicidal observation status
	superoxide dismutase		
	surgical officer of the day		
SODA	Severity of Dyspepsia Assessment	SOSOB	sit on side of bed
SODAS	spheriodal oral drug absorption system	SOT	solid organ transplant something other than stream of thought
SOE	source of embolism		
SOFA	sepsis-related organ failure assessment	SOTP	Sex-Offender Treatment Provider
	Sequential Organ Failure Assessment (score)	SOW	Scope of Work
		SP	sacrum to pubis
SOFAS	Social and Occupational Functioning Assessment Scale		sequential pulse serum protein shoulder press
SOG	suggestive of good		silent period (related to electromyographic responses)
SOGS	South Oaks Gambling Screen		
SOH	sexually oriented hallucinations		spastic dysphonia speech
SoHx	social history		Speech Pathologist
SOI	slipped on ice		spinal
	sudden overwhelming infection		spouse stand and pivot
	surgical orthotopic implantation (implant)		stand pivot status post *Streptococcus pneumoniae*
	syrup of ipecac		
SOL	solution		sulfadoxine; pyrimethamine (Fansidar)
	space occupying lesion		
SOL I	special observations level one (there are also SOL II and SOL III)		systolic pressure
		sp	species
SOM	secretory otitis media	S/P	status post
	serous otitis media		suprapubic
	somatization	SP 1	suicide precautions number 1
SOMI	sterno-occipital mandibular immobilizer	SP 2	suicide precautions number 2
SONK	spontaneous osteonecrosis of the knee	SPA	albumin human (formerly known as salt-poor albumin)
Sono	sonogram		
SONP	solid organs not palpable		scintillation proximity assay
SOOL	spontaneous onset of labor		

S

	serum prothrombin activity	SPEC	specimen
	sheep pulmonary adenomatosis		streptococcal pyrogenic exotoxins C
	single photon absorptiometry	Spec Ed	special education
	Speech Pathology and Audiology	SPECT	single-photon emission computed tomography
	stimulation produced analgesia	SPEEP	spontaneous positive end-expiratory pressure
	student physician's assistant	SPEP	serum protein electrophoresis
	subperiosteal abscess	SPET	single-photon emission tomography
	suprapubic aspiration	SPF	semipermeable film
SpA	spondyloarthropathy		S-phase fraction
SP-A	surfactant-specific protein A		split products of fibrin
SPAC	satisfactory postanesthesia course		sun protective factor
		sp fl	spinal fluid
SPAG	small-particle aerosol generator	SPG	scrotopenogram
			sphenopalatine ganglion
SPAMM	spatial modulation of magnetization	SpG	specific gravity
SPBE	saw palmetto berry extract	SPH	severely and profoundly handicapped
SPBI	serum protein bound iodine		sighs per hour
SPBT	suprapubic bladder tap		spherocytes
SPC	saturated phosphatidylcholine	SPHERO	spherocytes
		SPI	speech processor interface
	sclerosing pancreatocholangitis		surgical peripheral iridectomy
	single-point cane	SPIA	solid phase immunoabsorbent assay
	statistical process control		
	Summary of Product Characteristics	SPIF	spontaneous peak inspiratory force
	suprapubic catheter	SPIFE	serum protein and immunofixation electrophoresis (system)
SPCA	serum prothrombin conversion accelerator (factor VII)		
		S-PIN	Steinmann pin
SPCT	simultaneous prism and cover test	SPINK1	serine protease inhibitor Kazal type 1
SPD	subcorneal pustular dermatosis	SPK	simultaneous pancreas-kidney (transplant)
	Supply, Processing, and Distribution (department)		single parent keeping (baby)
	suprapubic drainage		superficial punctate keratitis
SPE	saw palmetto extract	SPL	sound pressure level
	serum protein electrophoresis		superior parietal lobule
	solid-phase extraction	SPL®	Staphylococcal Phage Lysate
	superficial punctate erosions	SPLATTT	split anterior tibial tendon transfer
SPEB	streptococcal pyrogenic exotoxins B	SPM	scanning probe microscopy

S

	second primary malignancy		status post surgery
			stiff-person syndrome
SPM96	statistical parametric mapping 96		systemic progressive sclerosis
SPMA	spinal progressive muscle atrophy	SPSU	straight partial sit-up
		SPT	second primary tumors
SPMD	scapuloperoneal muscular dystrophy		skin prick test
			standing pivot transfer
SPMDs	semipermeable membrane devices		supportive periodontal therapy
SPME	solid-phase microextraction		suprapubic tenderness
		SP TAP	spinal tap
SPMI	severely and persistently mentally ill	SPTL	spontaneous preterm labor
		SPTs	second primary tumors
SPMSQ	Short Portable Mental Status Questionnaire		single-patient trials
SPN	solitary pulmonary nodule	SP TUBE	suprapubic tube
	student practical nurse	SPTX	static pelvic traction
	superficial peroneal nerve	SPU	short procedure unit
SPNK	single parent not keeping (baby)	SPVR	systemic peripheral vascular resistance
SPO	status postoperative	SPX	smallpox vaccine, not otherwise specified
SpO2	oxygen saturation by pulse oximeter		
		SPXv	smallpox vaccine (vaccinia virus)
spont	spontaneous		
SponVe	spontaneous ventilation	SQ	status quo
SPP	Sexuality Preference Profile		subcutaneous (this is a dangerous abbreviation, use subcut)
	single presentation phenotype		
		Sq CCa	squamous cell carcinoma
	super packed platelets	SQE	subcutaneous emphysema
	suprapubic prostatectomy	SQM	square meter(s)
spp	species	SQUID	superconducting quantum interference device
SPQ	Schizotypal Personality Questionnaire		
		SQV	saquinavir (Fortovose; Invirase)
SPR	surface plasmon resonance		
		SR	screen
SPRAS	Sheehan Patient Rated Anxiety Scale		sedimentation rate
			see report
SP-RIA	solid-phase radioimmunoassay		senior resident
			service record
SPR-MS	surface plasmon resonance mass spectrometry		side rails
			sinus rhythm
			slow release
SPROM	spontaneous premature rupture of membrane		smooth-rough
			social recreation
SPS	shoulder pain and stiffness		stretch reflex
	simple partial seizure		superior rectus
	sodium polyethanol sulfonate		sustained release
			sustained response
	sodium polystyrene sulfonate (Kayexalate; SPS®)		suture removal
			system review
		S/R	strong/regular (pulse)

S

S&R	seclusion and restraint		single room occupancy
	smooth and rough		smallest region of overlap
^{89}Sr	strontium 89		sustained-release oral
SRA	serotonin release assay	SROA	sports-related
	steroid-resistant asthma		osteoarthritis
SRAN	surgical resident	SROCPI	Self-Rating Obsessive-
	admission note		Compulsive Personality
SRBC	sheep red blood cells		Inventory
	sickle red blood cells	SROM	serous right otitis media
SRBOW	spontaneous rupture of		spontaneous rupture of
	bag of waters		membrane
SRC	sclerodermal renal crisis	SRP	scaling and root planing
SRCC	sarcomatoid renal cell		(dental)
	carcinoma		septorhinoplasty
SRCS	Division of Surveillance,		stapes replacement
	Research, and		prosthesis
	Communication	SRR	surgical recovery room
	Support (FDA)	SRS	Silver-Russell syndrome
SRD	service-related disability		somatostatin receptor
	smallest real difference		scintigraphy
	sodium-restricted diet	s̄RS	without redness or
SRE	sex and relationships		swelling
	education	SRS-A	slow-reacting substance of
	skeletal related event		anaphylaxis
SRF	somatotropin releasing	SRSV	small round structured
	factor		viruses
	subretinal fluid	SRT	sedimentation rate test
SRF-A	slow-releasing factor of		sleep-related tumescence
	anaphylaxis		speech reception threshold
SRGVHD	steroid-resistant graft-		speech recognition
	versus-host disease		threshold
SRH	signs of recent		stereotactic radiotherapy
	hemorrhage		surfactant replacement
SRI	serotonin reuptake		therapy
	inhibitor		sustained release
SRICU	surgical respiratory		theophylline
	intensive care unit	SRU	side rails up
SRIF	somatotropin-release	SRUS	solitary rectal ulcer
	inhibiting factor		syndrome
	(somatostatin; Zecnil)	SRVC	subcutaneous reservoir
SRK	smooth-rod Kaneda		and ventricular
	(implant)		catheter
SRMD	stress-related mucosal	SR ↑ X2	both siderails up
	damage	SS	half (this is a dangerous
SRMS	sustained-release		abbreviation as it is not
	morphine sulfate		understood or read as
SRMs	specified risk materials		sliding scale)
SR/NE	sinus rhythm, no ectopy		sacral sulcus
SRNV	subretinal		sacrosciatic
	neovascularization		saline soak (sodium
SRNVM	subretinal neovascular		chloride 0.9%)
	membrane		saline solution (0.9%
SRO	sagittal ramus osteotomy		sodium chloride)

S

saliva sample
salt sensitivity (sensitive)
salt substitute
serotonin syndrome
serum sickness
sickle cell
single-session (treatment)
single-strength (as compared to double-strength)
Sjögren syndrome
sliding scale (this is a dangerous abbreviation as it is not understood or read as one half)
slip sent
Social Security
social service
somatostatin (Zecnil)
stainless steel
steady state
step stool
subaortic stenosis
susceptible
suprasciatic (notch)
symmetrical strength

S/S Saturday and Sunday
sprain/strain

SS# Social Security number

S & S shower and shampoo
signs and symptoms
sitting and supine
sling and swathe
soft and smooth (prostate)
support and stimulation
swish and spit
swish and swallow

SSA sagittal split advancement
salicylsalicylic acid (salsalate)
Sjögren syndrome antigen A
Social Security Administration
specific surface area
Subjective Symptoms Assessment (profile)
sulfasalicylic acid (test)

SSADH succinic semialdehyde dehydrogenase

SSAs standard sedative agents

SSBP sitting systolic blood pressure

SSC sign symptom complex
silver sulfadiazine and chlorhexidine
Similac® and special care
Special Services for Children
stainless steel crown
standard straight cane

SSc systemic sclerosis (scleroderma)

SSCA single shoulder contrast arthrography

SSCP single-stranded conformational polymorphism
substernal chest pain

SSCr stainless steel crown

SSCU surgical special care unit

SSCVD sterile spontaneous controlled vaginal delivery

SSD serosanguineous drainage
sickle cell disease
silver sulfadiazine (Silvadene)
Social Security disability
source to skin distance

SSDI Social Security disability income

ss DNA single-stranded desoxyribonucleic acid

SSE saline solution enema (0.9% sodium chloride)
skin self-examination
soapsuds enema
subacute spongiform encephalopathy
systemic side effects

SSEH spontaneous spinal epidural hematoma

SSEPs somatosensory evoked potentials

SSF subscapular skinfold

SSG sodium stibogluconate
sublabial salivary gland

SSHL sudden sensorineural hearing loss

SSI sliding scale insulin
Social Skills Inventory
sub-shock insulin
superior sector iridectomy
Supplemental Security Income

S

	surgical site infection	SSRs	simple sequence repeats
SSKI	saturated solution of potassium iodide	SSS	layer upon layer
			scalded skin syndrome
SSL	second stage of labor		Scandinavian Stroke Scale
	subtotal supraglottic laryngectomy		Sepsis Severity Score
			Severity Scoring System (Dart Snakebite)
SSLF	sacrospinous ligament fixation		short stay service (unit)
SSLR	seated straight leg raise		sick sinus syndrome
SSM	short stay medical		skin and skin structures
	skin-sparing mastectomy		Spanish-speaking
	skin surface microscopy		sometimes
	superficial spreading melanoma		sphincter-saving surgery
			Stanford Sleepiness Scale
SSN	severely subnormal		sterile saline soak
	Social Security number	SSSB	sagittal split setback
SSNB	suprascapular nerve block	SSSDW	significant sharp, spike, or delta waves
SSO	second surgical opinion		
	sequence-specific oligonucleotide	SSSE	self-sustained status epilepticus
	short stay observation (unit)	SSSIs	skin and skin structure infections
	Spanish speaking only	SSSS	staphylococcal scalded skin syndrome
SSOP	Second Surgical Opinion Program		
	sequence-specific oligonucleotide probe	SSSs	small short spikes (encephalography)
SSP	sequence-specific primer	SST	sagittal sinus thrombosis
	short stay procedure (unit)		Simple Shoulder Test
	superior spermatic plexus		somatostatin (Zecnil)
	supragingival scaling and prophylaxis (dental)	SSTI	skin and skin structure infections
SSPA	staphylococcal-slime polysaccharide antigens	SSU	short stay unit
		SSX	sulfisoxazole acetyl
		S/SX	signs/symptoms
SSPE	subacute sclerosing panencephalitis	ST	esotropic
			sacrum transverse
SSPG	steady-state plasma glucose		Schiotz tonometry
SSPL	saturation sound pressure level		Schirmer Test (dry-eye test)
			shock therapy
SSPU	surgical short procedure unit		sinus tachycardia
			skin tear
SSQ	Staring Speel Questionnaire		skin test
			slight trace
SSR	Sleep Self-Reporting		slow-twitch
	substernal retractions		smokeless tobacco
	sympathetic skin response		sore throat
SSRFC	surrounding subretinal fluid cuff		spasmodic torticollis
			speech therapist
SSRI	selective serotonin reuptake inhibitor		speech therapy
			sphincter tone
SSRP	subgingival scaling and root planing (dental)		split thickness

	spondee threshold		slow-transit constipation
	station (obstetrics)		soft tissue calcification
	stomach		special treatment center
	straight		stimulate to cry
	strength training		stroke treatment center
	stress testing		subtotal colectomy
	stretcher		sugar tongue cast
	subtotal	ST CLK	station clerk
	Surgical Technologist	STD	sexually transmitted
	survival time		disease(s)
	synapse time		short-term disability
S & T	sulfamethoxazole and		skin test dose
	trimethoprim (SMZ-		skin to tumor distance
	TMP or SMX-TMP)		sodium tetradecyl
STA	second trimester abortion		sulfate
	spike-triggered averaging	STD TF	standard tube feeding
	staphylococcus vaccine,	STE	ST-segment elevation
	not otherwise	STEAM	stimulated-echo
	specified		acquisition mode
	superficial temporal artery	STEC	shiga toxin-producing
STA_aur	*Staphylococcus aureus*		*Escherichia coli*
	vaccine	STEM	scanning transmission
stab.	polymorphonuclear		electron microscopic
	leukocytes (white blood	STEMI	ST-segment elevation
	cells, in nonmature		myocardial infarction
	form)	Stereo	steropsis
STAI	State-Trait Anxiety	STEPS	The System for
	Inventory		Thalidomide Educating
STAI-I	State-Trait-Anxiety		and Prescribing
	Index—I		Safety
STA-MCA	superficial temporary	STET	single photon emission
	artery-middle cerebral		tomography
	artery (anastomosis;		submaximal treadmill
	bypass)		exercise test
STAPES	stapedectomy	STETH	stethoscope
staph	*Staphylococcus aureus*	STF	special tube feeding
STA_SPL	staphylococcus vaccine,		standard tube feeding
	bacteriophage lysate	STG	short-term goals
STAT	immediately (or as		split-thickness graft
	defined by the		superior temporal gyri
	institution)	STH	soft tissue hemorrhage
	signal transducers and		somatotrophic hormone
	activators of		subtotal hysterectomy
	transcription		supplemental thyroid
STATINS	HMG-CoA reductase		hormone
	inhibitors	STHB	said to have been
STAXI	State-Trait Anger	STI	sexually transmitted
	Expression Inventory		infection
STB	stillborn		signal transduction
STBAL	standing balance		inhibitor((s)
ST BY	stand by		soft tissue injury
STC	serum theophylline		structured treatment
	concentration		interruption(s)

S

	sum total impression	STPI	State-Trait Personality Inventory
	systolic time interval		
STI-571	imatinib mesylate (Gleevec)	STPS	Short-Term Performance Status
STILLB	stillborn	STPT	second-trimester pregnancy termination
STIR	short TI (tau) inversion recovery	STR	scotopic threshold response
STIs	sexually transmitted infections		short tandem repeat
	systolic time intervals		sister
STJ	scapulothoracic joint		small tandem repeat
	subtalar joint		stretcher
STK	streptokinase	Strab	strabismus
STL	sent to laboratory	strep	streptococcus
	serum theophylline level		streptomycin
STLE	St. Louis encephalitis	STRICU	shock/trauma/respiratory intensive care unit
STLI	subtotal lymphoid irradiation	Str Post MI	strictly posterior myocardial infarction
STLOM	swelling, tenderness, and limitation of motion	STS	serologic test for syphilis
STLV	simian T-lymphotrophic viruses		short-term survivors
			slide thin slab
STM	scanning tunneling microscope		sodium tetradecyl sulfate
			sodium thiosulfate
	short-term memory		soft tissue sarcoma
	soft tissue mobilization		soft tissue swelling
	sternocleidomastoideus		somatostatin (Zecnil)
	streptomycin		standard threshold shift (audiology)
STMS	Short Test of Mental Status		staurosporine
STMT	Seat Movement		Surgical Technology Student
STN	subtalar neutral		
	subthalamic nucleus	STSG	split thickness skin graft
STNI	subtotal nodal irradiation	STSS	streptococcal-induced toxic shock syndrome
STNM	surgical evaluative staging of cancer		
STNR	symmetrical tonic neck reflex	STS-SPT	simple two-step swallowing provocation test
S to	sensitive to	STT	scaphoid, trapezium trapezoid
STOP	sensitive, timely, and organized programs (battered spouses)		serial thrombin time
			skin temperature test
			soft tissue tumor
STORCH	syphilis, toxoplasmosis, other agents, rubella, cytomegalovirus, and herpes (maternal infections)		subtotal thyroidectomy
		STT#1	Schirmer tear test one
		STT#2	Schirmer tear test two
		STTb	basal Schirmer tear test
STP	short-term plans	STTOL	standing tolerance
	sodium thiopental	STU	shock trauma unit
	step training progression		surgical trauma unit
		STV	short-term variability
STPD	standard temperature and pressure—dry	STV+	short-term variability-present

S

STV 0	short-term variability-absent	SULF-PRIM	sulfamethoxazole and trimethoprim
STV inter	short-term variability-intermittent	SUN	serum urea nitrogen
STX	stricture	SUNDS	sudden unexplained nocturnal death syndrome
STZ	streptozocin (Zanosar)	SUO	syncope of unknown origin
SU	sensory urgency		
	Somogyi units	SUP	stress ulcer prophylaxis
	stasis ulcer		superior
	stroke unit		supination
	sulfonylurea		supinator
	supine		symptomatic uterine prolapse
Su	Sunday		
S/U	shoulder/umbilicus	SUPAC	Scale-Up and Post Approval Change
S&U	supine and upright		
SUA	serum uric acid	supp	suppository
	single umbilical artery	SUR	suramin (Metaret)
SUB	Skene urethra and Bartholin glands		surgery
			surgical
Subcu	subcutaneous	Surgi	Surgigator
SUBCUT	subcutaneous	SUUD	sudden unexpected, unexplained death
Subepi M Inj	subepicardial myocardial injury		
		SUV	standard uptake variable
SUBL	sublingual	SUVs	standard uptake values
SUB-MAND	submandibular	SUX	succinylcholine
			suction
sub q	subcutaneous (this is a dangerous abbreviation since the q is mistaken for every, when a number follows)	SUZI	subzonal insertion
		SV	scimitar vein
			seminal vesical
			severe
			sigmoid volvulus
SUCC	succinylcholine		single ventricle
SUCT	suction		single vessel
SUD	sudden unexpected death		snake venom
SuDBP	supine diastolic blood pressure		stock volume
			subclavian vein
SUDEP	sudden unexpected (unexplained) death in epilepsy	Sv	sievert (radiation unit)
		SV40	simian virus 40
		SVA	small volume admixture
SUDS	Subjective Unit of Distress (Disturbance) (Discomfort) Scale	SVAS	supravalvular aortic stenosis
		SVB	saphenous vein bypass
	sudden unexplained death syndrome	SVBG	saphenous vein bypass graft
SUF	symptomatic uterine fibroids	SVC	slow vital capacity
			subclavian vein compression
SUI	stress urinary incontinence		
	suicide		superior vena cava
SUID	sudden unexplained infant death	SVCO	superior vena cava obstruction
SUIOS	Simplified Urinary Incontinence Outcome Score	SVC-RPA	superior vena cava and right pulmonary artery (shunt)

S

SVCS	superior vena cava syndrome	SW	sandwich
			sea water
SVD	singular value decomposition (analysis)		seriously wounded
			shallow walk (aquatic therapy)
SVD	single-vessel disease		short wave
	spontaneous vaginal delivery		Social Worker
			stab wound
	structural valve deterioration (dysfunction)		sterile water
			swallowing reflex
SVE	sterile vaginal examination	S&W	soap and water
		S/W	somewhat
	Streptococcus viridans endocarditis	SWA	Social Work Associate
		SWAP	short-wavelength automated perimetry
	subcortical vascular encephalopathy	SWAT	skin wound assessment and treatment
SV&E	suicidal, violent, and eloper	SWD	short wave diathermy
		SWFI	sterile water for injection
SVG	saphenous vein graft	SWG	standard wire gauge
SVH	subjective visual horizontal (test)	SWI	sterile water for injection
			surgical wound infection
SVI	seminal vesicle invasion	S&WI	skin and wound isolation
	stroke volume index	SWL	shock wave lithotripsy
S VISC	serum viscosity	SWMA	segmental wall-motion abnormalities
SVL	severe visual loss		
SVN	small volume nebulizer	SWO	superficial white onychomycosis
SVO	small vessel occlusion		
SVO$_2$	mixed venous oxygen saturation	SWOG	Southwest Oncology Group
SVOO	systemic ventricular outflow obstruction	SWOT	strengths, weaknesses, opportunities, threats (analysis)
SVP	spontaneous venous pulse		
SVPB	supraventricular premature beat	SWP	small whirlpool
		SWR	surface wrinkling retinopathy
SVPC	supraventricular premature contraction		surgical waiting room
SV/PP	stroke volume/pulse pressure	SWS	sheltered workshop
			slow-wave sleep
SVR	supraventricular rhythm		social work service
	sustained virological response		student ward secretary
			Sturge-Weber syndrome
	systemic vascular resistance	SWSD	shift-work sleep disorder
		SWT	stab wound of the throat
SVRI	systemic vascular resistance index		shuttle-walk test
		SWU	septic work-up
SVT	superficial vein thrombosis	SWW	static wall walk (aquatic therapy)
	supraventricular tachycardia	Sx	signs
			surgery
	symptom validity test(s)		symptom
SVVD	spontaneous vertex vaginal delivery	SXA	single-energy x-ray absorptiometry

SXR	skull x-ray
SYN	synovial
SYN-D	synthadotin
SYN Fl	synovial fluid
SYPH	syphilis
SYR	syrup
SYS BP	systolic blood pressure
SZ	schizophrenic
	seizure
	suction
SZN	streptozocin (Zanosar)

T

T	inverted T wave
	tablespoon (15 mL) (this is a dangerous abbreviation)
	taenia
	temperature
	tender
	tension
	tesla (unit of magnetic flux density in radiology)
	testicles
	testosterone
	thoracic
	thymine
	Toxoplasma
	trace
	transcribed
t	teaspoon (5 mL) (this is a dangerous abbreviation)
T+	increase intraocular tension
T−	decreased intraocular tension
2,4,5-T	2,4,5-trichlorophenoxyacetic acid
$T°$	temperature
$T_{1/2}$	half-life
T_1	tricuspid first sound
T_2	tricuspid second sound
T-2	dactinomycin, doxorubicin, vincristine, and cyclophosphamide
T_3	triiodothyronine (liothyronine)
T3	transurethral thermo-ablation therapy (Targis)
	Tylenol with codeine 30 mg (this is a dangerous abbreviation)
$T_{3/4}$ind	triiodothyronine to thyroxine index
T_4	levothyroxine
	thyroxine

T

345

T4	CD4 (helper-inducer cells)		tetracaine, Adrenalin® and cocaine
T-7	free thyroxine factor		total arterial compliance
T-10	methotrexate, calcium leucovorin rescue, doxorubicin, cisplatin, bleomycin, cyclophosphamide, and dactinomycin		tibial artery catheter
			total abdominal colectomy
			total allergen content
			triamicinolone cream
		TACC	thoracic aortic cross-clamping
$T_1...T_{12}$	thoracic nerve 1 through 12	TACE	transarterial chemoembolization
	thoracic vertebra 1 through 12	TACI	total anterior cerebral infarct
TA	Takayasu arteritis temperature axillary temporal arteritis	tac-MRA	timed arterial compression magnetic resonance angiography
	temporal artery tendon Achilles	TACT	tuned aperture computed tomography
	therapeutic abortion tibialis anterior (muscle)	TAD	thoracic asphyxiant dystrophy
	tracheal aspirate traffic accident		transverse abdominal diameter
	tricuspid atresia truncus arteriosus	TADAC	therapeutic abortion, dilation, aspiration, and curettage
Ta	tonometry applanation	
T&A	tonsillectomy and adenoidectomy	TADC	tumor-associated dendritic cells
	tonsils and adenoids	TAE	transcatheter arterial embolization
T(A)	axillary temperature	
TA1	thymosin alpha-1	TAF	tissue angiogenesis factor
TA-55	stapling device	TAG	triacylglycerol
TAA	Therapeutic Activities Aide		tumor-associated glycoprotein
	thoracic aortic aneurysm total ankle arthroplasty transverse aortic arch triamcinolone acetonide	TAGA	term, appropriate for gestational age
			term, average gestational age
	tumor-associated antigen (antibodies)	TA-GVHD	transfusion-associated graft-versus-host disease
TAAA	thoracoabdominal aortic aneursym	TAH	total abdominal hysterectomy
TAB	tablet		total artificial heart
	therapeutic abortion total androgen blockade triple antibiotic (bacitracin, neomycin, and polymyxin—this is a dangerous abbreviation)	TAHBSO	total abdominal hysterectomy, bilateral salpingo-oophorectomy
		TAHL	thick ascending limb of Henle loop
		T Air	air puff tonometry
		TAKE	Targeting Abnormal Kinetic Effects
TAC	docetaxel (Taxotere), doxorubicin (Adriamycin), and cyclophosphamide	TAL	tendon Achilles lengthening
			total arm length

T

T ALCON	Alcon® tonometry		treatment administration record
T-ALL	T-cell acute lymphoblastic leukemia		treatment authorization request
TALP	total alkaline phosphatase	TARA	total articular replacement arthroplasty
TAML	therapy-related acute myelogenous leukemia	TART	tenderness, asymmetry, restricted motion, and
t-AML	therapy-related acute myeloid leukemia		tissue texture changes tumorectomy and
TAM	tamoxifen (Novaldex)		radiotherapy
	teenage mother	TAS	therapeutic activities
	total active motion		specialist
	tumor-associated macrophages		Thrombolytic Assessment System
TAN	treatment-as-needed		transabdominal sutures
	Treatment Authorization Number		turning against self typical absence seizures
	tropical ataxic neuropathy	TAT	tandem autotransplants
TANF	Temporary Assistance for Needy Families		tell a tale tetanus antitoxin
TANI	total axial (lymph) node irradiation		thematic apperception test thrombin-antithrombin III
TAO	thromboangitis obliterans		complex
	troleandomycin		'til all taken
TAP	tone and positioning		total adipose tissue
	tonometry by applanation		transactivator of
	transabdominal preperitoneal (laparoscopic hernia repair)		transcription transplant-associated thrombocytopenia
	transesophageal atrial paced		turnaround time tyrosine aminotransferase
	trypsinogen activation peptide	TATT	tired all the time
	tumor-activated prodrug	TAU	tumescence activity units
TAPP	transabdominal preperitoneal polypropylene (mesh-plasty)	TAUC	target area under the curve time-averaged urea concentration
T APPL	applanation tonometry	TAUSA	thrombolysis and
TAPVC	total anomalous pulmonary venous connection		angioplasty in unstable angina
		TAX	cefotaxime (Claforan)
TAPVD	total anomalous pulmonary venous drainage		paclitaxel (Taxol)
		TB	Tapes for the Blind terrible burning
TAPVR	total anomalous pulmonary venous return		thought broadcasting toothbrush total base
TAR	thoracic aortic rupture thrombocytopenia with absent radius		total bilirubin total body tuberculosis
	total ankle replacement	TBA	to be absorbed
	total anorectal reconstruction		to be added to be administered

347

	to be admitted	TBNA	transbronchial needle aspiration
	to be announced		treated but not admitted
	to be arranged		
	to be assessed	TBNa	total-body sodium
	total body (surface) area	TBO	toluidine blue O
TBAGA	term birth appropriate for gestational age	TBOCS	Tale-Brown Obsessive-Compulsive Scale
T-bar	tracheotomy bar (a device used in respiratory therapy)	TBP	thyroxine-binding protein toe blood pressure total-body phosphorus
TBARS	thiobarbituric acid reactive substances		total-body protein tuberculous peritonitis
TBB	transbronchial biopsy	TBPA	thyroxine-binding prealbumin
TBC	to be cancelled		
	total-blood cholesterol	TBR	total-bed rest
	total-body clearance	TBRF	tick-borne relapsing fever
	tuberculosis	TBS	tablespoon (15ml)(this is a dangerous abbreviation)
TBD	to be determined		
TBE	tick-borne encephalitis		tachycardia-bradycardia syndrome
	to be evaluated		
TBE$_e$	tick-borne encephalitis, eastern subtype (Far eastern encephalitis, Russian spring-summer e., Taiga e.) vaccine		The Bethesda System (reporting cervical and vagina cytology)
			total-serum bilirubin
T-berg	Trendelenburg (position)	TBSA	total-body surface area
TBEV	tick-borne encephalitis virus		total-burn surface area
		tbsp	tablespoon (15 mL)
TBE$_w$	tick-bone encephalitis, western subtype (Central European encephalitis) vaccine	TBT	tolbutamide test tracheal bronchial toilet
			transbronchoscopic balloon tipped
TBF	total-body fat		
TBG	thyroxine-binding globulin	TBUT	tear break-up time (dry-eye test)
TBI	tick-borne illness(es)	TBV	thiotepa, bleomycin, and vinblastine
	toothbrushing instruction		
	total-body irradiation		total-blood volume
	traumatic brain injury		transluminal balloon valvuloplasty
T bili	total bilirubin		
TBK	total-body potassium	TBW	total-body water
tbl	tablespoon (15 mL)	TBZ	thiabendazole (Mintezol)
TBLB	transbronchial lung biopsy		
TBLC	term birth, living child	TC	paclitaxel (Taxol) and cisplatin
TBLF	term birth, living female		
TBLI	term birth, living infant		tai chi (exercise program)
TBLM	term birth, living male		team conference
TBM	tracheobronchomalacia		telephone call
	tuberculous meningitis		terminal cancer
	tubule basement membrane		testicular cancer
			thioguanine and cytarabine
TBMg	total-body magnesium		
TBN	total-body nitrogen		thoracic circumference

T

	throat culture
	tissue culture
	tolonium chloride
	tonic-clonic
	tonsillar coblation
	total cholesterol
	total communication
	to (the) chest
	tracheal collar
	trauma center
	true conjugate
	tubocurarine
Tc	technetium
T/C	telephone call
	ticarcillin-clavulanic acid (Timentin)
	to consider
3TC	lamivudine (Epivir)
TC7	Interceed®
T&C	turn and cough
	type and crossmatch
T&C#3	Tylenol with 30 mg codeine
TCA	thioguanine and cytarabine
	tissue concentrations of antibiotic(s)
	trichloroacetic acid
	tricuspid atresia
	tricyclic antidepressant
	tumor chemosensitivity assay
	tumor clonogenic assays
TCABG	triple coronary artery bypass graft
TCAD	transplant-related coronary-artery disease
	tricyclic antidepressant
TCAR	tiazofurin
TCB	to call back
	tumor cell burden
TCBS agar	thiosulfate-citrate-bile salt-sucrose agar
TCC	transitional cell carcinoma
TCCB	transitional cell carcinoma of bladder
TC/CL	ticarcillin-clavulanate (Timentin)
TcCO$_2$	transcutaneous carbon dioxide
TCD	T-cell depleted
	transcerebellar diameter

	transcranial Doppler (ultrasonography)
	transverse cardiac diameter
	transcystic duct
TCDB	turn, cough, and deep breath
TCDD	tetrachlorodibenzo-p-dioxin (dioxin)
^{99m}Tc DTPA	technetium Tc 99m pentetate
TCE	tetrachloroethylene
	total-colon examination
	toxicity composite endpoint
	transcatheter embolotherapy
T cell	small lymphocyte
TCES	transcranial electrical stimulation
^{99m}TcGHA	technetium Tc 99m gluceptate
TCH	paclitaxel (Taxol), carboplatin, and trastuzumab (Herceptin)
	turn, cough, hyperventilate
^{99m}Tc-HAS	technetium Tc 99m-labeled human serum albumin
TCHRs	traditional Chinese herbal remedies
TCI	target-control infusion
	to come in
TCID	tissue culture infective dose
TCIE	transient cerebral ischemic episode
TCL	tibial collateral ligament
	transverse carpal ligament
TCM	tissue culture media
	traditional Chinese medicine
	transcutaneous (oxygen) monitor
^{99m}Tc-MAA	technetium Tc 99m albumin microaggregated
TCMH	tumor-direct cell-mediated hypersensitivity
TCMS	transcranial cortical magnetic stimulation

T

TCMZ	trichlormethiazide (Naqua)	tone decay
TCN	tetracycline	total disability
	triciribine phosphate (tricyclic nucleoside)	transdermal
		transverse diameter
TCNS	transcutaneous nerve	travelers' diarrhea
	stimulator	treatment discontinued
TCNU	tauromustine	Td	tetanus-diphtheria toxoids

TCMZ   trichlormethiazide
            (Naqua)
TCN   tetracycline
        triciribine phosphate
            (tricyclic nucleoside)
TCNS   transcutaneous nerve
            stimulator
TCNU   tauromustine
TcO₂   transcutaneous oxygen
            pressure
TcO₄⁻   pertechnetate
TCOM   transcutaneous oxygen
            monitor
T Con   temporary conservatorship
TCP   thrombocytopenia
        transcutaneous pacing
        tranylcypromine (Parnate)
        tumor control probability
TCPC   total cavopulmonary
            connection
TcPCO₂ transcutaneous carbon
            dioxide
TcPO₂   transcutaneous oxygen
⁹⁹ᵐTcPYP technetium Tc 99m
            pyrophosphate
TCR   T-cell receptor
TCRE   transcervical resection of
            the endometrium
TCRFTA temperature-controlled
            radiofrequency tissue
            ablation
TCS   tonic-clonic seizure
⁹⁹ᵐTcSC technetium Tc 99m sulfur
            colloid
TCT   thyrocalcitonin
        tincture
        transcatheter therapy
        triple combination tablet
            (abacavir, lamivudine,
            and zidovudine)
            (Trizivir)
TCU   transitional care unit
TCVA   thromboembolic cerebral
            vascular accident
TD   Takayasu disease
        tardive dyskinesia
        temporary disability
        terminal device
        test dose
        tetanus-diphtheria toxoids
            (pediatric use)
        tidal volume
        tolerance dose

tone decay
total disability
transdermal
transverse diameter
travelers' diarrhea
treatment discontinued
Td   tetanus-diphtheria toxoids
            (adult type)
TDAC   tumor-derived activated
            cell (cultures)
TDD   telephone device for the
            deaf
        thoracic duct drainage
        total daily dose
TDE   total daily energy
            (requirement)
TDF   tenofovir disoproxil
            fumarate (Virend)
        testis determining factor
        total-dietary fiber
        tumor dose fractionation
TDI   tolerable daily intake
        toluene diisocyanate
TDK   tardive diskinesia
TDL   thoracic duct lymph
TDLN   tumor-draining lymph
            nodes
TDM   therapeutic drug
            monitoring
TDMAC   tridodecylmethyl
            ammonium chloride
TDN   totally digestible nutrients
        transdermal nitroglycerin
TDNTG   transdermal nitroglycerin
TDNWB   touchdown
            nonweightbearing
TdP   torsades de pointes
TDPDS   temporomandibular
            disorder pain
            dysfunction syndrome
TDPWB   touchdown partial
            weight-bearing
TdR   thymidine
TDS   Teacher Drool Scale
        traveler's diarrhea
            syndrome
TDS   three times a day (United
            Kingdom)
TDT   tentative discharge
            tomorrow
        transmission
            disequilibrium test
        Trieger Dot Test

T

350

	tumor doubling time		transluminal extraction-endarterectomy catheter
TdT	terminal deoxynucleotidyl transferase		triethyl citrate
TDW	target dry weight	T&EC	trauma and emergency center
TDWB	touch down weight bearing	TECA	titrated extract of *Centella asiatica*
TDx®	fluorescence polarization immunoassay	TECAB	totally endoscopic (off-pump) coronary artery bypass grafting
TE	echo time	TED	thromboembolic disease
	tennis elbow		thyroid eye disease
	terminal extension	TEDS	thromboembolic disease stockings
	tooth extraction		transesophageal echo-Doppler system
	toxoplasmic encephalitis		Treatment Episode Data Set
	trace elements (chromium, copper, iodine, manganese, selenium, molybdenum andzinc)	TEE	total energy expended
	tracheoesophageal		transnasal endoscopic ethmoidectomy
	transesophageal echocardiography		transesophageal echocardiography
	transrectal electroejaculation	TEF	tracheoesophageal fistula
*t*E	total expiratory time	TEG	thromboelastogram (thromboelastography)
T/E	testosterone to epitestosterone ratio	TEH	theophylline, ephedrine, and hydroxyzine
T&E	testing and evaluation	TEI	therapeutic equivalence interchange
	training and evaluation		total episode of illness
	trial and error		transesophageal imaging
TEA	thromboendarterectomy	TEL	telemetry
	Time and Extent Application (FDA)		telephone
	total elbow arthroplasty	tele	telemetry
	transluminal extraction atherectomy	TEM	temozolomide (Temodar)
TEAE	treatment-emergent adverse event		transanal endoscopic microsurgery
TEAP	transesophageal atrial pacing		transmission electron microscopy
TEB	thoracic electrical bioimpedance	TEMI	transient episodes of myocardial ischemia
TEBG	testosterone-estradiol binding globulin	TEMP	temperature
TeBG	testeosterone binding globulin		temporal
TeBIDA	technetium 99m trimethyl 1-bromo-imono diacetic acid		temporary
		TEN	tension (intraocular pressure)
TEC	thromboembolic complication		toxic epidermal necrolysis
	total eosinophil count	TEN®	Total Enteral Nutrition
	toxic *Escherichia coli*	TENS	transcutaneous electrical nerve stimulation
	transient erythroblasto-penia of childhood	TEOAE	transient evoked otoacous-tic emission (test)

T

TEP	total endoprosthesis	TF	tactile fremitus
	total extraperitoneal (laparoscopic hernia repair)		tail flick (reflex)
			tetralogy of Fallot
			tibiofemoral
	tracheoesophageal puncture		to follow
			tube feeding
	tubal ectopic pregnancy	TFA	topical fluoride application
TEQ	toxic equivalents		
TER	terlipressin		trans fatty acids
	total elbow replacement		trifluoroacetic acid
	total energy requirement	TFB	trifascicular block
	transurethral electroresection	TFBC	The Family Birthing Center
TERB	terbutaline	TFC	thoracic fluid content
TERC	Test of Early Reading Comprehension		time to following commands
TERM	full-term	TFCC	triangular fibrocartilage complex
	terminal		
TERT	human telomerase reverse transcriptase (also hTRT)	TFF	tangential flow filtration
			trefoil factor family (peptides)
	tertiary	TF-Fe	transferrin-bound iron
	total end-range time	TFI	total fluid intake
TES	therapeutic electrical stimulation		treatment-free interval
		TFL	tensor fasciae latae
	thoracic endometriosis syndrome		transnasal fiberoptic laryngoscopy
	thoracic endoscopic sympathectomy		trimetrexate, fluorouracil, and leucovorin
	treatment emergent symptoms		trunk-forward lean
		TFM	transverse friction massage
TESA	testicular sperm aspiration		
TESE	testicular sperm extraction	TFO	triplex-forming oligonucleotide
TESI	thoracic epidural steroid injection	TFOs	triplex-forming oligonucleotides
TESS	Toronto Extremity Salvage Score	TFPI	tissue-factor pathway inhibitor
	treatment emergent signs and symptoms	TFR	total fertility rate
	Treatment Emergent Symptom Scale	TFT	thin-film transistor
			thumb-finding test
TET	transcranial electrostimulation therapy		trifluridine (trifluorothymidine)
		TFTs	thyroid function tests
	treadmill exercise test	TG	total gym
TETE	too early to evaluate		triglycerides
TETig	tetanus immune globulin	Tg	thyroglobulin
TEU	token economy unit	6-TG	thioguanine
TEV	talipes equinovarus (deformity)	TGA	Therapeutic Goods Administration (Australia)
TEVAP	transurethral electrovaporization of the prostate		third-generation antidepressant

	transient global amnesia	THAL	thalassemia
	transposition of the great arteries		thalidomide (Thalomid)
TGAR	total graft area rejected	THAT	Toronto Hospital Alertness Test
TGB	tiagabine (Gabatril)	THBI	thyroid hormone binding index
TGCE	temperature gradient capillary electrophoresis	THBR	thyroid hormone-binding ratio
TGCT	testicular germ cell tumor(s)	THAM®	tromethamine
TGD	thyroglossal duct	THBO$_2$	topical hyperbaric oxygen
	tumor growth delay	THC	tetrahydrocannabinol (dronabinol)
TGDC	thyroglossal duct cyst		thigh circumference
TGE	transmissible gastroenteritis		transhepatic cholangiogram
TGFA	triglyceride fatty acid	THCT	triple-phase helical computer tomography
TGF	transforming growth factor	TH-CULT	throat culture
TGF-β	transforming growth factor-beta	tHcy	total homocysteine
		THE	total-head excursion
TGGE	temperature-gradient gel electrophoresis		transhepatic embolization
TGR	tenderness, guarding, and rigidity	Ther Ex	therapeutic exercise
		THF	thymic humoral factor
TGS	tincture of green soap	THG	tetrahydrogestrinone
TGs	triglycerides	THg	total mercury
TGT	thromboplastin generation test	THI	transient hypogamma-globinemia of infancy
TGTL	total glottic transverse laryngectomy	THKAFO	trunk-hip-knee-ankle-foot orthosis
TGV	thoracic gas volume	THKAFO-LU	lockable joints using trunk-hip-knee-ankle-foot orthosis
	transposition of great vessels		
TGXT	thallium-graded exercise test	THL	transvaginal hydrolaparoscopy
TGZ	troglitazone (Rezulin)	THLAA	tubular hypoplasia left aortic arch
TH	thrill	THP	take home packs
	thyroid hormone		total hip prosthesis
	total hysterectomy		transhepatic portography
Th	thorium		trihexyphenidyl (Artane)
	Thursday	THR	target heart rate
T&H	type and hold		thrombin receptor
TH1	T helper cell, type 1		total hip replacement
TH2	T helper cell, type 2		training heart rate
THA	tacrine (tetrahydroacridine; Cognex)	THRL	total hip replacement, left
	total hip arthroplasty	THRR	total hip replacement, right
	transient hemispheric attack		transient hyperemic response ratio
THAA	thyroid hormone autoantibodies	THS	Tolosa-Hunt syndrome
	tubular hypoplasia aortic arch	THTV	therapeutic home trial visit

T

THV	therapeutic home visit		three times a night (this is a dangerous abbreviation)
TI	terminal ileus		
	therapeutic index		tubulointerstitial nephritis
	thought insertion	tinct	tincture
	time following inversion pulse (radiology)	TIND	Treatment Investigational New Drug (application)
	transischial	TINEM	there is no evidence of malignancy
	transverse diameter of inlet		
	tricuspid incompetence	TIP	toxic interstitial pneumonitis
	tricuspid insufficiency		
TIA	transient ischemic attack		tubularized incised plate (urethroplasty)
TIB	tibia		
TIBC	total iron-binding capacity	TIPS	transvenous intrahepatic portosystemic shunt (stent-shunt)
tib-fib	tibia and fibula		
TIC	paclitaxel (Taxol), ifosfamide, and cisplain		
		TIPSS	transjugular intrahepatic portosystemic shunt (stent)
	trypsin-inhibitor capacity		
TICOSMO	trauma, infection, chemical/drug exposure, organ systems, stress, musculoskeletal, and other (prompts used during history taking for possible etiologies of problems)		
		TIRFM	total-internal reflection microscopy
		TIS	tumor in situ
		TISS	Therapeutic Intervention Scoring System
		TIT	Treponema (pallidum) immobilization test
TICS	diverticulosis		triiodothyronine (liothyronine)
TICU	thoracic intensive care unit		
		TIUP	term intrauterine pregnancy
	transplant intensive care unit		
		TIVA	total intravenous anethesia
	trauma intensive care unit	TIVC	thoracic inferior vena cava
t.i.d.	three times a day	+tive	positive
TIDM	three times daily with meals	TIW	three times a week (this is a dangerous abbreviation)
TIE	transient ischemic episode		
TIF	tracheal intubation fiberscope	TJ	tendon jerk
			triceps jerk
TIG	tetanus immune globulin	TJA	total joint arthroplasty
TIH	tumor-inducing hypercalcemia	TJC	tender joint count
		TJN	tongue jaw neck (dissection)
TKI	tyrosine kinase inhibitor		
TIL	tumor-infiltrating lymphocytes		twin-jet nebulizer
		TJR	total joint replacement
%tile	percentile	TK	thymidine kinase
TIMI	Thrombolysis in Myocardial Infarction (studies)		toxicokinetics
		TKA	total knee arthroplasty
			tyrosine kinase activity
TIMP	tissue inhibitor of metalloproteinase	TKD	tokodynamometer
		TKE	terminal knee extension
TIN	testicular intraepithelial neoplasia	TKIC	true knot in cord
		TKNO	to keep needle open

T

TKP	thermokeratoplasty	TLP	transitional living program
	total knee prosthesis	TLR	target lesion reintervention
TKO	to keep open		tonic labyrinthine reflex
TKR	total knee replacement	TLS	tumor lysis syndrome
TKRL	total knee replacement, left	TLSO	thoracic lumbar sacral orthosis
TKRR	total knee replacement, right	TLSSO	thoracolumbosacral spinal orthosis
TKVO	to keep vein open	TLT	tonsillectomy
TL	team leader	TLTBI	treatment of latent
	thoracolumbar		tuberculosis infection
	total laryngectomy	TLV	threshold limit value
	transverse line		total lung volume
	trial leave	TM	temperature by mouth
	tubal ligation		tetrathiomolybdate
T/L	terminal latency		thalassemia major
Tl	thallium		Thayer-Martin (culture)
TLA	translumbar arteriogram (aortogram)		thyromegaly
			Tibetan Medicine
	transverse ligament of atlas		trabecular meshwork
			trademark (unregistered)
TLAC	triple lumen Arrow catheter		transcendental meditation
TL BLT	tubal ligation, bilateral		treadmill
TLC	tender loving care		tropical medicine
	therapeutic lifestyle changes		tumor
			tympanic membrane
	thin layer chromatography	T & M	type and crossmatch
	titanium linear cutter	TMA	thrombotic
	T-lymphocyte choriocarcinoma		microangiopathy
			tissue microarray
	total lung capacity		trained medication aid
	total lymphocyte count		transcription mediated
	transitional living center		amplification
	triple lumen catheter		transmetatarsal amputation
TLD	thermoluminescent dosimeter		trimethylamine
		T/MA	tracheostomy mask
TLE	temporal lobe epilepsy	TMAS	Taylor Manifest Anxiety
TLFB	timeline follow back (interview)		Scale
		TMA-uria	trimethylaminuria
TLH	total laparoscopic hysterectomy	T_{max}	temperature maximum
		t_{max}	time of occurrence for
TLI	total lymphoid irradiation		maximum (peak) drug
	translaryngeal intubation		concentration
TLIF	thoracolumbar intervertebral fusion	TMB	tetramethylberizidine
			therapeutic back massage
	translumbar interbody fusion		transient monocular blindness
TLK	thermal laser keratoplasty		trimethoxybenzoates
TLM	thalidomide (Thalomid)	TMC	transmural colitis
	torn lateral meniscus		Transtheoretical Model of
TLNB	term living newborn		Change
TLOA	temporary leave of absence		trapeziometacarpal
			triamcinolone

T

TMCA	trimethylcolchicinic acid	TMS	transcranial magnetic stimulation
TMCN	triamcinolone	TMSI	Task Management Strategy Index
TMD	temporomandibular dysfunction (disorder)	TMST	treadmill stress test
	treating physician	TMT	tarsometatarsal
t-MDS	therapy-related myelodysplastic syndrome		teratoma with malignant transformation
			treadmill test
TME	thermolysin-like metalloendopeptidase		tympanic membrane thermometer
	total mesorectal excision	TMTC	too many to count
TMET	treadmill exercise test	TMTX	trimetrexate (Neutrexin)
TMEV	Theiler murine encephalomyelitis virus	TMUGS	Tumor Marker Utility Grading Scale
TMG	trimegestone	TMX	tamoxifen (Novaldex)
TMH	trainable mentally handicapped	TMZ	temazepam (Restoril)
			temozolomide (Temodar)
TMI	threatened myocardial infarction	TN	normal intraocular tension
	transmandibular implant		team nursing
	transmural infarct		temperature normal
T>MIC	time above minimum inhibitory concentration		tree nut
			trigeminal neuralgia
TMJ	temporomandibular joint	T&N	tension and nervousness
TMJD	temporomandibular joint dysfunction		tingling and numbness
		TNA	total nutrient admixture
TMJS	temporomandibular joint syndrome	TNAB	transthoracic needle biopsy
		TNB	term newborn
TML	tongue midline		transnasal butorphanol
	treadmill		transrectal needle biopsy (of the prostate)
TMLR	transmyocardial laser revascularization		Tru-Cut® needle biopsy
		TNBP	transurethral needle biopsy of prostate
TMM	torn medial meniscus		
	total muscle mass	TND	term, normal delivery
Tmm	McKay-Marg tension	TNDM	transient neonatal diabetes mellitus
TMNG	toxic multinodular goiter		
TMO	transcaruncular medial orbitotomy	TNF	tumor necrosis factor
		TNF-bp	tumor necrosis factor binding protein
TMP	thallium myocardial perfusion	TNG	nitroglycerin
	transmembrane pressure		toxic nodular goiter
	trimethoprim	TNI	total nodal irradiation
TMP/SMZ	trimethoprim and sulfamethoxazole (correct name is sulfamethoxazole and trimethoprin; SMZ-TMP)	TnI	troponin I
		TNKase®	tenecteplase
		TNM	primary tumor, regional lymph nodes, and distant metastasis (used with subscripts for the staging of cancer)
TMR	trainable mentally retarded	t-NNT	threshold number needed to treat
	transmyocardial revascularization	TNR	tonic neck reflex

T

356

TNS	transcutaneous nerve stimulation (stimulator)	TOFMS	time-of-flight mass spectrometry
	transient neurologic symptoms	TOGV	transposition of the great vessels
	Tullie-Niebörg syndrome	TOH	throughout hospitalization
TNT	thiotepa, mitoxantrone (Novantrone), and paclitaxel (Taxol)	TOI	Trial Outcome Index
		TOL	tolerate
			trial of labor
	triamcinolone and nystatin	TOLD	Test of Language Development
TnT	troponin T	TOM	therapeutic outcomes monitoring
TNTC	too numerous to count		
TNU	tobacco nonuser		tomorrow
TNY	trichomonas and yeast		transcutaneous oxygen monitor
TO	old tuberculin		
	telephone order	ToM	theory-of-mind
	time off	Tomo	tomography
	tincture of opium (warning: this is NOT paregoric)	TON	tonight
		TOP	termination of pregnancy
			Topografov (virus)
	total obstruction		topotecan (Hycamtin)
	transfer out	TOP-8	Treatment Outcome PTSD (post-traumatic stress disorder) (scale)
T(O)	oral temperature		
T/O	time out		
T&O	tubes and ovaries	TOPO	topotecan (Hycamtin)
TOA	time of arrival	TOPO 1	topoisermerase
	tubo-ovarian abscess	TOPS	Take Off Pounds Sensibly
TOAA	to affected areas	TOPV	trivalent oral polio vaccine
TOB	tobacco		
	tobramycin	TOR	toremifene (Faneston)
TOC	table of contents	TORB	telephone order read back
	test-of-cure (post-therapy visit)	TORC	Test of Reading Comprehension
	total occlusal convergence	TORCH	toxoplasmosis, others (other viruses known to attack the fetus), rubella, cytomegalovirus, and herpes simplex (maternal viral infections)
	total organic carbon		
TOCE	transcatheter oily chemoembolization		
TOCO	tocodynamometer		
TOD	intraocular pressure of the right eye		
	target organ damage		
	target-organ disease	TORP	total ossicular replacement prosthesis
	time of death		
	time of departure	TOS	intraocular pressure of the left eye
	tubal occlusion device		
TOE	transoesophageal echocardiography (United Kingdom and other countries)		thoracic outlet syndrome
		TOT BILI	total bilirubin
		TOTM	trioctyltrimellitate
		TOV	telephone order verified
TOF	tetralogy of Fallot		trial of void
	time of flight (radiology)	TOW	time off work
	total of four	TOWL	Test of Written Language
	train-of-four		

T

TOX	toxoplasmosis (*Toxo-plasma gondii*) vaccine	TPD$_{HP}$	typhoid vaccine, heat and phenol inactivated, dried
TOXO	toxoplasmosis		
TP	teaching physician	TPD$_{VI}$	typhoid vaccine, *Vi* capsular polysaccharide
	temperature and pressure		
	temporoparietal	TPE	therapeutic plasma exchange
	tender point		
	therapeutic pass		total placental estrogens
	ThinPrep Pap (test)		total protective environment
	thought process		
	thrombophlebitis	T-penia	thrombocytopenia
	thymidine phosphorylase	TPF	docetaxel (Taxotere), cisplatin (Platinol AQ), and fluorouracil
	time to progression		
	Todd paralysis		
	toe pressure		trained participating father
	toilet paper	TPH	thromboembolic pulmonary hypertension
	total protein		
	"T" piece		trained participating husband
	treating physician		
	trigger point	TPHA	*Treponema pallidum* hemagglutination
T:P	trough-to-peak ratio		
T & P	temperature and pulse	T PHOS	triple phosphate crystals
	turn and position	TPI	*Treponema pallidum* immobilization
TPA	alteplase, recombinant (tissue plasminogen activator) (Activase)		
			triose phosphate isomerase
	temporary portacaval anastomosis	TPIT	trigger point injection therapy
	third-party administrator	t$_{pk}$	time to peak
	tissue polypeptide antigen	TPL	thromboplastin
	total parenteral alimentation	T plasty	tympanoplasty
		TPLSM	two-photon laser-scanning microscope
TPAL	term infant(s), premature infant(s), abortion(s), living children		
		TPM	temporary pacemaker
			topiramate (Topamax)
TPB	Theory of Planned Behavior	TPMT	thiopurine methyltransferase
TPC	target plasma concentration	TPN	total parenteral nutrition
		TPO	thrombopoietin
	tender-point count		thyroid peroxidase
	total patient care		trial prescription order
	touch preparation cytology	TPP	thiamine pyrophosphate
		TpP	thrombus precursor protein
TPD	tropical pancreatic diabetes		
		TP & P	time, place, and person
	typhoid vaccine, not otherwise specified	TPPN	total peripheral parenteral nutrition
TPD$_a$	typhoid vaccine, attenuated live (oral Ty21a strain)	TPPS	Toddler-Preschooler Postoperative Pain Scale
TPD$_{AKD}$	typhoid vaccine, acetone-killed and dried (U.S. military)	TPPV	trans pars plana vitrectomy
		TPR	temperature

T

358

	temperature, pulse, and respiration	TRACH	tracheal
			tracheostomy
	total peripheral resistance	TRAFO	tone-reducing ankle/foot
TPRI	total peripheral resistance index		orthosis
		TRAIL	tumor-necrosis-factor-related apoptosis-inducing ligand
T PROT	total protein		
TPS	tender point score		
	typhus (*rickettsiae* sp.) vaccine	TRALI	transfusion-associated lung injury
tPSA	total prostate-specific antigen	TRAM	transverse rectus abdominis myocutaneous (flap)
TPT	time to peak tension		
	topotecan (Hycamtin)		transverse rectus abdominum muscle
	transpyloric tube		
	treadmill performance test		Treatment Response Assessment Method
*t*PTEF	time to peak tidal expiratory flow	TRAMP	transversus and rectus abdominis musculo-peritoneal (flap)
TPU	tropical phagedenic ulcer		
T-putty	Theraputty	TRANCE	tumor necrosis factor–related activation-induced cytokine
TPVA	tibioperoneal vessel angioplasty		
TPVR	total peripheral vascular resistance		
		TRANS	transfers
TPZ	tirapazamine	Trans D	transverse diameter
TQM	total quality management	TRANS Rx	transfusion reaction
TR	therapeutic recreation	TRAP	tartrate-resistant (leukocyte) acid phophatase
	time to repeat		
	time to repetition (radiology)		Telomeric Repeat Amplification Protocol
	tincture		
	to return		thrombospondin-related anonymous protein
	trace		
	transfusion reaction		total radical-trapping antioxidant parameter
	transplant recipients		
	trapezius		trapezium
	treatment		trapezius muscle
	tremor	TRAS	transplant renal artery stenosis
	tricuspid regurgitation		
	tumor registry	TRB	return to baseline
T(R)	rectal temperature	TRBC	total red blood cells
T & R	tenderness and rebound	TRC	tanned red cells
	treated and released	TRD	tongue-retaining device
	turn and reposition		total-retinal detachment
TRA	therapeutic recreation associate		traction retinal detachment
			treatment-related death
	to run at		treatment-resistant depression
	tumor regression antigen		
TRAb	thyrotropin-receptor antibody	TRDN	transient respiratory distress of the newborn
TRAC	traction	TREC	T-cell receptor-rearrangement excision circles
TRACE	time-resolved amplified cryptate emission		

Tren	Trendelenburg		the real symptom
TRF	terminal restriction fragment	TRT	tangential radiation therapy
TRH	protirelin (thyrotropin-releasing hormone) (Relefact TRH®; Thypinone®)		testosterone replacement therapy
			thermoradiotherapy
TRI	transient radicular irritation		thoracic radiation therapy
			tinnitus retraining therapy
	trimester		treatment-related toxicity
TriA	tricuspid atresia	TR/TE	time to repetition and time to echo in spin (echo sequence of magnetic resonance imaging)
T₃RIA	triiodothyronine level by radioimmunoassay		
TRIAC	triiodothyroacetic acid		
TRIC	trachoma inclusion conjunctivitis	T₃RU	triiodothyronine resin uptake
TRICH	*Trichomonas*		
TRICKS	time-resolved imaging contrast kinetics	TRUS	transrectal ultrasonography
TRIG	triglycerides	TRUSP	transrectal ultrasonography of the prostate
TRISS	Trauma Related Injury Severity Score		
TR-LSC	time-resolved liquid scintillation counting	TRUST	toluidine red unheated serum test
TRM	transplant-related mortality	TRZ	triazolam (Halcion)
	treatment-related mortality	TS	Tay-Sachs (disease)
TRM-SMX	trimethoprim-sulfamethoxazole (correct name is sulfamethoxazole and trimethoprin; SMZ-TMP; SMX-TMP)		telomerase
			temperature sensitive
			test solution
			thoracic spine
			throat swab
			thymidylate synthase
tRNA	transfer ribonucleic acid		timed samplings
TRNBP	transrectal needle biopsy prostate		toe signs
			Tourette syndrome
TRND	Trendelenburg (position)		transsexual
			Trauma Score
TRNG	tetracycline-resistant *Neisseria gonorrhoeae*		tricuspid stenosis
			triple strength
TRO	to return to office		tuberous sclerosis
TROFO	trofosfamide		Turner syndrome
TROM	torque range of motion	T/S	trimethoprim/sulfamethoxazole (correct name is sulfamethoxazole and trimethoprim)
	total range of motion		
TRP	tubular reabsorption of phosphate		
TRP-1	tyrosine-related protein-1		
TRPS	trichorhinophalangeal syndrome (types I, II, and III)	T&S	type and screen
		Ts	Schiotz tension
			T suppressor cell
TrPs	trigger points	TSAb	thyroid stimulating antibodies
TRPT	transplant		
TRS	Therapeutic Recreation Specialist	TSA	toluenesulfonic acid
			total shoulder arthroplasty

	tryptone soya (blood) agar	TSIs	tobramycin solution for inhalation (TOBI®) thymidylate synthase inhibitors
	tumor-specific antigen		
	type-specific antibody	T-skull	trauma skull
	tyramine signal amplification	TSM	two-spotted spider mite
TSAR®	tape surrounded Appli-rulers	tsp	teaspoon (5 mL)
		TSP	thrombospondin
TSAS	Total Severity Assessment Score		total serum protein
			tropical spastic paraparesis
TSAT	transferrin saturation		
TSB	total serum bilirubin	TSPA	thiotepa
	trypticase soy broth	T-spine	thoracic spine
TSBB	transtracheal selective bronchial brushing	TSR	total shoulder replacement
		TSS	total serum solids
TSC	technetium sulfur colloid		toxic shock syndrome
	theophylline serum concentration		transsphenoidal surgery
			tumor score system
	total symptom complex	TSST	toxic shock syndrome toxin
	tuberous sclerosis complex		
		TST	titmus stereocuity test
T-score	number of standard deviations from the average bone mineral density (BMD) of a 25-30 year old woman		total sleep time
			trans-scrotal testosterone
			treadmill stress test
			tuberculin skin test(s)
TSD	target to skin distance	TSTA	tumor-specific transplantation antigens
	Tay-Sachs disease		
	total sleep deprivation	TSTM	too small to measure
	T-(tumor) stage downstaging	TT	testicular torsion
			Test Tape®
TSDP	tapered steroid dosing package		tetanus toxoid
			thiotepa (Thioplex)
TSE	targeted systemic exposure		thoracostomy tube
			thrombin time
	testicular self-examination		thrombolytic therapy
	total skin examination		thymol turbidity
	transmissible spongiform encephalopathy		tilt table
			tilt testing
			tonometry
TSEBT	total skin electron beam therapy		total thyroidectomy
			transit time
T set	tracheotomy set		transtracheal
TSF	tricep skin fold (thickness)		treponemal test
			tuberculin tested
TSGA	term, small gestational age		tuberculoid leprosy
			twitch tension
TSGs	tumor suppressor genes		tympanic temperature
TSH	thyroid-stimulating hormone	T-T	time-to-time
		T/T	trace of ____/ trace of ____
TSH-RH	thyrotropin-releasing hormone		
		T&T	tobramycin and ticarcillin
TSI	thyroid stimulating immunoglobulin		touch and tone

T

	tympantomy and tube (insertion)	TTP	tender to palpation
TT4	total thyroxine		tender to pressure
TTA	total toe arthroplasty		thrombotic thrombocytopenic purpura
	transtracheal aspiration		time to pregnancy
TTAT	toe touch as tolerated		time to tumor progression
TTC	transtracheal catheter		time-to-progression
TTD	tarsal tunnel decompression	TTP/HUS	thrombotic thrombocytopenic purpura and hemolytic-uremic syndrome
	temporary total disability		
	total tumor dose		
	transverse thoracic diameter	TTR	time in therapeutic range
TTDE	touch-tone data entry		transthyretin
	transthoracic color Doppler echocardiography		triceps tendon reflex
		TTS	tarsal tunnel syndrome
			temporary threshold shift
TTDM	thallim threadmill		through the skin
TTDP	time-to-disease progression		transdermal therapeutic system
TTE	transthoracic echocardiography		transfusion therapy service
	trial terminated early		
t test	Student's t-test	TTs	tympanostomy tubes
TTF	time-to-treatment failure	TTT	tilt-table test
TTGE	timed-temperature gradient electrophoresis		tolbutamide tolerance test
			total tourniquet time
TTI	Teflon tube insertion		transpupillary thermotherapy
	total time to intubate		
	transfer to intermediate		turn-to-turn transfusion
TTII	thyrotropin-binding inhibitory immunoglobulins	TTTS	twin-twin transfusion syndrome
		TTUTD	tetanus toxoid up-to-date
TTJV	transtracheal jet ventilation	TTV	total tumor volume
			transfusion-transmitted virus
TTM	total tumor mass		
	transtelephonic monitoring	TTVP	temporary transvenous pacemaker
	trichotillomania		
TTN	time to normalization	TTWB	touch-toe weight bearing
	transient tachypnea of the newborn	TTx	thrombolytic therapy
		TU	Todd units
TTNA	transthoracic needle aspiration		transrectal ultrasound
			transurethral
TTNB	transient tachypnea of the newborn		tuberculin units
			tumor
TTND	time to nondetectable	Tu	Tuesday
TTO	tea tree oil	1-TU	1 tuberculin unit
	time trade-off	5-TU	5 tuberculin units
	to take out	250-TU	250 tuberculin units
	transfer to open	TUB	tuberculosis vaccine, not BCG
	transtracheal oxygen		
TTOD	tetanus toxoid outdated	TUBS	traumatic, unidirectional instability and Bankart lesion
TTOT	transtracheal oxygen therapy		

TUDS	temporary ureteral drainage system		temporary visit
			thyroid volume
TUE	transurethral extraction		tidal volume
TUF	total ultrafiltration		tonic vergence
TUG	timed Up and GO (test)		transvenous
	total urinary gonadotropin		trial visit
TUIBN	transurethral incision of bladder neck		*Trichomonas vaginalis*
			tricuspid value
TUIP	transurethral incision of the prostate	T/V	touch-verbal
		TVC	triple voiding cystogram
TUL	tularemia (*Francisella tularensis*) vaccine		true vocal cord
		TVc	tricuspid valve closure
TULIP®	transurethral ultrasound-guided laser-induced prostatectomy (system)	TVD	triple vessel disease
		TVDALV	triple vessel disease with an abnormal left ventricle
TULIPS	touch-up and loop incorporated primers (an alternative PCR technique)	TVF	tactile vocal fremitus
			target vessel failure
			true vocal fold
		TVH	total vaginal hysterectomy
TUMT	transurethral microwave thermotherapy	TVI	time velocity integral
		TVN	tonic vibration response
TUN	total urinary nitrogen	TVP	tensor veli palatini (muscle)
TUNA	transurethral needle ablation		transvenous pacemaker
TUNEL	terminal deoxynucleotidyl transferase-mediated dUTP-biotin nick-end labeling		transvesicle prostatectomy
		TVR	tricuspid valve replacement
		TVRSS	total vasomotor rhinitis symptom score
TUPR	transurethral prostatic resection	TVS	transvaginal sonography
			transvenous system
TUR	transurethral resection		trigemino-vascular system
T₃UR	triiodothyronine uptake ratio	TVSC	transvaginal sector scan
		TVT	tension-free vaginal tape
TURB	transurethral resection of the bladder		transvaginal taping
			transvaginal tension-free
	turbidity	TVU	total volume of urine
TURBN	transurethral resection bladder neck		transvaginal ultrasonography
TURBT	transurethral resection bladder tumor	TVUS	transvaginal ultrasonography
TURP	transurethral resection of prostate	TW	talked with
			tapwater
TURV	transurethral resection valves		test weight
			thought withdrawal
TURVN	transurethral resection of vesical neck		*Trophermyma whippleii*
			T-wave
TUTL	transuterine tubal lavage	T1WI	T1 weighted image (magnetic resonance imaging term for short repetition time and short echo time)
TUU	transureterourerostomy		
TUV	transurethral valve		
TUVP	transurethral vaporization of the prostate		
TV	television		

T

T2WI	T2 weighted image (magnetic resonance imaging term for long repetition time and long echo time)	TXE	Timoptic-XE®
		TXL	paclitaxel (Taxol) (this is a dangerous abbreviation as it can be read as TXT)
TW2	Tanner-Whitehouse mark 2 (bone-age assessment)	TXM	type and crossmatch
		TXS	type and screen
5TW	five times a week (this is a dangerous abbreviation)	TXT	docetaxel (Taxotere) (this is a dangerous abbreviation as it can be read as TXL)
TWA	time-weighted average total wrist arthroplasty T-wave alternans	TY	tympanic
		T & Y	trichomonas and yeast
TWAR	*Chlamydia pneumoniae*	TYCO #3	Tylenol with 30 mg of codeine (#1=7.5 mg, #2=15 mg and #4=60 mg of codeine present)
T-wave	part of the electrocardiographic cycle, representing a portion of ventricular repolarization		
		Tyl	Tylenol (acetaminophen) tyloma (callus)
TWB	total weight bearing	TYMP	tympanogram
TWD	total white and differential count	TYR	tyrosine
		TZ	temozolomide (Temodar) transition zone
TWE	tapwater enema		
TWETC	tapwater enema 'til clear	TZD	thiazolidinedione
		TZDs	thiazolidinediones
TWG	total weight gain	TZM	temozolomide (Temodar)
TWH	transitional wall hyperplasia		
TWHW ok	toe walking and heel walking all right		
TWI	tooth-wear index T-wave inversion		
TWiST	time without symptoms of progression or toxicity		
TWR	total wrist replacement		
TWSTRS	Toronto Western Spasmodic Torticollis Rating Scale		
TWT	timed walking test		
TWWD	tap water wet dressing		
Tx	therapist therapy traction transcription transfuse transplant transplantation treatment tympanostomy		
T & X	type and crossmatch		
TXA$_2$	thromboxane A$_2$		
TXB$_2$	thromboxane B$_2$		

T

U

U   Ultralente Insulin®
units (this is the most dangerous abbreviation—spell out "unit")
unknown
upper
uranium
urine

Ⓤ   Kosher
U/1   1 finger breadth below umbilicus
1/U   1 finger over umbilicus
U/   at umbilicus
24U   24-hour urine (collection)
U100   100 units per milliliters
UA   umbilical artery
unauthorized absence
uncertain about
unstable angina
upper airway
upper arm
uric acid
urinalysis
UABD   upper airway bronchodilation
UAC   umbilical artery catheter
under active
upper airway congestion
UA/C   uric acid to creatinine (ratio)
UAD   upper airway disease
UADT   upper aerodigestive tract
UAE   urinary albumin excretion
uterine artery embolization
UACEs   unplanned acute care encounters
UAER   urinary albumin excretion rate
UAL   umbilical artery line
up *ad lib*
UA&M   urinalysis and microscopy
UA/NSTEMI   unstable angina and non-ST-segment elevation myocardial infarction
UAO   upper airway obstruction
UAP   upper abdominal pain
UAPD   Union of American Physicians and Dentists

UAPF   upon arrival patient found
UAPs   unlicensed assistive personnel
U-ARM   upper arm
UARS   upper airway resistance syndrome
UAS   upstream activating sequence
UASA   upper airway sleep apnea
UASQ   Unstable Angina Symptoms Questionnaire
UAT   up as tolerated
UAVC   univentricular atrioventricular connection
UBAs   urethral bulking agents
UBC   University of British Columbia (brace)
UBD   universal blood donor
UBE   upper body ergometer
UBF   unknown black female
uterine blood flow
UBI   ultraviolet blood irradiation
UBM   unknown black male
UBO   unidentified bright object
UBT ^{13}C-urea breath test
uterine balloon therapy
UBW   usual body weight
UC   ulcerative colitis
umbilical cord
unchanged
unconscious
Unit clerk
United Church of Christ
urea clearance
urinary catheter
urine culture
usual care
uterine contraction
U&C   urethral and cervical
usual and customary
UCAD   unstable coronary artery disease
UCB   umbilical cord blood
unconjugated bilirubin (indirect)
Unicorn Campbell Boy (orthotics)
UCBT   unrelated cord-blood transplant

U

365

UCD	urine collection device	UDN	updraft nebulizer
	usual childhood diseases	UDO	undetermined origin
UCE	urea cycle enzymopathy	UDP	unassisted diastolic
UCF	unexplained chronic		pressure
	fatigue	UDPGT	uridinediphospho-
UCG	urinary chorionic		glucuronyl transferase
	gonadotropins	UDS	unconditioned stimulus
UCHD	usual childhood diseases		urine drug screen
UCHI	usual childhood illnesses	UDT	undescended testicle(s)
UCHS	uncontrolled hemorrhagic	UE	under elbow
	shock		undetermined etiology
UCI	urethral catheter in		upper extremity
	usual childhood illnesses	U & E	urea and electrolytes (see
UCL	uncomfortable loudness		page 392)
	level	UEBW	ultrasound estimated
UCLP	unilateral cleft lip and		bladder weight
	palate	UEC	uterine endometrial
UCN	urocortin		carcinoma
UCN-01	7-hydroxystaurosporin	UEDs	unilateral epileptiform
UCO	urethral catheter out		discharges
UCP	umbilical cord prolapse	UES	undifferentiated
	urethral closure pressure		embryonal sarcoma
UCPs	urine collection pads		upper esophageal
UCR	unconditioned reflex		sphincter
	unconditioned response	UESEP	upper extremity
	usual, customary, and		somatosensory evoked
	reasonable (fees)		potential
UCP-3	uncoupling protein −3	UESP	upper esophageal
UCRE	urine creatinine		sphincter pressure
UCRP	universal coagulation	UF	ultrafiltration
	reference plasma		until finished
UCS	unconscious	UFC	urinary free cortisol
UC&S	urine culture and	UFF	unusual facial features
	sensitivity	UFFI	urea formaldehyde foam
UCTD	undifferentiated		insulation
	connective tissue	UFH	unfractionated heparin
	disease	UFN	until further notice
UCVA	uncorrected visual	UFO	unflagged order
	acuity		unidentified foreign
UCX	urine culture		object
UD	as directed	UFOV	useful field of view
	ulnar deviation	UFR	ultrafiltration rate
	unit dose	UFT	uracil and tegafur
	urethral dilatation	UFV	ultrafiltration volume
	urethral discharge	UG	until gone
	urodynamics		urinary glucose
	uterine distension		urogenital
u.d.	as directed	UGA	under general anesthesia
UDC	uninhibited detrusor		urogenital atrophy
	(muscle) capacity	UGCR	ultrasound-guided
	usual diseases of childhood		compression repair
UDCA	ursodeoxycholic acid	UGDP	University Group
	(Ursodiol)		Diabetes Project

UGH	uveitis, glaucoma, and hyphema (syndrome)	UITN	Urinary Incontinence Treatment Network
UGI	upper gastrointestinal series	UJ	universal joint (syndrome)
		UK	United Kingdom
UGIB	upper gastrointestinal bleeding		unknown
			urine potassium
UGIH	upper gastrointestinal hemorrhage		urokinase
		UK IC	urokinase intracoronary
UGIS	upper gastrointestinal series	UKE	unknown etiology
		UKNDS	United Kingdom Neurological Disability Score
UGIT	upper gastrointestinal tract		
UGI w/SBFT	upper gastrointestinal (series) with small bowel follow through	UKO	unknown origin
		UL	Unit Leader
			upper left
UGK	urine, glucose, and ketones		upper lid
			upper limb
UGP	urinary gonadotropin peptide		upper lobe
		U/L	upper and lower
UGTI	ultrasound-guided thrombin injection	U & L	upper and lower
		ULBW	ultra low birth weight (between 501 and 750 g)
UGVA	ultrasound-guided vascular access		
UH	umbilical hernia	ULDT	ultra low-dose therapy
	unfavorable history	ULLE	upper lid, left eye
	University Hospital	ULN	upper limits of normal
UHBI	upper hemibody irradiation	ULPA	ultra-low particulate air
		ULQ	upper left quadrant
UHDDS	Uniform Hospital Discharge Data Set	ULRE	upper lid, right eye
		ULSB	upper left sternal border
UHDRS	Unified Huntington Disease Rating Scale	ULTT1	upper limb tension test 1 (median nerve)
		ULTT2a	upper limb tension test 2a (medial nerve)
UHDs	ulcer-healing drugs		
UHMWPE	ultra-high molecular weight polyethylene	ULTT2b	upper limb tension test 2b (radial nerve)
UHP	University Health Plan	ULTT3	upper limb tension test 3 (ulnar nerve)
UI	urinary incontinence		
UIB	Unemployment Insurance Benefits	ULYTES	electrolytes, urine
		UM	unmarried
UIBC	unbound iron binding capacity		utilization management
		Umb A Line	umbilical artery line
	unsaturated iron binding capacity		
		Umb V Line	umbilical venous line
UID	once daily (this is a dangerous abbreviation, spell out "once daily")		
		umb ven	umbilical vein
		UMCD	uremic medullary cystic disease
UIEP	urine (urinary) immunoelectrophoresis	UMLS	Unified Medical Language System
UIP	usual interstitial pneumonitis (pneumonia)		
		UMN	upper motor neuron (disease)
UIQ	upper inner quadrant	UN	undernourished

U

	urinary nitrogen	UPO	metastatic carcinoma of
UNA	urinary nitrogen		unknown primary
	appearance		origin
UNa	urine sodium	UPOR	usual place of residence
unacc	unaccompanied	UPP	urethral pressure profile
UNC	uncrossed	UPPP	uvulopalatopharyngo-
UNDEL	undelivered		plasty
UNDP	United Nations	U/P ratio	urine to plasma ratio
	Development Program	UPS	ubiquitin-dependent
UNE	ulnar neuropathy at the		proteasomal system
	elbow		ubiquitin-proteasome
	urinary norepinephrine		system
UNG	ointment	UPSC	uterine papillary serous
UNHS	universal newborn		carcinoma
	hearing screening	UPSIT	University of
UNK	unknown		Pennsylvania Smell
UNL	upper normal levels		Identification Test
UNOS	United Network for	UPT	uptake
	Organ Sharing		urine pregnancy test
UN/P	unpatched eye	UR	unrelated
UN/P OD	unpatched right eye		upper respiratory
UN/P OS	unpatched left eye		upper right
UNS	unsatisfactory		urinary retention
UNSAT	unsatisfactory		utilization review
UO	under observation	URA	unilateral renal
	undetermined origin		agenesis
	ureteral orifice	URAC	Utilization Review
	urinary output		Accreditation
UONx	unilateral optic nerve		Commission
	transection	UR AC	uric acid
UOP	urinary output	URAS	unilateral renal artery
UOQ	upper outer quadrant		stenosis
Uosm	urinary osmolality	URD	undifferentiated
✓ up	check up		respiratory disease
UP	unipolar		unrelated donor
	ureteropelvic	URE	Uniform Rules of
U/P	urine to plasma		Evidence
	(creatinine)	URG	urgent
UPC	unknown primary	URI	upper respiratory infection
	carcinoma	URIC A	uric acid
UPD	uniparental disomy	url	unrelated
UPDRS	Unified Parkinson Disease	UR&M	urinalysis, routine and
	Rating Scale		microscopic
UPEP	urine protein	URO	urology
	electrophoresis	UROB	urobilinogen
UPG	uroporphyrinogen	UROD	ultra-rapid opiate
UPIN	unique physician		detoxification [under
	(provided)		anesthesia]
	identification number	UROL	Urologist
UPJ	ureteropelvic junction		urology
UPLIF	unilateral posterior	URQ	upper right quadrant
	lumbar interbody fusion	URR	urea reduction ratio
UPN	unique patient number	URS	ureterorenoscopy

U

URSB	upper right sternal border		United States Navy
URT	upper respiratory tract	USO	unilateral salpingo-oophorectomy
	uterine resting tone	USOGH	usual state of good health
URTI	upper respiratory tract infection	USOH	usual state of health
US	ultrasonography	USP	unassisted systolic pressure
	unit secretary		
	United States of America		United States Pharmacopeia
USA	unit services assistant	USPHS	United States Public Health Service
	United States Army		
	United States of America	USS	Upshaw-Schulman syndrome
	unstable angina		
USAF	United States Air Force	USUCVD	unsterile uncontrolled vaginal delivery
USAMRIID	United States Army Medical Research Institute of Infectious Diseases	USVMD	urine specimen volume measuring device
		UT	upper thoracic
USAN	United States Adopted Names	UTA	urinary tract anomaly
		UTC	urinary tract calculi
USAP	unstable angina pectoris	UTD	unable to determine
			up to date
USB	upper sternal border	*ut dict*	as directed
USC	uterine serous carcinoma	UTF	usual throat flora
U-SCOPE	ureteroscopy	UTI	urinary tract infection
USCVD	unsterile controlled vaginal delivery	UTL	unable to locate
		UTM	urinary-tract malformations
USDA	United States Department of Agriculture	UTMDACC	University of Texas M.D. Anderson Cancer Center
USED-CARP	**u**reterosigmoidostomy, **s**mall bowel fistula, **e**xtra chloride, **d**iarrhea, **c**arbonic anhydrase inhibitors, **a**drenal insufficiency, **r**enal tubular acidosis, and **p**ancreatic fistula (common causes of nonanion gap metabolic acidosis)	UTO	unable to obtain
			upper tibial osteotomy
		UTP	uridine triphosphate
		UTR	untranslated region
		UTS	ulnar tunnel syndrome
			ultrasound
		U/U−	uterine fundus at umbilicus (usually modified as number of finger breadths below)
USG	ultrasonography		
	urine specific gravity	U/U+	uterine fundus at umbilicus (usually modified as number of finger breadths above)
USH	United Services for Handicapped		
	usual state of health		
USI	urinary stress incontinence	UUD	uncontrolled unsterile delivery
USM	ultrasonic mist	UUN	urinary urea nitrogen
USMC	United States Marine Corps	UUTI	uncomplicated urinary tract infections
USMLE	United States Medical Licensing Examination	UV	ultraviolet
USN	ultrasonic nebulizer		ureterovesical

U

	urine volume
UVA	ultraviolet A light
	ureterovesical angle
UVB	ultraviolet B light
UVBI	ultra-violet blood irradiation
UVC	umbilical vein catheter
	ultraviolet C light
UVEB	unifocal ventricular ectopic beat
UVGI	ultraviolet germicidal irradiation
UVH	univentricular heart
UVIB	ultra-violet irradiation of blood
UVJ	ureterovesical junction
UVL	ultraviolet light
	umbilical venous line
UVR	ultraviolet radiation
UVT	unsustained ventricular tachycardia
UV-VIS	ultraviolet-visible (spectrometer)
U/WB	unit of whole blood
UW	unilateral weakness
UWF	unknown white female
UWM	unknown white male
	unwed mother
UXO	unexploded ordnance

U

V

V	five
	gas volume
	minute volume
	vaccinated
	vagina
	vein
	ventricular
	verb
	verbal
	vertebral
	very
	Viagra (sildenafil citrate) as in "vitamin V"
	viral
	vision
	vitamin
	vomiting
$\dot{V}$	ventilation (L/min)
+V	positive vertical divergence
V1	fifth cranial nerve, ophthalmic division
V2	fifth cranial nerve, maxillary division
V3	fifth cranial nerve, mandibular division
V_1 to V_6	precordial chest leads
VA	vacuum aspiration
	valproic acid
	ventriculoatrial
	vertebral artery
	Veterans Administration
	visual acuity
V_A	alveolar gas volume
V&A	vagotomy and antrectomy
VAAESS	Vaccine-Associated Adverse Events Surveillance System (Canada)
VAB	variable atrial blockage
	vinblastine, dactinomycin (actinomycin D), bleomycin
VABS	Vineland Adaptive Behavior Scales
VAC	vacuum-assisted closure (dressings)
	ventriculoarterial conduction

	vincristine, dactinomycin (actinomycin D), and cyclophosphamide
	vincristine, doxorubicin (Adriamycin), and cyclophosphamide
VA cc	distance visual acuity with correction
VA ccl	near visual acuity with correction
VACE	*Vitex agnus-castus* extract (Chaste tree berry extract)
VAC EXT	vacuum extractor
VAC$_{ig}$	vaccinia immune globulin
VACO	Veterans Administration Central Office
VACTERL	vertebral, anal, cardiac, tracheal, esophageal, renal, and limb anomalies
VAD	vascular (venous) access device
	ventricular assist device
	vertebral artery dissection
	Veterans Administration Domiciliary
	vincristine, doxorubicin (Adriamycin), and dexamethasone
VaD	vascular dementia
VADCS	ventricular atrial distal coronary sinus
VADRIAC	vincristine, doxorubicin (Adriamycin), and cyclophosphamide
VAE	venous air embolism
VAERS	Vaccine Adverse Events Reporting System
VAFD	vascular access flush device
VAG	vagina
VAG HYST	vaginal hysterectomy
VAH	Veterans Administration Hospital
VAHBE	ventricular atrial His bundle electrocardiogram
VAHRA	ventricular atrial height right atrium
VAI	vertebral artery injury

VAIN	vaginal intraepithelial neoplasia
VALE	visual acuity, left eye
VALI	ventilator-associated lung injury
VAMC	Veterans Affairs Medical Center
VAMP®	venous-arterial management protection system
VAMS	Visual Analogue Mood Scale
VANCO/P	vancomycin-peak
VANCO/T	vancomycin-trough
VAOD	visual acuity, right eye
VAOS	visual acuity, left eye
VA OS LP with P	visual acuity, left eye, left perception with projection
VAP	venous access port
	ventilator-associated pneumonia
	vincristine, asparaginase, and prednisone
VAPCS	ventricular atrial proximal coronary sinus
VAPP	vaccine-associated paralytic poliomyelitis
VAR	variant
	varicella (chickenpox) (*varicella zoster* virus) vaccine
VARE	visual acuity, right eye
VARig	varicella-zoster immune globulin
VAS	vasectomy
	vascular
	Visual Analogue Scale (Score)
VASC	Visual-Auditory Screen Test for Children
VA sc	distance visual acuity without correction
VA scl	near visual acuity without correction
VASPI	Visual Analogue Self Assessment Scales For Pain Intensity
VAS RAD	vascular radiology
VAT	ventilatory anaerobic threshold
	vertebral artery test
	video-assist thoracoscopy

V

	visceral adipose tissue	VC	color vision
VATER	vertebral, anal, tracheal, esophageal, and renal anomalies		etoposide (VePesid) and carboplatin
			pulmonary capillary blood volume
VATH	vinblastine, doxorubicin (Adriamycin), thiotepa, and fluoxymesterone (Halotestin)		vena cava
			verbal cues
			vincristine
VATS	video assisted thoracic surgery		virtual colonoscopy
			vital capacity
VAVD	vacuum-assisted venous drainage		vocal cords
			voluntary cough
VAX-D	vertebral axial decompression	V&C	vertical and centric (a bite)
		VCA	vasoconstrictor assay
VB	Van Buren (catheter)	VCAM	vascular cell adhesion molecule
	venous blood		
	vinblastine (Velban)	VCAP	vincristine, cyclophospha-mide, doxorubicin (Adriamycin), and prednisone
	vinblastine and bleomycin		
	virtual bronchoscopy		
VB$_1$	first voided bladder specimen	Vcc	vision with correction
		VCCA	velocity common carotid artery
VB$_2$	second midstream bladder specimen		
		VCD	vocal cord dysfunction
VB$_3$	third voided urine specimen	VCDR	vertical cup-to-disk ratio
		VCE	vaginal cervical endocervical (smear)
VBAC	vaginal birth after cesarean		
		VCF	Vaginal Contraception Film™
VBAI	vertebrobasilar artery insufficiency		
		VCFS	velo-cardio-facial syndrome
VBAP	vincristine, carmustine (BiCNU), doxorubicin (Adriamycin), and prednisone		
		VCG	vectorcardiography
			voiding cystogram
		vCJD	variant Creutzfeldt-Jakob disease
VBC	vinblastine, bleomycin, and cisplatin		
		VCO	ventilator CPAP oxyhood
VBG	venous blood gas	V$_{CO_2}$	carbon dioxide output
	vertical banded gastroplasty	VCPR	veterinarian-client-patient relationship
VBGP	vertical banded gastroplasty	VCR	video cassette recorder
			vincristine sulfate (Oncovin)
VBI	vertebrobasilar insufficiency		
		VCT	venous clotting time
VBL	vinblastine (Velban)		voluntary counselling and testing
VBM	vinblastine, bleomycin, and methotrexate		
		VCTS	vitreal corneal touch syndrome
	voxel-based morphometry		
VBP	vinblastine, bleomycin, and cisplatin	VCU	voiding cystourethrogram
		VCUG	vesicoureterogram
VBR	ventricular brain ratio		voiding cystourethrogram
VBS	vertebral-basilar system	VCV	volume-control ventilation
	videofluoroscopic barium swallow (evaluation)	VD	venereal disease
			vessel disease

V

viral diarrhea
voided
voiding diary
volume of distribution
V_D deadspace volume
V_d volume of distribution
V&D vomiting and diarrhea
1-VD one-vessel disease
VDA venous digital angiogram
visual discriminatory acuity
VDAC vaginal delivery after cesarean
VDC vincristine, doxorubicin, and cyclophosphamide
VDD atrial synchronous ventricular inhibited pacing
VDDR I vitamin D dependency rickets type I
VDDR II vitamin D dependency rickets type II
VDE vasodilatory edema
VDEPT virus-directed enzyme prodrug therapy
VDG venereal disease–gonorrhea
Vdg voiding
VDH valvular disease of the heart
VDJ variable diversity joining
VDL vasodepressor lipid
visual detection level
VDO varus derotational osteotomy
VD or M venous distention or masses
VDP vinblastine, dacarbazine, and cisplatin (Platinol AQ)
VDPCA variable-dose patient-controlled analgesia
VDR vitamin D receptor (gene)
VDRF ventilator dependent respiratory failure
VDRL Venereal Disease Research Laboratory (test for syphilis)
VDRR vitamin D-resistant rickets
VDRS Verdun Depression Rating Scale
VDS vasodepressor syncope
venereal disease—syphilis

vindesine (Eldisine)
VDT video display terminal
VD/VT dead space to tidal volume ratio
VE vaginal examination
vertex
Vietnam era
virtual endoscopy
visual examination
vitamin E
vocational evaluation
V_E minute volume (expired)
V/E violence and eloper
VEA ventricular ectopic activity
viscoelastic agent
VEB ventricular ectopic beat
VEC vecuronium (Norcuron)
velocity-encoded cine
VECG vector electrocardiogram
VED vacuum erection device
vacuum extraction delivery
ventricular ectopic depolarization
VEE Venezuelan equine encephalitis
VEE_a Venezuelan equine encephalitis vaccine, attenuated live
VEE_I Venezuelan equine encephalitis vaccine, inactivated
VEF visually evoked field
VEG vegetation (bacterial)
VEGF vascular endothelial growth factor
VeIP vinblastine (Velban), ifosfamide, and cisplatin (Platinol AQ)
VEMP vestibular evoked myogenic potentials
VENC velocity encoding value (radiology)
VENT ventilation
ventilator
ventral
ventricular
VEP visual evoked potential
VER ventricular escape rhythm
visual evoked responses
VERDICT Veterans Evidence-based Research Dissemination Implementation Center

V

VERP	ventricular effective refractory period	VGAD	vein of Galen aneurysmal dilatation
VERT	velocity-enhanced resistance training	VGAM	vein of Galen aneurysmal malformation
VES	ventricular extrasystoles	VGB	vigabatrin (Sabril)
	video-endoscopic surgery	VGE	viral gastroenteritis
	vitamin E succinate	VGH	very good health
VESS	video endoscopic swallowing study	VGKC	voltage-gated potassium channel
VET	veteran	VGM	vein graft myringoplasty
	Veterinarian	VGPO	volume-guaranteed pressure option
	veterinary		
VF	left leg (electrode)	VH	vaginal hysterectomy
	ventricular fibrillation		Veterans Hospital
	vertical float (aquatic therapy)		viral hepatitis
			visual hallucinations
	visual field		vitreous hemorrhage
	vocal fremitus		von Herrick (grading system)
VFC	Vaccines for Children (program)	VH I	very narrow anterior chamber angles
VFCB	vertical flow clean bench		
VFD	ventilator-free days	VH II	moderately narrow anterior chamber angles
	visual fields		
VFFC	visual fields full to confrontation	VH III	moderately wide open anterior chamber angles
VFI	visual fields intact	VH IV	wide open anterior chamber angles
	Visual Functioning index	VHD	valvular heart disease
V. Fib	ventricular fibrillation		vascular hemostatis device
VFL	vinflunine	VHF	viral hemorrhagic fever
VFMI	vocal fold motion impairment	VHI	Voice Handicap Index
		VHL	von Hippel-Lindau disease (complex)
VFP	vertical float progression (aquatic therapy)		
	vitreous fluorophotometry	VHP	vaporized hydrogen peroxide
	vocal fold paralysis	VI	six
VFPN	Volu-feed premie nipple		velocity index
VFR	visiting friends and relatives (possible contacts for communicable diseases)		volume index
		via	by way of
		vib	vibration
		VIBS	Victim's Information Bureau Service
VFRN	Volu-feed regular nipple		
VFSS	videofluoroscopic swallowing study	VICA	velocity internal carotid artery
VFT	venous filling time	VICP	Vaccine Injury Compensation Program
	ventricular fibrillation threshold	Vi CPs	typhoid Vi (capsular) polysaccharide vaccine (Typhim Vi)
VG	vein graft		
	ventricular gallop		
	ventrogluteal	VID	videodensitometry
	very good	VIG	vaccinia immune globulin
V&G	vagotomy and gastroenterotomy		vinblastine, ifosfamide, and gallium nitrate

VIH	human immunodeficiency virus (Spanish and French abbreviation)	VKA	vitamin K antagonists
		VKC	vernal keratoconjunctivitis
VIN	vulvar intraepithelial neoplasm	VKDB	vitamin K deficiency bleeding
VIP	etopside (VePesid), ifosfamide, and cisplatin (Platinol AQ)	VKH	Vogt-Koyanagi-Harada disease
		VL	left arm (electrode)
	vasoactive intestinal peptide		vial
			viral load
	vasoactive intracorporeal pharmacotherapy		visceral leishmaniasis (kala-azar)
		VLA	very-late antigen
	Vattikuti Institute prostatectomy	VLAD	variable life-adjusted display
	very important patient	VLAP	vaporization laser ablation of the prostate
	vinblastine, ifosfamide, and cisplatin (Platinol)		
		VLBW	very low birth weight (less than 1500 g)
	voluntary interruption of pregnancy		
		VLBWPN	very low birth weight preterm neonate
VIPomas	vasoactive intestinal peptide-secreting tumors		
		VLCAD	very-long-chain acyl coenzyme A dehydrogenase
VIQ	Verbal Intelligence Quotient (part of Wechsler tests)		
		VLCD	very low calorie diet
		VLCFA	very-long-chain fatty acids
VIS	Vaccine Information Statement		
		VLDL	very-low-density lipoprotein
	Visual Impairment Service		
		VLE	vision left eye
VISA	vancomycin-intermediate-resistant *Staphylococcus aureus*	VLH	ventrolateral nucleus of the hypothalamus
		VLM	visceral larva migrans
VISC	vitreous infusion suction cutter	VLP	virus-like particle
		VLPP	Valsalva lead-point pressure
VISI	Vaccine Identification Standards Initiative		
		VLR	vastus lateralis release
	volar intercalated segmental instability	VM	venous malformation
			ventilated mask
VISN	Veterans Integrated Service Networks		ventimask
			Venturi mask
VISs	Vaccine Information Statements		vestibular membrane
		VM 26	teniposide (Vumon)
VIT	venom immunotherapy	VMA	vanillylmandelic acid
	vital	VMATs	Veterinary Medical Assistance Teams
	vitamin		
	vitreous	VMCP	vincristine, melphalan, cyclophosphamide, and prednisone
Vitamin	see individual letters such as R, V, etc.		
VIT CAP	vital capacity	VMD	Doctor of Veterinary Medicine (DVM)
VIU	visual internal urethrotomy		
			vertical maxillary deficiency
VIZ	namely		
V-J	ventriculo-jugular (shunt)	VME	vertical maxillary excess

V

VMH	ventromedial hypothalamus		variegate porphyria
			venipuncture
VMI	vendor-managed inventory		venous pressure
	visual motor integration		ventriculoperitoneal
VMO	vaccinia melanoma oncolysate		visual perception
			voiding pressure
	vastus medialis oblique	V & P	vagotomy and pyloroplasty
VMR	vasomotor rhinitis		
VMS	vanilla milkshake		ventilation and perfusion
VN	visiting nurse	VP-16	etoposide
VNA	Visiting Nurses' Association	VPA	valproic acid
			ventricular premature activation
VNB	vinorelbine (Navelbine)		
VNC	vesicle neck contracture		vigorous physical activity
VNS	vagal nerve stimulation	V-Pad	sanitary napkin
VNTR	variable number of tandem repeats	VPB	ventricular premature beat
		VPC	ventricular premature contractions
VO	verbal order		
	visual observation	VPD	ventricular premature depolarization
VO₂	oxygen consumption		
VOCAB	vocabulary	VPDC	ventricular premature depolarization contraction
VOCOR	vaso-occlusive crisis		
	void on-call to operating room		
		VPDF	vegetable protein diet plus fiber
VOCs	volatile organic compounds		
		VPDs	ventricular premature depolarizations
VOCTOR	void on-call to operating room		
		VPI	velopharyngeal incompetence
VOD	veno-occlusive disease		
	vision right eye		velopharyngeal insufficiency
VOE	vascular occlusive episode		
		VPL	ventro-posterolateral
VO₂I	oxygen consumption index	VPLN	vaccine-primed lymph node (cells)
VOL	Valuation of Life	VPLS	ventilation-perfusion lung scan
	volume		
	voluntary	VPM	venous pressure module
VOM	vomited	VPR	virtual patient record
VOO	continuous ventricular asynchronous pacing		volume pressure response
		VPS	valvular pulmonic stenosis
VOOD	vesico-outlet obstructive disease		
			ventriculoperitoneal shunt
VOR	vestibular ocular reflex	VPT	vascularized patellar tendon
VORB	verbal order read back		
VOS	vision left eye		vibration perception threshold
VOSS	visual observation shivering score		
		VQ	ventilation perfusion
VOT	Visual Organization Test	VR	right arm (electrode)
VOU	vision both eyes		valve replacement
VOV	verbal order verified		venous resistance
VP	etoposide (VePesid) and cisplatin (Platinol AQ)		ventricular rhythm
			verbal reprimand
	vagal paraganglioma		vocational rehabilitation

V

376

V₃R··V₆R	right sided precordial leads	VSLI	vincristine sulfate liposomal injection
VRA	visual reinforcement audiometry	VSMC	vascular smooth muscle cell
	visual response audiometry	VSN	vital signs normal
		VSO	vertical subcondylar oblique
VRB	vinorelbine (Navelbine)	VSOK	vital signs normal
VRC	vocational rehabilitation counselor	VSP	vertical stabilization program
VRE	vancomycin-resistant enterococci	VSQOL	Vital Signs Quality of Life
	vision right eye	VSR	venous stasis retinopathy
VREF	vancomycin-resistant *Enterococcus faecium*		ventricular septal rupture
VRI	viral respiratory infection	VSS	variable spot scanning
VRL	ventral root, lumbar		visual sexual stimulation
	vinorelbine (Navelbine)		vital signs stable
VRP	vocational rehabilitation program	V_SS	apparent volume of distribution
VRS	viral rhinosinusitis	VSSAF	vital signs stable, afebrile
VRSA	vancomycin-resistant *Staphylococcus aureus*	VST	visual search task
		VSULA	vaccination scar, upper left arm
VRT	variance of resident time	VSV	vesicular stomatitis virus
	ventral root, thoracic	VT	validation therapy
	vertical radiation topography		ventricular tachycardia
	Visual Retention Test	V_t	tidal volume
	vocational rehabilitation therapy	VTA	ventral tegmentum area
		VTBI	volume to be infused
VRTA	Vocational Rehabilitation Therapy Assistant	v. tach.	ventricular tachycardia
		VTE	venous thromboembolism
VRU	ventilator rehabilitation unit	VTEC	verotoxin-producing *Escherichia coli*
VS	vagal stimulation	VTED	venous thromboembolic disease
	vegetative state	VT-NS	ventricular tachycardia nonsustained
	versus *(vs)*		
	very sensitive	VTOP	voluntary termination of pregnancy
	visit		
	visited	VTP	voluntary termination of pregnancy
	vital signs (temperature, pulse, and respiration)	VTS	Volunteer Transport Service
VSADP	vocational skills assessment and development program	VT-S	ventricular tachycardia sustained
		VTSRS	Verdun Target Symptom Rating Scale
VSBE	very short below elbow (cast)	VT/VF	ventricular tachycardia/fibrillation
VSD	ventricular septal defect	VTX	vertex
	vesicosphincter dyssynergia	VU	venous ulcer
VSGP	vertical supranuclear gaze palsy		vesicoureteral (reflux)
VSI	visual motor integration	V/U	verbalize understanding

V

VUC	voided-urine cytology
VUD-BMT	volunteer unrelated-donor bone marrow transplantation
VUJ	vesico ureteral junction
VUR	vesicoureteric reflux
VV	vaccina virus
	varicose veins
	vulvar vestibulitis
V-V	ventriculovenous (shunt)
V&V	vulva and vagina
V/V	volume to volume ratio
VVB	venovenous bypass
VVC	vulvovaginal candidiasis
VVD	vaginal vertex delivery
VVETP	Vietnam Veterans Evaluation and Treatment Program
VVFR	vesicovaginal fistula repair
VVI	venous valvular insufficiency
V/VI	grade 5 on a 6 grade basis
VVI	ventricular demand pacing
VVIR	ventricular demand inhibited pacemaker (V = chamber paced-ventricle, V = chamber sensed-ventricle, I = response to sensing-inhibited, R = programmability–rate modulation)
VVL	varicose veins ligation
	verruca vulgaris of the larynx
VVOR	visual-vestibulo-ocular-reflex
VVR	ventricular response rate
VVS	vasovagal syncope
	vulvar vestibulitis syndrome
VVs	varicose veins
VVT	ventricular synchronous pacing
VW	vessel wall
VWD	ventral wall defect
vWD	von Willebrand disease
vWF	von Willebrand factor
VWM	ventricular wall motion
V_x	vaccination
	vitrectomy

V-XT	V-pattern exotropia
VY	surgical replacement flap
VZ	varicella zoster
VZIG	varicella zoster immune globulin
VZV	varicella zoster virus

V

W

W	wash	WALK	weight-activated locking knee (prosthesis)
	watts	WAM	white adult male
	wearing glasses	WAP	wandering atrial pacemaker
	Wednesday	WAPRT	whole-abdominopelvic radiation therapy
	week	WARI	wheezing associated respiratory infection
	weight	WAS	whiplash-associated disorders
	well		Wiskott-Aldrich syndrome
	West (as in the location e.g. 2W, is second floor, West wing)	WASO	wakefulness after sleep onset
	white	WASP	Wiskott-Aldrich syndrome protein
	widowed	WASS	Wasserman test
	wife	WAT	word association test
	with	WB	waist belt
	work		weight bearing
W-1	insignificant (allergies)		well baby
W-3	minimal (allergies)		Western blot
W-5	moderate (allergies)		whole blood
W-7	moderate-severe (allergies)	WBACT	whole-blood activated clotting time
W-9	severe (allergies)	WBAT	weight bearing as tolerated
W 22	Central Institute for the Deaf 22 Word List	WBC	weight bearing with crutches
WA	when awake		well baby clinic
	while awake		white blood cell (count)
	White American	WBCT	whole-blood clotting time
	wide awake	WBD	weeks by dates (for gestational age)
	with assistance	WBE	weeks by examination (for gestational age)
W-A	Wyeth-Ayerst Laboratories		whole-body extract
W & A	weakness and atrophy	WBGD	whole-body glucose disposal
W or A	weakness or atrophy	WBH	weight-based heparin (dosing)
WACH	wedge adjustable cushioned heel		whole-body hyperthermia
WAF	weakness, atrophy, and fasciculation	WBI	whole-bowel irrigation
	white adult female	W Bld	whole blood
WAGR	Wilm tumor, aniridia, genitourinary malformations, and mental retardation (syndrome)	WBN	wellborn nursery
		WBNAA	whole-brain N-acetylaspartate
WAIS	Wechsler Adult Intelligence Scale	WBOS	wide base of support
		WBPTT	whole-blood partial thromboplastin time
WAIS-R	Wechsler Adult Intelligence Scale-Revised	WBQC	wide-base quad cane
WAL	Wyeth-Ayerst Laboratories	WBR	whole-body radiation

W

WBRT	whole-brain radiotherapy
WBS	weeks by size (for gestational age)
	whole body scan
	Williams-Beuren syndrome
WBTF	Waring Blender tube feeding
WBTT	weight bearing to tolerance
WBUS	weeks by ultrasound
WBV	whole blood volume
WC	ward clerk
	ward confinement
	warm compress
	wet compresses
	wheelchair
	when called
	white count
	whooping cough
	will call
	workers' compensation
WCA	work capacity assessment
WCC	well-child care
	white cell count
WCE	white coat effect
	work capacity evaluation
WCH	white coat hypertension
WCHE	well-child health examination
WC/LC	warm compresses and lid scrubs
WCM	whole cow's milk
WCS	work capacity specialist
WCST	Wisconsin Card Sorting Test
WCT	wide-complex tachycardia
WD	ward
	well developed
	well differentiated
	wet dressing
	Wilson disease
	word
	working distance
	wound
W/D	warm and dry
	withdrawal
W → D	wet to dry
W4D	Worth four-dot (test for fusion)
WDCC	well-developed collateral circulation
WDF	white divorced female

WDHA	watery diarrhea, hypokalemia, and achlorhydria
WDHH	watery diarrhea, hypokalemia, and hypochlorhydria
WDL	within defined limits
WDLL	well-differentiated lymphocytic lymphoma
WDM	white divorced male
WDS	word discrimination score
WDTC	well-differentiated thyroid cancer
WDWG	well dressed, well groomed
WDWN-AAF	well-developed, well-nourished African-American female
WDWN-BM	well-developed, well-nourished black male
WDWN-WF	well-developed, well-nourished white female
WDXRF	wavelength-dispersive x-ray fluorescence
WE	weekend
	wide excision
W/E	weekend
WEBINO	wall-eyed bilateral internuclear ophthalmoplegia
WE-D	withdrawal-emergent dyskinesia
WEE	Western equine encephalitis
WEMINO	wall-eyed monocular internuclear ophthalmoplegia
WEP	weekend pass
WESR	Westergren erythrocyte sedimentation rate
	Wintrobe erythrocyte sedimentation rate
WEUP	willful exposure to unwanted pregnancy
WF	well flexed
	wet film
	white female
W/F	weakness and fatigue
WFB	wooden foreign body
WFE	Williams flexion exercises

W

W FEEDS	with feedings		walk-in
WFH	white-faced hornet	W/I	within
WFI	water for injection	W+I	work and interest
WFL	within full limits	WIA	wounded in action
	within functional limits	WIC	Women, Infants, and
WFLC	white female living child		Children (program)
WFNS	World Federation of	WID	widow
	Neurosurgical Societies		widower
	(grade or scale)	WIED	walk-in emergency
WF-O	will follow in office		department
WFR	wheel-and-flare reaction	WIP	work in progess
WG	Wegener granulomatosis	WIQ	Walking Impairment
WGA	wheat germ agglutinin		Questionnaire
WH	walking heel (cast)	WIS	Ward Incapacity Scale
	well healed		Wister Institute
	well hydrated	WISC	Wechsler Intelligence
	work hardening (physical		Scale for Children
	therapy)	WISC-R	Wechsler Intelligence
WHA	warmed humidified air		Scale for Children-
WHAS	Women's Health		Revised
	Assessment Scale	WIT	water-induced
WHI	Women's Health Initiative		thermotherapy
WHIM	Worts, Hypogammaglobu-	WK	week
	linamia, Infections,		work
	and Myelokathexis	WKI	Wakefield Inventory
	(syndrome)	WKS	Wernicke-Korsakoff
WHIS	War Head-Injury Score		Syndrome
WHNR	well-healed, no residuals	WL	waiting list
WHNS	well-healed, no sequelae		wave length
	well-healed,		weight loss
	nonsymptomatic	WLE	wide local excision
WHO	World Health	WLM	working level months
	Organization	WLQ	Work Limitation
	wrist-hand orthosis		Questionnaire
WHOART	World Health	WLS	weight-loss surgery
	Organization Adverse		wet lung syndrome
	Reaction Terms	WLT	waterload test
	(Terminology)	WM	wall motion
WHOQOL-100	World Health		warm, moist
	Organization Quality of		wet mount
	Life 100-Item		white male
	(instrument)		white matter
WHP	whirlpool		whole milk
WHPB	whirlpool bath		working memory
WHR	ratio of waist to hip	WMA	wall motion abnormality
	circumference	WMD	warm moist dressings
WHV	woodchuck hepatitis virus		(sterile)
WHVP	wedged hepatic venous		weapons of mass
	pressure		destruction
WH/WD	withholding/withdrawal		weighted mean
	(of life support)		differences
WHZ	wheezes	WMF	white married female
WI	ventricular demand pacing	WMFT	Wolf Motor Function Test

W

WMI	wall motion index
	weighted mean index
WML	white matter lesions (cerebral)
WMLC	white male living child
WMM	white married male
WMP	warm moist packs (unsterile)
	weight management program
WMS	Wechsler Memory Scale
	Wilson-Mikity syndrome
WMT	Word Memory Test
WMX	whirlpool, massage, and exercise
WN	well nourished
WND	wound
WNE	West Nile encephalitis
WNF	well-nourished female
	West Nile fever
WNL	within normal limits
WNL x 4	upper and lower extremities within normal limits
WNLS	weighted nonlinear least squares
WNM	well-nourished male
WNR	within normal range
WNt^{50}	Wagner-Nelson time 50 hours
WNV	West Nile virus
WO	weeks old
	wide open
	written order
W/O	water-in-oil
	without
WOB	work of breathing
WOCF	worst observation carried forward
WOCN	Wound, Ostomy and Continence Nurses (Society)-formerly known as the International Association for Enterostomal Therapy (IEAT)
WOMAC	Western Ontario and McMaster Universities Osteoarthritis Index
WOP	without pain
W or A	weakness or atrophy
WORD	Wechsler objective reading dimensions
WORLD/ DLROW	a test used in mental status examinations (patient is asked to spell WORLD backwards)
WP	whirlpool
WPAI	Work Productivity and Activity Impairment (Questionnaire)
WPBT	whirlpool, body temperature
WPCs	washed packed cells
WPFM	Wright peak flow meter
WPOA	wearing patch on arrival
WPP	Wechsler Preschool and Primary Scale of Intelligence
WPPSI	Wechsler Preschool and Primary Scale of Intelligence
WPPSI-R	WPPSI revised
WPR	written progress report
WPS	Worker Protection Standard
WPV	within-person variability
WPW	Wolff-Parkinson-White (syndrome)
WR	Wassermann reaction
	wrist
WRA	with-the-rule astigmatism
WRAIR	Walter Reed Army Institute of Research
WRAMC	Walter Reed Army Medical Center
WRARU	Walter Reed AFRIMS (Armed Forces Research Institute of Medical Sciences) Research Unit
WRAT	Wide Range Achievement Test
WRAT-R	The Wide Range Achievement Test, Revised
WRBC	washed red blood cells
WRC	washed red (blood) cells
WRIOT	Wide Range Interest-Opinion Test (for career planning)
WRL	World Reference Laboratory for Foot-and-Mouth Disease (Institute for Animal Health, Survey, United Kingdom)

W

WRN	Werner syndrome protein	WWidF	white widowed female
WRT	weekly radiation therapy	WWidM	white widowed male
	with respect (regards) to	WWTP	wastewater treatment plant
WRUED	work-related upper-extremity disorder	WWW	World Wide Web
		WYOU	women years of usage
WS	walking speed		
	ward secretary		
	watt seconds		
	Werner syndrome		
	West syndrome		
	Williams syndrome		
	work simplification		
	work simulation		
	work status		
W&S	wound and skin		
WSCP	Williams Syndrome Cognitive Profile		
WSEP	Williams syndrome, early puberty		
WSepF	white separated female		
WSepM	white separated male		
WSF	white single female		
WSLP	Williams syndrome, late puberty		
WSM	white single male		
WSO	white superficial onychomycosis		
WSOC	water-soluble organic compounds		
WSP	wearable speech processor		
WSW	women who have sex with women		
WT	walking tank		
	walking training		
	weight (wt)		
	wild type		
	Wilms tumor		
	wisdom teeth		
0WT	zero work tolerance		
W-T-D	wet to dry		
WTP	willingness to pay		
WTS	whole tomography slice		
W/U	work-up		
WV	whispered voice		
W/V	weight-to-volume ratio		
WW	Weight Watchers		
	wheeled walker		
WWI	World War One		
WWII	World War Two		
W/W	weight-to-weight ratio		
W Ø W	wet-to-wet		
WWAC	walk with aid of cane		
WW Brd	whole wheat bread		

W

X

X	break
	capecitabine (Xeloda)
	(This is a dangerous abbreviation)
	cross
	crossmatch
	exophoria for distance
	Ecstasy (methylenedioxymethamphetamine; MDMA)
	extra
	female sex chromosome
	start of anesthesia
	ten
	times
	xylocaine
$\bar{x}$	except
	mean
X′	exophoria at 33 cm
X^2	chi-square
X+#	xyphoid plus number of fingerbreadths
X3	orientation as to time, place and person
X-ALD	X-linked adrenoleukodystrophy
XBT	xylose breath test
XC	excretory cystogram
XCF	aortic cross clamp off
XCO	aortic cross clamp on
XD	times daily
X&D	examination and diagnosis
X2d	times two days
XDP	xeroderma pigmentosum
Xe	xenon
^{133}Xe	xenon, isotope of mass 133
XeCl	xenon chloride
XeCT	xenon-enhanced computed tomography
X-ed	crossed
XEM	xonics electron mammography
XES	x-ray energy spectrometer
XFER	transfer

XFS	exfoliation syndrome
XGP	xanthogranulomatous pyelonephritis
XI	eleven
XII	twelve
XIP	x-ray in plaster
XKO	not knocked out
XL	extended release (once a day oral solid dosage form)
	extra large
	forty
XLA	X-linked infantile agammaglobulinemia
X-leg	cross leg
XLFDP	cross-linked fibrin degradation products
XLH	X-linked hypophosphatemia
XLJR	X-linked juvenile retinoschisis
XLMR	X-linked mental retardation
XLP	X-linked proliferative (syndrome)
XLRS	X-linked retinoschisis
XM	crossmatch
X-mat.	crossmatch
XMG	mammogram
XML	extensible markup language
XMM	xeromammography
XMR	magnetic resonance and X-rays
XMT	cross matched
XNA	xenoreactive natural antibodies
XOM	extraocular movements
XOP	x-ray out of plaster
XP	xeroderma pigmentosum
XR	x-ray
XRF	x-ray fluorescence
XRT	radiation therapy
XS	excessive
X-SCID	X-linked severe combined immunodeficiency disease
XS-LIM	exceeds limits of procedure
XT	exotropia
	extract
	extracted

X(T')	intermittent exotropia at 33 cm
X(T)	intermittent exotropia
XTLE	extratemporal-lobe epilepsy
XU	excretory urogram
XULN	times upper limit of normal
XV	fifteen
3X/WK	three times a week
XX	normal female sex chromosome type
	twenty
XX/XY	sex karyotypes
XXX	thirty
XY	normal male sex chromosome type
XYL	xylose
XYLO	lidocaine (Xylocaine)

Y

Y	male sex chromosome
	year
	yellow
YAC	yeast artificial chromosome
YACs	yeast artificial chromosomes
YACP	young adult chronic patient
YAG	yttrium aluminum garnet (laser)
YAS	youth action section (police)
Yb	ytterbium
YBOCS	Yale-Brown Obsessive-Compulsive Scale
Yel	yellow
YEPQ	Yale Eating Patterns Questionnaire
YF	yellow fever
YFH	yellow-faced hornet
YFI	yellow fever immunization
YHL	years of healthy life
YJV	yellow jacket venom
Y2K	year 2,000
YLC	youngest living child
YLD	years of life with disability
YLL	years of life lost
YMC	young male Caucasian
YMRS	Young Mania Rating Scale
Y/N	yes/no
YO	years old
YOB	year of birth
YOD	year of death
YORA	younger-onset rheumatoid arthritis
YPC	YAG (yttrium aluminum garnet) posterior capsulotomy
YPLL	years of potential life lost before age 65
yr	year
YSC	yolk sac carcinoma
YTD	year to date
YTDY	yesterday

Z

Z	impedance
	pyrazinamide [part of tuberculosis regimen, see RHZ(E/S)/HR]
ZAL	zaleplon (Sonata)
ZAP	zoster-associated pain
ZDV	zidovudine (Retrovir)
Z-E	Zollinger-Ellison (syndrome)
ZEEP	zero end-expiratory pressure
ZES	Zollinger-Ellison syndrome
Z-ESR	zeta erythrocyte sedimentation rate
ZIFT	zygote intrafallopian (tube) transfer
ZIG	zoster serum immune globulin
ZIP	zoster immune plasma
ZMC	zygomatic
	zygomatic maxillary compound (complex)
Zn	zinc
ZnO	zinc oxide
ZnOE	zinc oxide and eugenol
ZnPc	zinc phthalocyanine
ZnPP	zinc protoporphyrin
ZNS	zonisamide (Zonegran)
ZOI	zone of inhibition
ZOOM	Guarana
ZOT	zonula occludens toxin
ZPC	zero point of charge
	zopiclone
z-Plasty	surgical relaxation of contracture
ZPO	zinc peroxide
ZPP	zinc protoporphyrin
ZPT	zinc pyrithione
ZSB	zero stools since birth
ZSR	zeta sedimentation rate
ZSRDS	Zung Self-Rating Depression Scale

Z

Chapter 6

Symbols and Numbers

Symbols

↑	above		to and from
	alive		unchanging
	elevated	↓↓	flexor
	greater than		plantar response
	high		(Babinski)
	improved		testes descended
	increase		
	rising	↑↑	extensor
	up		extensor response
	upper		(positive Babinsky)
			testes undescended
↑g	increasing		
		‖	parallel
↓	dead		parallel bars
	decrease	√	check
	depressed		flexion
	diminished		
	down	√'d	checked
	falling		
	lower	√'ing	checking
	lowered		
	normal plantar	#	fracture
	reflex		number
	restricted		pound
			weight
↓g	decreasing		
		∴	therefore
→	causes to	∵	because
	greater than	Δ scan	delta scan (computed
	progressing		tomography scan)
	results in		
	showed	+	plus
	to the right		positive
	transfer to		present
←	less than	−	absent
	resulted from		minus
	to the left		negative
↔	same as	/	extend
	stable		extended

387

/	slash mark signifying per, and, over, as a blood pressure of 160 over 100, or with (this is a dangerous symbol as it is mistaken for a one)
±	either positive or negative
	no definite cause
	plus or minus
	very slight trace
∟	right lower quadrant
Γ	right upper quadrant
⌐	left upper quadrant
⌐	left lower quadrant
>	greater than (can be confused with <, use "greater than")
	left ear-bone conduction threshold
≥	greater than or equal to
<	caused by
	less than (can be confused with >, use "less than")
	right ear-bone conduction threshold
≤	less than or equal to
≮	not less than
≯	not more than
∨	above
	diastolic blood pressure
	increased
	below
	systolic blood pressure
≠	not equal to
≅	approximately equal to
=	equal
	equal to
′	feet
	minutes (as in 30′)
″	inches
	seconds
~	about
	approximately
	difference
≈	approximately equal to

≡	identical
×	left ear-air conduction threshold
	ten
]	left ear-masked bone conduction threshold
[	right ear-masked bone conduction
△	right ear-masked air conduction threshold
	change
○	threshold
	reversible
?	questionable
—	not tested
Ø	no
	none
	without
⊙	start of an operation
⊗	end of anesthesia
@	at
i̇	one
ii̇	two
♂	male
♀	female
♂♂	gay
♀♀	lesbian
■	deceased male
●	deceased female
□	living male
	left ear-masked air conduction threshold
○	living female
	respiration
	right ear-air conduction threshold
◇	sex unknown
(□)	adopted living male
*	birth
†	dead
	death
♀	standing
○—<	recumbent position
♀	sitting position
♥	heart

388

Numbers (Arabic and Roman)

1/2 and 1/2	half Dakin solution and half glycerin
1°	first degree primary
1:1	one-to-one (individual session with staff)
2°	second degree secondary
2×2	gauze dressing folded 2″×2″
222	aspirin, caffeine, and codeine (8 mg) tablets (Canada)
282	aspirin, caffeine, codeine, and meprobamate (Canada)
3°	tertiary third degree
3×	three times
4×4	gauze dressing folded 4″×4″
5+2	5 days of cytarabine and 2 days of daunorubicin leukemia therapy
642	propoxyphene tablets (Canada)
7+3	7 days of cytarabine and 3 days of daunorubicin leukemia therapy
Serial 7's	a mental status examination (starting with 100, count backward by 7's)
24°	twenty-four hours (24 hr is safer as the ° is seen as a zero)
777	Ortho Novum 777® (a triphasic oral contraceptive)
1500	Health Insurance Claim Form HCFA 1500
1,000	one thousand (1×10^3)
10,000	ten thousand (1×10^4)
100,000	one hundred thousand (1×10^5)
1,000,000	one million (1×10^6)
10,000,000	ten million (1×10^7)
100,000,000	one hundred million (1×10^8)
1,000,000,000	one billion (1×10^9)
i	one (Roman numerals are dangerous expressions and should not be used because they are not universally understood)
ii	two
iii	three
iiii	four
iv	four (this is a dangerous abbreviation as it is read as intravenous, use 4)
v	five
vi	six
vii	seven
viii	eight
ix	nine
x	ten
xi	eleven
xii	twelve
XL	forty extended release dosage form

Greek Letters

A α	alpha
β B	beta
Γ γ	gamma
Δ δ	anion gap change delta delta gap prism diopter temperature trimester
E ε	epsilon
Z ζ	zeta
H η	eta
Θ θ	negative theta
I ι	iota
K κ	kappa
Λ λ	lambda

389

M μ	micro
	mu
N ν	nu
Ξ ξ	xi
O o	omicron
Π π	pi
P ρ	rho
Σ σ	sigma
	sum of
	summary
T τ	tau
Y υ	upsilon

Φ φ	phenyl
	phi
	thyroid
X χ	chi
Ψ ψ	psi
	psychiatric
Ω ω	omega

Miscellaneous

liver, kidneys, and spleen negative, no masses, or tenderness

Chapter 7

Tables and Lists

Numbers and letters for teeth

Two adult numbering systems and a deciduous system are shown. The adult systems are shown as numbers, whereas deciduous teeth are lettered. The system commonly used in the U.S. is 1 to 32 (shown in bold face type).

1 (18)   upper right 3rd molar
2 (17) (A)   upper right 2nd molar
3 (16) (B)   upper right 1st molar
4 (15)   upper right 2nd bicuspid
5 (14)   upper right 1st bicuspid
6 (13) (C)   upper right canine (eyetooth)
7 (12) (D)   upper right lateral incisor
8 (11) (E)   upper right central incisor
9 (21) (F)   upper left central incisor
10 (22) (G)   upper left lateral incisor
11 (23) (H)   upper left canine
12 (24)   upper left 1st bicuspid
13 (25)   upper left 2nd bicuspid
14 (26) (I)   upper left 1st molar
15 (27) (J)   upper left 2nd molar
16 (28)   upper left 3rd molar

17 (38)   lower left 3rd molar
18 (37) (K)   lower left 2nd molar
19 (36) (L)   lower left 1st molar
20 (35)   lower left 2nd bicuspid
21 (34)   lower left 1st bicuspid
22 (33) (M)   lower left canine
23 (32) (N)   lower left lateral incisor
24 (31) (O)   lower left central incisor
25 (41) (P)   lower right central incisor
26 (42) (Q)   lower right lateral incisor
27 (43) (R)   lower right canine
28 (44)   lower right 1st bicuspid
29 (45)   lower right 2nd bicuspid
30 (46) (S)   lower right 1st molar
31 (47) (T)   lower right 2nd molar
32 (48)   lower right 3rd molar

UPPER																	UPPER
	1	**2**	**3**	**4**	**5**	**6**	**7**	**8**	**9**	**10**	**11**	**12**	**13**	**14**	**15**	**16**	
	18	17	16	15	14	13	12	11	21	22	23	24	25	26	27	28	
Right	A	B			C	D	E	F	G	H			I	J			**Left**
	T	S			R	Q	P	O	N	M			L	K			
	48	47	46	45	44	43	42	41	31	32	33	34	35	36	37	38	
	32	**31**	**30**	**29**	**28**	**27**	**26**	**25**	**24**	**23**	**22**	**21**	**20**	**19**	**18**	**17**	
LOWER																	LOWER

Laboratory Test Panels*

	Cl CO₂ K Na	BUN Ca Creat Gluc	Alb Alk P AST(SGOT) ALT(SGPT) T Bili TP	ANA ESR RF Ur Ac	Calc LDL HDL T Chol Trig VLDL	Alb Phos	HAAb, IgM Ab HbcAb, IgM Ab HbsAG HCAb
Lytes (electrolyte panel)	X						
BMP (basic metabolic panel) or MBP, MPB	X	X					
CMP (comprehensive metabolic panel)	X	X	X				
HFP (hepatic function panel)			X plus D Bili				
AP (arthritis panel)				X			
LP (lipid Panel)					X		
RFP (renal function panel)	X	X				X	
AHP (acute hepatitis panel)							X

*These can vary from institution to institution and from year to year

Abbreviation Key

Ab-antibody
Alb-albumin
Alk P-alkaline phosphate
ALT (SGPT)-alanine aminotransferase
  (serum glutamate pyruvate)
ANA-antinuclear antibody
AST (SGOT)-aspartate-aminotransferase
  (serum glutamate oxaloacetic transaminase)
BUN-blood urea nitrogen
Ca-calcium
Calc LDL-calculated low-density lipoprotein
LDL-low density lipoprotein

Cl-chloride
CO₂-carbon dioxide
Creat-creatinine
D Bili-direct bilirubin
ESR-erythrocyte sedimentation rate
Gluc-glucose
HAAb-hepatitis A antibody
HBcAb-hepatitis B core antibody
HBsAg-hepatitis B surface antigen
HCAb-hepatitis C antibody
HDL-high-density lipoprotein

IgM-immunoglobulin M
K-potassium
Na-sodium
Phos-phosphate
RF-rheumatoid factor
T Bili-total bilirubin
T Chol-total cholesterol
TP-total protein
Trig-triglycerides
Ur Ac-uric acid
VLDl-very low-density lipoprotein

See text for meaning of the abbreviations shown

Complete Blood Count

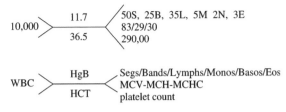

$$10,000 \diagdown \begin{array}{c} 11.7 \\ 36.5 \end{array} \diagup \begin{array}{l} \text{50S, 25B, 35L, 5M 2N, 3E} \\ \text{83/29/30} \\ \text{290,00} \end{array}$$

$$\text{WBC} \diagdown \begin{array}{c} \text{HgB} \\ \text{HCT} \end{array} \diagup \begin{array}{l} \text{Segs/Bands/Lymphs/Monos/Basos/Eos} \\ \text{MCV-MCH-MCHC} \\ \text{platelet count} \end{array}$$

Electrolyte Panel

142	99	sodium	chloride
4.7	25	potassium	carbon dioxide

Blood Gases

7.4/80/48/98/25 $pH/PO_2/PCO_2/\% \ O_2$ saturation/bicarbonate

Obstetrical shorthand

$$\frac{2 \ cm | 80\%}{-2 \ Vtx} \qquad 2 \ cm = \text{dilation of cervix}$$

80% = degree of cer-   Vtx = vertex; presen-
    vix effacement   tation of fetus,
                               (breech = Br)

−2 = station; distance
    above (−) or
    below (+) the
    spine of the ischium measured in cm

Reflexes

Reflexes are usually graded on a 0 to 4+ scale. The designations +, ++, +++, and ++++ should not be used.

4+   may indicate disease
      often associated with clonus
      very brisk, hyperactive
3+   brisker than average
      possibly but not necessarily indicative of disease
2+   average
      normal
1+   low normal
      somewhat diminished
0   may indicate neuropathy
      no response

Muscle strength[1]

0—No muscular contraction detected
1—A barely detectable flicker or trace of contraction
2—Active movement of the body part with gravity eliminated
3—Active movement against gravity
4—Active movement against gravity and some resistance
5—Active movement against full resistance without evident fatigue. This is
      normal muscle strength

Pulse[1]

0   completely absent
+1   markedly impaired (or 1+)
+2   modereately impaired (or 2+)
+3   slightly impaired (or 3+)
+4   normal (or 4+)

Gradation of intensity of heart murmurs[1]

1/6 or I/VI	may not be heard in all positions very faint, heard only after the listener has "tuned in"
2/6 or II/VI	quiet, but heard immediately upon placing the stethoscope on the chest
3/6 or III/VI	moderately loud
4/6 or IV/VI	loud
5/6 or V/VI	very loud, may be heard with a stethoscope partly off the chest (thrills are associated)
6/6 or VI/VI	may be heard with the stethoscope entirely off the chest (thrills are associated)

Tonsil Size

0   no tonsils
1   less than normal
2   normal
3   greater than normal
4   touching

Metric Prefixes and Symbols

Prefix	Symbol	
tera-	T	1,000,000,000,000 or (10^{12}) one trillion
giga-	G	1,000,000,000 or (10^9) one billion
mega-	M	1,000,000 or (10^6) one million
kilo-	k	1,000 or (10^3) one thousand
hecto-	h	100 or (10^2) one hundred
deka-	da	10 or (10^1) ten
deci-	d	0.1 or (10^{-1}) one-tenth
centi-	c	0.01 or (10^{-2}) one-hundredth
milli-	m	0.001 or (10^{-3}) one-thousandth
micro-	μ	0.000,001 or (10^{-6}) one-millionth
nano-	n	0.000,000,001 or (10^{-9}) one-billionth
pico-	p	0.000,000,000,000,001 or (10^{-12}) one-trillionth
femto-	f	0.000,000,000,000,001 or (10^{-15}) one-quadrillionth
atto-	a	0.000,000,000,000,000,001 or (10^{-18}) one-quintillionth

Apothecary symbols (Should never be used)

The symbols presented below are for informational use. The apothecary system should *not* be used. Only the metric system should be used. The methods of expressing the symbols, the meanings, and the equivalence are not the classic ones, nor are they accurate, but reflect the usual intended meanings when used by some older physicians in writing prescription directions.

Symbol	Meaning	Symbol	Meaning
ʒ or ʒ ī	dram, teaspoonful, (5 mL)	℥ or ℥ ī	ounce, (30 mL)
		gr	grain (approximately 60 mg)
ʒ ī ī	two drams, 2 teaspoonfuls, (10 mL)	♏	minim (approximately 0.06 mL)
℥ s̄s̄	half ounce, tablespoonful, (15 mL)	gtt	drop

Reference
1. Adopted from Bates B. Bates' guide to physical examinations and history taking, 8th ed. Philadelphia: Lippincott Williams and Wilkins; 2003.

\#

PDA Versions are Available

See pricing and ordering information in the pricing section on page 461.

Multi-User Site Licenses are Available

Medical facilities can substitute their own "Do Not Use" list of dangerous abbreviations for the one present. This list would be controlled by the facility. Demonstrations and pricing information are available by calling 1 888 333 1862 or 1 215 442 7430 or via an e-mail request to ev@neilmdavis.com

Additions, Corrections, and Suggestions are Welcomed

Please send them via any means shown below:

Neil M Davis
2049 Stout Drive, B-3
Warminster PA 18974-3861

FAX 1 888 333 4915 or 1 215 442 7432
Email med@neilmdavis.com
Web site www.medabbrev.com

Thank you for your help in the past.

Have You Used the Web-Version of This Book?

- It is instantaneously searchable for the meanings of abbreviations
- It is reverse searchable (search for all the abbreviations containing a particular word)
- Each month, about 80 new entries are added

See the preface (page vii) for access instructions. A two-year, single-user access is included in the purchase price of the book.

Chapter 8

Cross-Referenced List of Generic and Brand Drug Names

L isted below is a cross-referenced index of generic and brand drug names. Generic names begin with a lower case letter while brand names begin with a capital letter. This partial list consists of frequently prescribed and new drugs.

The meanings of abbreviated and coded drug names can be found in Chapter 5 (Lettered Abbreviations and Acronyms).

Complete indices of United States drug names can be found in current editions of Drug Facts and Comparisons[1] and the American Drug Index[2]. A complete list of world-wide names may be found in Martindales.[3] These and other references should be used to determine the equivalence of products, strengths, and dosage forms. Although several products may be listed under one generic name they may differ in strength, dosage form, or concentration available, as is the case with estradiol transdermal (Climara, Estraderm, and Vivelle).

Some products are marketed without a brand name, as in the case of thioguanine. In such cases only the generic name is listed. When a product is often prescribed and/or labeled generically, the generic name is shown in italics.

The following abbreviations are used in this listing:

EC	enteric coated	SR	sustained release tablets or capsules (and other forms of extended release)
HCl	hydrochloride		
IM	intramuscular		
IV	intravenous	susp	suspension
inj	injection	(W)	withdrawn or discontinued from US market
oint	ointment		
ophth	ophthalmic	(WA)	withdrawn or discontinued from US market but available under different name from another manufacturer
soln	solution		

A

abacavir sulfate	Ziagen
abarelix	Plenaxis
Abbokinase	urokinase
abciximab	ReoPro
Abelcet	amphotericin B lipid complex
Abilify	aripiprazole
acamprosate calcium	Campral
acarbose	Precose
Accolate	zafirlukast
AccuNeb	albuterol inhalation soln
Accupril	quinapril HCl
Accuretic	quinapril; hydrochlorothiazide
Accutane	isotretinoin
Accuzyme	papain; urea oint
acebutolol HCl	Sectral
Aceon	perindopril erbumine
acetaminophen	paracetamol Tylenol
acetaminophen 300 mg with Codeine Phosphate (15, 30, and 60 mg)	Phenaphen with Codeine (#2, 3, and 4) (WA) Tylenol with Codeine (#2, 3, and 4)
acetazolamide	Diamox
acetohexamide	Dymelor
acetohydroxamic acid	Lithostat
acetylcholine ophth	Miochol E
acetylcysteine	Mucomyst
Achromycin (WA)	tetracycline HCl
Aciphex	rabeprazole sodium
acitretin	Soriatane
Acora	argatroban
Acthar	corticotropin
ActHIB/Tripedia	*Haemophilus b* conjugate vaccine reconstituted with

	diphtheria and tetanus toxoids and acellular pertussis vaccine adsorbed
Acthrel	corticorellin ovine triflutate
Actifed	triprolidine HCl; pseudoephedrine HCl
Actigall	ursodiol
Actimmune	interferon gamma 1-b
Actiq	fentanyl oral transmucosal
Activase	alteplase, recombinant
Activella (WA)	norethindrone acetate; estradiol
Actonel	risedronate sodium
Actos	pioglitazone HCl
Acular	ketorolac tromethamine ophth
acyclovir	Zovirax
Adalat	nifedipine
Adalat CC	nifedipine SR
adalimumab	Humira
adapalene	Differin
Adapin	doxepin HCl
Adderall	amphetamine; dextroamphetamine mixed salts
adefovir dipivoxil	Hepsera Preveon
Adenocard	adenosine
adenosine	Adenocard
Adrenalin	epinephrine
Adriamycin	doxorubicin HCl
Advair Diskus	fluticasone propionate; salmeterol inhalation powder
Advicor	lovastatin; niacin
Advil	ibuprofen
AeroBid	flunisolide
Afrin nasal spray	oxymetazoline HCl
agalsidase beta	Fabrazyme

Agenerase	amprenavir
Aggrastat	tirofiban HCl
Aggrenox	aspirin; extended-release dipyridamole
Agrylin	anagrelide HCl
Akineton	biperiden
Alamast	pemirolast potassium ophth soln
alatrofloxacin mesylate IV	Trovan inj
albendazole	Albenza
Albenza	albendazole
albumin human	Albuminar Albutein Buminate Plasbumin
albumin (human), sonicated	Albunex
Albuminar	albumin human
Albunex	albumin (human), sonicated
Albutein	albumin human
albuterol	AccuNeb Proventil salbutamol Ventolin
albuterol SR	Proventil Repetabs Volmax
albuterol sulfate inhalation aerosol	Proventil HFA
Aldactazide	spironolactone; hydrochloro-thiazide
Aldactone	spironolactone
Aldara	imiquimod cream
aldesleukin	Proleukin
Aldomet	methyldopa
Aldoril	methyldopa; hydrochloro-thiazide
Aldurazyme	laronidase
alefacept	Amevive
alemtuzumab	Campath
alendronate sodium	Fosamax
Alesse	levonorgestrel; ethinyl estradiol
Alfenta	alfentanil HCl
alfentanil HCl	Alfenta
alfuzosin	UroXatral
alglucerase	Ceredase
Alimta	pemetrexed disodium
alitretinoin	Panretin
Allegra	fexofenadine HCl
Alinia	nitazoxanide
Alkeran	melphalan
allopurinol	Zyloprim
almotriptan malate	Axert
Alocril	nedocromil ophth soln
Alomide	lodoxamide tromethamine ophth soln
Alora	estradiol transdermal
alosetron	Lotronex
Aloxi	palonosetron HCl
Alphagan	brimonidine tartrate ophth
alpha$_1$-proteinase inhibitor (human)	Prolastin
alprazolam	Xanax
alprostadil	Caverject Edex Prostin VR
alprostadil urethral suppository	Muse
Alrex	loteprednol etabonate ophth susp
Altace	ramipril
alteplase, recombinant	Activase
alteplase (for catheter occlusions)	Cathflo Activase
altretamine	Hexalen
aluminum acetate	Domeboro
aluminum carbonate	Basaljel
aluminum hydroxide	Amphojel
aluminum hydroxide; magnesium hydroxide	Maalox

Alupent	metaproterenol sulfate	amlodipine besylate; atorvastatin calcium	Caduet
Alustra	hydroquinone topical susp		
amantadine HCl	Symmetrel	amlodipine besylate; benazepril HCl	Lotrel
Amaryl	glimepiride		
Ambien	zolpidem tartrate		
AmBisome	liposomal amphotericin B	ammonium lactate lotion	AmLactin
amcinonide	Cyclocort	amobarbital sodium	Amytal
Amerge	naratriptan HCl		
Amevive	alefacept	amoxapine	Asendin
Amicar	aminocaproic acid	*amoxicillin*	Amoxil
Amidate	etomidate		Trimox
amifostine	Ethyol		Wymox
amikacin sulfate	Amikin	amoxicillin; clavulanic acid	Augmentin
Amikin	amikacin sulfate		
amiloride HCl	Midamor	amoxicillin; clavulanate potassium SR	Augmentin XR
amiloride; hydro-chlorothiazide	Moduretic		
amino acid inj	Aminosyn Travasol TrophAmine	Amoxil	amoxicillin
		amphetamine resins (W)	Biphetamine (W)
amino acid with electrolytes in dextrose with calcium inj (various concentrations)	Clinimix E	amphetamine; dextroamphet-amine mixed salts	Adderall
		Amphojel	aluminum hydroxide
aminocaproic acid	Amicar	Amphotec	amphotericin B cholesteryl sulfate
aminocaproic acid gel	Caprogel	amphotericin B	Fungizone
aminogluteth-imide	Cytadren	amphotericin B cholesteryl sulfate	Amphotec
aminolevulinic acid HCl topical soln	Levulan Kerastick		
		amphotericin B lipid complex	Abelcet
aminophylline	aminophylline	*ampicillin*	Principen
aminosalicylic acid	Paser	ampicillin sodium; sulbactam sodium	Unasyn
Aminosyn	amino acid inj		
amiodarone HCl	Cordarone	amprenavir	Agenerase
amitriptyline HCl	Elavil Endep	amrinone (former name)	inamrinone (new name)
AmLactin	ammonium lactate lotion	amsacrine	Amsidyl
		Amsidyl	amsacrine
amlexanox oral paste	Aphthasol	Amvisc	sodium hyaluronate
amlodipine besylate	Norvasc		

Amytal	amobarbital sodium
Anadrol-50	oxymetholone
Anafranil	clomipramine HCl
anagrelide HCl	Agrylin
anakinra	Kineret
Anaprox	naproxen sodium
anastrozole	Arimidex
Anbesol	benzocaine
Ancef	cefazolin sodium
Ancobon	flucytosine
Androderm	testosterone transdermal system
AndroGel	testosterone gel
Androgel-DHT	dihydro-testosterone transdermal
Anectine	succinylcholine chloride
Anexsia	hydrocodone bitartrate; acetaminophen
Angiomax	bivalirudin
Ansaid	flurbiprofen
Antabuse	disulfiram
Antagon	ganirelix acetate
antihemophilic factor (recombinant)	Kogenate ReFacto
Antilirium	physostigmine salicylate
antipyrine otic	Auralgan
antithrombin III (human)	Thrombate III
antithymocyte globulin, (rabbit)	Thymoglobulin
Antivert	meclizine
Antizol	fomepizole
Anturane	sulfinpyrazone
Anzemet	dolasetron mesylate
Aphthasol	amlexanox oral paste
Apidra	insulin glulisine [rDNA origin]
A.P.L.	chorionic gonadotropin
apligraf	Graftskin
Aplisol	tuberculin skin test
Apokyn	apomorphine HCl inj
apomorphine HCl	Uprima
apomorphine HCl inj	Apokyn
Aposyn	exisulind
aprepitant	Emend
Apresazide	hydralazine HCl; hydrochloro-thiazide
Apresoline	hydralazine HCl
aprotinin	Trasylol
AquaMEPHY-TON	phytonadione
Aralen	chloroquine phosphate
Aramine	metaraminol bitartrate
Aranesp	darbepoetin
Arava	leflunomide
arbutamine HCl	GenEsa
arcitumomab	CEA-Scan
ardeparin sodium (W)	Normiflo (W)
Arduan	pipecuronium bromide
Aredia	pamidronate disodium
Arestin	minocycline HCl dental microspheres
Arfonad (W)	trimethaphan camsylate (W)
argatroban	argatroban
arginine HCl	R-Gene
Aricept	donepezil HCl
Arimidex	anastrozole
aripiprazole	Abilify
Aristocort	triamcinolone acetonide
Arixtra	fondaparinux sodium
Aromasin	exemestane
arsenic trioxide	Trisenox
Artane (W)	trihexyphenidyl HCl (W)
Arthrotec	diclofenac; misoprostol
Asacol	mesalamine
Asendin	amoxapine
Aslera	prasterone
asparaginase	Elspar

aspirin 325 mg with codeine phosphate (30 and 60 mg)	Empirin with codeine #3 and #4	Aurolate	gold sodium thiomalate
aspirin buffered	Bufferin	aurothioglucose	Solganal
aspirin EC	Ecotrin	Avalide	irbesartan; hydro-chlorothiazide
Astelin	azelastine HCl nasal spray	Avandamet	rosiglitazone maleate; metformin HCl
astemizole (W)	Hismanal (W)		
Atacand	candesartan cilexetil	Avandia	Rosiglitazone maleate
Atarax	hydroxyzine HCl	Avanir	docosanol cream
atazanavir sulfate	Reyataz	Avapro	irbesartan
		Avastin	bevacizumab
atenolol	Tenormin	Avelox	moxifloxacin HCl
atenolol; chlorthalidone	Tenoretic	Aventyl	nortriptyline HCl
		Avinza	morphine sulfate tab SR
Atgam	lymphocyte imimmune globulin	Avita	tretinoin cream 0.025%
articaine; epinephrine	Septocaine	Avitene	collagen hemostat
		Avodart	dutasteride
aspirin; extended-release dipyridamole	Aggrenox	Avonex	interferon beta-la
		Axert	almotriptan malate
		Axid	nizatidine
Atacand HCT	candesartan cilexetil; hydrochloro-thiazide	azacitidine	Vidaza
		Azactam	aztreonam
		azatadine maleate	Optimine
		azathioprine	Imuran
Ativan	lorazepam	azelaic acid cream	Azelex
Atomoxetine HCl	Strattera		Finevin
atorvastatin calcium	Lipitor	azelastine HCl nasal spray	Astelin
atovaquone	Mepron	azelastine HCl ophth soln	Optivar
atovaquone; proguanil HCl	Malarone		
		Azelex	azelaic acid cream
atracurium besylate	Tracrium	azithromycin	Zithromax
		Azmacort	triamcinolone acetonide aerosol
Atridox	doxycycline hyclate gel		
Atromid-S	clofibrate	Azopt	brinzolamide ophth susp
atropine sulfate tablets	Sal-Tropine		
		aztreonam	Azactam
Atrovent	ipratropium bromide	Azulfidine	sulfasalazine
Augmentin	amoxicillin; clavulanic acid		
Augmentin XR	amoxicillin; clavulanate potassium SR	**B**	
		Baciguent	bacitracin ointment
Auralgan	antipyrine otic	bacitracin ointment	Baciguent
auranofin	Ridaura		

baclofen	Lioresal	benzocaine	Anbesol
Bactrim	sulfamethoxa-zole; trimeth-oprim		Hurricaine
			Orabase
			Orajel
Bactroban	mupirocin nasal ointment	benzocaine; tetracaine HCl	Cetacaine
BAL in Oil	dimercaprol	benztropine mesylate	Cogentin
Basaljel	aluminum carbonate	bepridil (W)	Vascor (W)
balsalazide disodium	Colazal	beractant	Survanta
		Berroca	vitamin B complex; folic acid; vitamin C
basiliximab	Simulect		
Baycol (W)	cerivastatin sodium (W)		
		Betadine	povidone iodine
BCG intravesical	Pacis TheraCys TICE BCG	17β-estradiol; norgestimate	Ortho-Prefest
becaplermin gel	Regranex	Betagan	levobunolol HCl
beclomethasone dipropionate	Beclovent		
	Beconase AQ Nasal	betaine anhydrous	Cystadane
	Qvar	betamethasone	Celestone
	Vancenase	betamethasone dipropionate	Diprosone
	Vancenase AQ Nasal		
	Vanceril	betamethasone; clotrimazole cream	Lotrisone
Beclovent	beclomethasone dipropionate		
Beconase AQ Nasal	beclomethasone dipropionate	betamethasone valerate (foam)	Luxiq
belladonna alkaloids; phenobarbital	Donnatal (W)	Betapace	sotalol
		Betaseron	interferon beta-1b
		betaxolol	Kerlone
Bellergal-S	phenobarbital; ergotamine; belladonna	betaxolol HCl ophth soln	Betoptic
Benadryl	diphenhydramine HCl	betaxolol HCl ophth susp	Betoptic S
benazepril HCl	Lotensin	betaxolol HCl; pilocarpine HCl ophth soln	Betoptic Pilo
BeneFix	factor IX, (recombinant)		
Benemid	probenecid	bethanechol chloride	Urecholine
Benicar	olmesartan medoxomil	Betoptic	betaxolol HCl ophth soln
Benicar HCT	olmesartan medoxomil; hydrochloro-thiazide	Betoptic Pilo	betaxolol HCl; pilocarpine HCl, ophth soln
bentoquatam	IvyBlock	Betoptic S	betaxolol HCl ophth suspension
Bentyl	dicyclomine HCl		
Benzamycin	erythromycin; benzoyl peroxide topical gel	bevacizumab	Avastin
		bexarotene gel	Targretin
		Bextra	valdecoxib

Bexxar	tositumomab and I-131 tositumomab	Bravelle	urofollitropin
		Brethaire	terbutaline sulfate aerosol
Biaxin	clarithromycin	Brethine	terbutaline sulfate tablets and inj
Biaxin XL	clarithromycin SR		
bicalutamide	Casodex		
Bicillin C-R	penicillin G benzathine; penicillin G procaine (for IM use only)	bretylium tosylate	Bretylol
		Bretylol	bretylium tosylate
		Brevibloc	esmolol HCl
Bicillin L-A	penicillin G benzathine (for IM use only)	Brevital Sodium	methohexital sodium
		Bricanyl	terbutaline sulfate tablets and inj
Bicitra	sodium citrate; citric acid	brimonidine tartrate ophth	Alphagan
BiCNU	carmustine		
Bilopaque	tyropanoate sodium	brinzolamide ophth suspension	Azopt
bimatoprost ophth soln	Lumigan		
		bromocriptine mesylate	Parlodel
biperiden	Akineton		
Biphetamine (W)	amphetamine resins (W)	brompheniramine maleate	Dimetane
bisacodyl	Dulcolax	brompheniramine maleate; phenylpropan- olamime	Dimetapp Extentabs
bismuth subsalicylate; metronidazole; tetracycline HCl	Helidac		
		Bronkometer	isoetharine HCl aerosol
bisoprolol fumarate; hydrochlorothi- azide	Ziac	Bronkosol	isoetharine HCl soln
		Bucladin-S	buclizine HCl
		buclizine HCl	Bucladin-S
bitolterol mesylate	Tornalate	budesonide capsule SR	Entocort EC
bivalirudin	Angiomax	budesonide inhalation powder	Pulmicort Turbuhaler
Blenoxane	bleomycin sulfate		
bleomycin sulfate	Blenoxane	budesonide nasal inhaler	Rhinocort
Blocadren	timolol maleate		
Boniva	ibandronate	Bufferin	aspirin buffered
bortezomib	Velcade	bumetanide	Bumex
bosentan	Tracleer	Bumex	bumetanide
B & O Supprettes	opium; belladonna suppositories	Buminate	albumin human
		Buphenyl	phenylbutyrate sodium
Botox	botulinum toxin type A	bupivacaine HCl	Marcaine HCl
		buprenorphine HCl	Subutex
botulinum toxin type A	Botox		
botulinum toxin type B	Myobloc	buprenorphine HCl; naloxone HCl	Suboxone

bupropion HCl	Wellbutrin
bupropion HCl SR	Wellbutrin SR
	Zyban
BuSpar	buspirone HCl
buspirone HCl	BuSpar
busulfan	Myleran
busulfan inj	Busulfex
Busulfex	busulfan inj
butabarbital sodium	Butisol
butalbital; acetaminophen; caffeine	Fioricet
butalbital; aspirin; caffeine	Fiorinal
butenafine HCl	Mentax
Butisol	butabarbital sodium
butoconazole nitrate vaginal cream	Gynazole
butorphanol tartrate inj	Stadol
butorphanol tartrate nasal spray	Stadol NS

C

cabergoline	Dostinex
Caduet	amlodipine besylate; atorvastatin calcium
Cafcit	caffeine citrate inj
Cafergot	ergotaminetartrate; caffeine
caffeine citrate inj	Cafcit
Calan SR	verapamil HCl SR
Calciferol	ergocalciferol
Calcimar	calcitonin
calcipotriene cream	Dovonex
calcitonin	Calcimar

calcitonin-salmon	Miacalcin
calcitriol	Rocaltrol
calcium carbonate	Os-Cal 500 Tums
calcium carbonate; vitamin D and K chewable	Viactiv
calfactant intratracheal susp	Infasurf
Campath	alemtuzumab
camphorated tincture of opium	paregoric
Campral	acamprosate calcium
Camptosar	irinotecan HCl
candesartan cilexetil	Atacand
candesartan cilexetil; hydrochlorothiazide	Atacand HCT
Cancidas	caspofungin acetate
Capastat Sulfate	capreomycin sulfate
capecitabine	Xeloda
Capital w/ Codeine Suspension	codeine phosphate; acetaminophen suspension
Capitrol	chloroxine
Capoten	captopril
capreomycin sulfate	Capastat Sulfate
Caprogel	aminocaproic acid gel
capromab pendetide	ProstaScint
captopril	Capoten
Carafate	sucralfate
carbachol	Isopto Carbachol
carbamazepine	Tegretol
carbamazepine SR	Carbatrol Tegretol-XR
carbamide peroxide otic	Debrox
Carbatrol	carbamazepine SR
carbenicillin	Geocillin

Carbex	selegiline	Cefizox	ceftizoxime sodium
Carbocaine	mepivacaine HCl	Cefobid	cefoperazone sodium
carboplatin	Paraplatin	cefonicid sodium (W)	Monocid (W)
Cardene	nicardipine HCl	cefoperazone sodium	Cefobid
Cardiolite	technetium Tc99m sestamibi	Cefotan	cefotetan
		cefotaxime sodium	Claforan
Cardiotec	technetium Tc-99m teboroxime kit	cefotetan	Cefotan
		cefoxitin sodium	Mefoxin
Cardizem	diltiazem HCl	cefpodoxime proxetil	Vantin
Cardizem CD	diltiazem HCl SR	cefprozil	Cefzil
Cardura	doxazosin mesylate	ceftazidime	Ceptaz
			Fortaz
carisoprodol	Soma		Tazicef
carmustine	BiCNU		Tazidime
carmustine implantable wafer	Gliadel	ceftibuten	Cedax
		Ceftin	cefuroxime axetil
Carnitor	levocarnitine		
Cartia XR	diltiazem HCl SR	ceftizoxime sodium	Cefizox
carvedilol	Coreg	ceftriaxone sodium	Rocephin
Casodex	bicalutamide		
caspofungin acetate	Cancidas	cefuroxime axetil	Ceftin
Cataflam	diclofenac potassium	cefuroxime sodium	Kefurox
			Zinacef
Catapres	clonidine HCl	Cefzil	cefprozil
Cathflo Activase	alteplase (for catheter occlusions)	Celebrex	celecoxib
		celecoxib	Celebrex
		Celestone	betamethasone
Caverject	alprostadil	Celexa	citalopram hydrobromide
CEA-SCAN	arcitumomab		
Ceclor	cefaclor	CellCept	mycophenolate mofetil
Cedax	ceftibuten		
CeeNu	lomustine	Cenestin	synthetic conjugated estrogens, A
cefaclor	Ceclor		
cefadroxil	Duricef		
Cefadyl (W)	cephapirin sodium	Centrum	vitamins; minerals
		cephalexin	Keflex
cefamandole nafate	Mandol	cephalexin HCl	Keftab
cefazolin sodium	Ancef Kefzol (WA)	cephalothin sodium (W)	Keflin (W)
cefdinir	Omnicef	cephapirin sodium (W)	Cefadyl (W)
cefditoren pivoxil	Spectracef	cephradine	Velosef
cefepime HCl	Maxipime	Cephulac	lactulose
cefixime (W)	Suprax (W)	Ceptaz	ceftazidime

406

Cerebyx	fosphenytoin sodium
Ceredase	alglucerase
Cerezyme	imiglucerase
cerivastatin sodium (W)	Baycol (W)
Cernevit-12	multivitamins for infusion
Cerubidine	daunorubicin HCl
Cervidil	dinoprostone vaginal insert
Cetacaine	benzocaine; tetracaine HCl
cetirizine HCl	Zyrtec
cetirizine HCL; pseudoephedrine HCl SR	Zyrtec-D
cetrorelix	Cetrotide
Cetrotide	cetrorelix
cetuximab	Erbitux
cevimeline HCl	Evoxac
Chirocaine	levobupivacaine
chloral hydrate	chloral hydrate
chlorambucil	Leukeran
chloramphenicol	Chloromycetin
chloramphenicol ophth	Chloroptic ophth
chlordiazepoxide HCl	Librium
chlordiazepoxide HCl; amitriptyline HCl	Limbitrol
chlorhexidine gluconate	Hibiclens PerioChip
chlorhexidine gluconate mouth rinse	Peridex
Chloromycetin	chloramphenicol
chloroprocaine HCl	Nesacaine
Chloroptic ophth	chloramphenicol ophth
chloroquine phosphate	Aralen
chlorothiazide	Diuril
chloroxine	Capitrol
chlorpheniramine maleate	Chlor-Trimeton
chlorpheniramine maleate SR	Teldrin
chlorpromazine	Thorazine
chlorpropamide	Diabinese

chlorthalidone	Hygroton
chlorthalidone; reserpine	Regroton
Chlor-Trimeton	chlorpheniramine maleate
chlorzoxazone 250 mg	Paraflex
chlorzoxazone 500 mg	Parafon Forte DSC
Cholebrine	iocetamic acid
Choledyl	oxtriphylline
cholestyramine	Questran
choline chloride inj	Intrachol
choline magnesium trisalicylate	Trilisate
Choloxin (W)	dextrothyroxine sodium (W)
chorionic gonadotropin	A.P.L.
choriogona- dotropin alfa	Ovidrel
Chronulac	lactulose
Chymodiactin	chymopapain
chymopapain	Chymodiactin
Cialis	tadalafil
Cibalith-S	lithium citrate
ciclopirox cream and lotion	Loprox
ciclopirox soln	Penlac Nail Lacquer
cidofovir	Vistide
cilostazol	Pletal
Ciloxan	ciprofloxacin ophth soln
cimetidine HCl	Tagamet
cinacalcet HCl	Sensipar
Cipro	ciprofloxacin HCl
ciprofloxacin HCl	Cipro
ciprofloxacin; hydrocortisone otic	Cipro HC Otic
ciprofloxacin ophth soln	Ciloxan
Cipro HC Otic	ciprofloxacin; hydrocortisone otic
cisapride (W)	Propulsid (W)
cisatracurium besylate	Nimbex

C
℞

407

cisplatin	Platinol AQ	clonazepam	Klonopin
citalopram hydrobromide	Celexa	clonidine HCl	Catapres
		clonidine HCl inj	Duraclon
cladribine	Leustatin	clopidogrel bisulfate	Plavix
Claforan	cefotaxime sodium	clorazepate dipotassium	Tranxene
Clarinex	desloratadine	Clorpactin WCS-90	oxychlorosene sodium
clarithromycin	Biaxin		
clarithromycin SR	Biaxin XL	clotrimazole	Gyne-Lotrimin Lotrimin Mycelex
Claritin	loratadine		
Claritin D	loratadine; pseudoephed-rine sulfate		
		clozapine	Clozaril
clemastine fumarate	Tavist	Clozaril	clozapine
		coagulation factor IX (recombinant)	BeneFix
Cleocin	clindamycin HCl		
clidinium (W) bromide	Quarzan (W)	coagulation factor VII a (recombinant)	NovoSeven
clidinium; chlordiaze-poxide	Librax		
		coal tar product	Zetar
		codeine phosphate; acetaminophen suspension	Capital w/ Codeine Suspension
Climara	estradiol transdermal		
clindamycin; benzoyl peroxide gel	BenzaClin		
		coenzyme Q10	UbiQGel
clindamycin HCl	Cleocin	Cogentin	benztropine mesylate
clindamycin phosphate pledgets	Clindets		
		Cognex	tacrine HCl
Clindets	clindamycin phosphate pledgets	Colace	docusate sodium
		Colazol	balsalazide disodium
Clinimix E	amino acid with electrolytes in dextrose with calcium inj (various concentrations)	ColBENEMID (W)	probenecid; colchicine (W)
		colchicine	colchicine
		colesevelam HCl	Welchol
		Colestid	colestipol HCl
		colestipol HCl	Colestid
Clinoril	sulindac	colistimethate sodium	Coly-Mycin M
clioquinol	Vioform		
clobetasol foam	Olux	colistin sulfate; hydrocortisone, and neomycin otic soln	Coly-Mycin S
clobetasol propionate gel	Clobevate		
		collagen hemostat	Avitene
Clobevate	clobetasol propionate gel	collagenase	Santyl
		Collyrium	tetrahydrozoline HCl ophth
clofibrate	Atromid-S		
Clomid	clomiphene citrate	Colomed	short chain fatty acids enema
clomiphene citrate	Clomid		
clomipramine HCl	Anafranil	Coly-Mycin M	colistimethate sodium

Coly-Mycin S	colistin sulfate; hydrocortisone, and neomycin otic soln	co-trimoxazole	Bactrim Cotrim Septra sulfamethoxazole; trimethoprim
CoLyte	polyethylene glycol-electrolyte soln	Coumadin	warfarin sodium
CombiPatch	norethindrone acetate; estradiol transdermal	Covera HS	verapamil HCl SR bedtime formulation
Combivent	ipratropium bromide; albuterol sulfate	Cozaar	losartan potassium
		Crestor	rosuvastatin calcium
Combivir	lamivudine; zidovudine	Crinone	progesterone gel
Compazine	prochlorperazine	Crixivan	indinavir
Comtan	entacapone	CroFab	crotalidae poly-valent immune fab (ovine)
Comvax	*Haemophilus b* conjugate; Hepatitis B vaccine	cromolyn sodium	Gastrocrom Nasalcrom Opticrom
Concerta	methylphenidate HCl SR	crotalidae polyvalent immune fab (ovine)	CroFab
Condylox	podofilox gel		
Copaxone	glatiramer acetate	crotamiton	Eurax
Cordarone	amiodarone HCl	Cubicin	daptomycin
		Cuprimine	penicillamine
Coreg	carvedilol	Curosurf	poractant alpha intratracheal susp
Corgard	nadolol		
Corlopam	fenoldopam mesylate		
Cortef	hydrocortisone	Cutivate	fluticasone propionate cream & ointment
corticorellin ovine triflutate	Acthrel		
corticotropin	Acthar	cyanocobalamin nasal gel	Nascobal
cortisone acetate	Cortone Acetate		
Cortone Acetate	cortisone acetate	cyclobenzaprine HCl	Flexeril
Cortrosyn	cosyntropin		
Corvert	ibutilide fumarate	Cyclocort	amcinonide
Cosmegen	dactinomycin	Cyclogyl	cyclopentolate HCl
Cosopt	dorzolamide HCl; timolol maleate ophth soln	cyclopentolate HCl	Cyclogyl
		cyclophosphamide	Cytoxan Neosar
cosyntropin	Cortrosyn	cycloserine	Seromycin
Cotazym	pancrelipase	cyclosporine	Sandimmune
Cotazym-S	pancrelipase EC	cyclosporine capsules (modified) and oral soln	Neoral
Cotrim	sulfamethoxazole; trimethoprim		

C
℞

cyclosporine capsules, (modified)	Gengraf	Darvon	propoxyphene HCl
cyclosporine ophth emulsion	Restasis	Darvon Compound 65	propoxyphene HCl; aspirin; caffeine
Cycrin	medroxyproges-terone acetate	daunorubicin citrate liposomal	DaunoXome
Cylert	pemoline		
Cymbalta	duloxetine HCl	daunorubicin HCl	Cerubidine
cyproheptadine HCl	Periactin	DaunoXome	daunorubicin citrate liposomal
Cystadane	betaine anhydrous		
Cystospaz-M	hyoscyamine sulfate SR	Daypro	oxaprozin
Cytadren	aminogluteth-imide	DDAVP	desmopressin acetate
cytarabine	Cytosar-U	Debrox	carbamide peroxide otic
cytarabine, liposomal inj	DepoCyt	Decadron	dexamethasone
Cytomel	liothyronine sodium	Deca-Durabolin	nandrolone decanoate
Cytosar-U	cytarabine	Declomycin	demeclocycline HCl
Cytotec	misoprostol	deferoxamine mesylate	Desferal
Cytovene	ganciclovir		
Cytoxan	cyclophosphamide	delavirdine mesylate	Rescriptor

D

		Delestrogen	estradiol valerate
		Deltasone	prednisone
		Demadex	torsemide
		demecarium bromide	Humorsol
dacarbazine	DTIC-Dome		
daclizumab	Zenapax	demeclocycline HCl	Declomycin
dactinomycin	Cosmegen		
Dalmane	flurazepam HCl	Demerol	meperidine HCl
dalteparin sodium	Fragmin	Demser	metyrosine
danaparoid sodium	Orgaran	Demulen	ethynodiol diacetate; ethinyl estradiol
danazol	Danocrine		
Danocrine	danazol	Denavir	penciclovir cream
Dantrium	dantrolene sodium	denileukin diftitox	Ontak
dantrolene sodium	Dantrium		
dapsone	dapsone	Depacon	valproate sodium inj
daptomycin	Cubicin	Depakene	valproic acid
Daranide	dichlorphena-mide	Depakote	divalproex sodium
Daraprim	pyrimethamine	Depakote ER	divalproex sodium SR
darbepoetin	Aranesp		
Darvocet-N 100	propoxyphene napsylate; acetaminophen	DepoCyt	cytarabine, liposomal inj

DepoDur	morphine sulfate extended-release liposome inj	dexrazoxane	Zinecard
Depo-Medrol	methylprednis-olone acetate SR	dextro-amphetamine sulfate	Dexedrine
Depo-Provera	medroxyproges-terone acetate SR	dextrothyroxine sodium (W)	Choloxin (W)
Depo-Testosterone	testosterone cypionate SR	D.H.E. 45	dihydroergot-amine mesylate inj
Desferal	deferoxamine mesylate	DiaBeta	glyburide
desflurane	Suprane	Diabinese	chlorpropamide
desipramine HCl	Norpramin	Diamox	acetazolamide
Desirudin	iprivask	Diapid (W)	lypressin (W)
desloratadine	Clarinex	Diastat	diazepam rectal gel
desmopressin acetate	DDAVP	diazepam	Valium
Desogen	desogestrel; ethinyl estradiol	diazepam emulsified inj	Dizac
desogestrel; ethinyl estradiol	Desogen Ortho-Cept	diazepam rectal gel	Diastat
desogestrel and ethinyl estradiol; ethinyl estradiol	Mircette	diazoxide	Hyperstat
		Dibenzyline	phenoxybenz-amine HCl
		dibucaine	Nupercainal
desonide	Tridesilon	dichlorphena-mide	Daranide
desoximetasone	Topicort	diclofenac gel	Solaraze
Desoxyn	methamphet-amine HCl	diclofenac potassium	Cataflam
Desyrel	trazodone HCl	diclofenac sodium	Voltaren
Detrol	tolterodine tartrate		
Detrol LA	tolterodine tartrate (SR)	diclofenac sodium; misoprostol	Arthrotec
dexamethasone	Decadron Hexadrol	diclofenac sodium SR	Voltaren-XR
dexchlorphenir-amine maleate SR	Polaramine Repetabs	dicloxacillin sodium	Dynapen
Dexedrine	dextroampheta-mine sulfate	dicyclomine HCl	Bentyl
		didanosine	Videx
		didanosine SR	Videx EC
dexfenfluramine HCl (W)	Redux (W)	Didronel	etidronate disodium
Dexferrum	iron dextran inj	diethylcarbama-zine citrate	Hetrazan
dexmedetomidine HCl inj	Precedex	diethylpropion HCl	Tenuate
		Differin	adapalene
dexmethyl-phenidate HCl	Focalin	diflorasone diacetate	Florone
		Diflucan	fluconazole
		diflunisal	Dolobid

Digibind	digoxin immune fab	Disalcid	salsalate
digoxin	Lanoxin	disopyramide phosphate	Norpace
digoxin capsules	Lanoxicaps	disulfiram	Antabuse
digoxin immune fab	Digibind	Ditropan	oxybutynin chloride
dihydroergotamine mesylate inj	D.H.E. 45	Diulo (WA)	metolazone
		Diuril	chlorothiazide
dihydroergotamine mesylate nasal spray	Migranol	divalproex sodium	Depakote
		divalproex sodium SR	Depakote ER
dihydrotestosterone transdermal	Androgel-DHT	Dizac	diazepam emulsified inj
Dilacor XR	diltiazem HCl SR	dobutamine HCl	Dobutrex
Dilantin	phenytoin	Dobutrex	dobutamine HCl
Dilaudid	hydromorphone HCl	docetaxel	Taxotere
diltiazem HCl	Cardizem	docosanol cream	Avanir
diltiazem HCl SR	Cardizem CD	docusate sodium	Colace
	Cartia XR	docusate sodium; casanthranol	Peri-Colace
	Dilacor XR		
	Tiazac	dofetilide	Tikosyn
diltiazem maleate SR	Tiamate	dolasetron mesylate	Anzemet
dimenhydrinate	Dramamine	Dolobid	diflunisal
dimercaprol	BAL in Oil	Dolophine	methadone HCl
Dimetane	brompheniramine maleate	Domeboro	aluminum acetate
dinoprostone gel	Prepidil	donepezil HCl	Aricept
dinoprostone vaginal insert	Cervidil	Donnatal (W)	belladonna alkaloids; phenobarbital
dinoprostone vaginal suppositories	Prostin E2		
		dopamine HCl	Intropin
Diovan	valsartan	Dopar	levodopa
Diovan HCT	valsartan; hydrochlorothiazide	Dopram	doxapram HCl
		dornase alpha	Pulmozyme
Dipentum	olsalazine sodium	dorzolamide HCl	Trusopt
diphenhydramine HCl	Benadryl	dorzolamide HCl; timolol maleate ophth soln	Cosopt
diphenoxylate HCl; atropine sulfate	Lomotil		
dipivefrin	Propine	Dostinex	cabergoline
Diprivan	propofol	Dovonex	calcipotriene cream
Diprosone	betamethasone dipropionate	doxacurium chloride	Nuromax
dipyridamole	Persantine	doxapram HCl	Dopram
dirithromycin	Dynabac		

D
℞

doxazosin mesylate	Cardura
doxepin HCl	Adapin
	Sinequan
doxepin HCl cream	Prudoxin
doxercalciferol	Hectorol
Doxil	doxorubicin, liposomal
doxorubicin HCl	Adriamycin
	Rubex
doxorubicin, liposomal	Doxil
doxycycline hyclate	Vibramycin
doxycycline hyclate 20 mg tab & cap	Periostat
doxycycline hyclate gel	Atridox
Dramamine	dimenhydrinate
Drisdol	ergocalciferol
Dristan Long Lasting	oxymetazoline HCl
Drixoral Syrup	pseudoephedrine HCl; bromphiramine maleate
dronabinol	Marinol
droperidol	Inapsine
drospirenone; ethinyl estradiol	Yasmin
drotrecogin alfa	Xigris
Droxia	hydroxyurea
DTIC-Dome	dacarbazine
Dulcolax	bisacodyl
duloxetine HCl	Cymbalta
Durabolin (W)	nandrolone phenpropionate (W)
Duraclon	clonidine HCl inj
Duragesic	fentanyl transdermal
Duramorph	morphine sulfate inj
Duranest	etidocaine HCl
Duricef	cefadroxil
dutasteride	Avodart
Dyazide	triamterene 37.5 mg; hydro-chlorothiazide 25 mg

Dymelor	acetohexamide
Dynabac	dirithromycin
DynaCirc	isradipine
Dynapen	dicloxacillin sodium
dyphylline	Lufyllin
Dyrenium	triamterene

E

EchoGen	perflenapent emulsion
echothiophate iodide (W)	Phospholine Iodide (W)
Ecotrin	aspirin EC
Edecrin	ethacrynic acid
edetate disodium	Endrate
Edex	alprostadil inj
edrophonium chloride	Tensilon
E.E.S. 400	erythromycin ethylsuccinate
efalizumab	Raptiva
efaproxiral	Efaproxyn
Efaproxyn	efaproxiral
efavirenz	Sustiva
Effexor	venlafaxine HCl
Effexor XR	venlafaxine HCl SR
eflornithine HCl cream	Vaniqa
Efudex	fluorouracil cream; soln
Elavil	amitriptyline HCl
Eldepryl	selegiline HCl
Eldisine	vindesine sulfate
Elestat	epinastine
eletriptan hydrobromide	Relpax
Elidel	pimecrolimus cream
Eligard	leuprolide acetate
Elitek	rasburicase
Elixophyllin	theophylline
Ellence	epirubicin HCl
Elmiron	pentosan polysulfate sodium
Elocon	mometasone furoate topical

D
R

Eloxatin	oxaliplatin	Entocort EC	budesonide
Elspar	asparaginase		capsule SR
Emadine	emedastine	epinastine	Elestat
	difumarate	epinephrine	Adrenalin
	opthth soln	epinephrine	Vaponefrin
Emcyt	estramustine	racemic	
	phosphate	epirubicin HCl	Ellence
	sodium	Epivir	lamivudine
emedastine	Emadine	Epivir HBV	lamivudine
difumarate		eplerenone	Inspra
opthth soln		epoetin alfa	Epogen
Emend	aprepitant		Procrit
EMLA Cream	lidocaine; prilo-	Epogen	epoetin alfa
	caine cream	epoprostenol	Flolan
Empirin with	aspirin 325 mg	sodium	
codeine #3	with codeine	eprosartan	Teveten
and #4	phosphate (30	mesylate	
	and 60 mg)	eprosartan	Teveten HCT
emtricitabine	Emtriva	mesylate;	
emtricitabine;	Truvada	hydrochloro-	
tenofovir		thiazide	
disoproxil		eptifibatide	Integrilin
Emtriva	emtricitabine	Epzicom	lamivudine;
E-Mycin	erythromycin		abacavir sulfate
enalapril maleate	Vasotec	Equanil (WA)	meprobamate
enalapril	Teczem	Erbitux	cetuximab
maleate;		Ergamisol (W)	levamisole
diltiazem			HCl (W)
malate		ergocalciferol	Calciferol
enalapril	Lexxel		Drisdol
maleate;		ergoloid	Hydergine
felodipine SR		mesylates	
enalapril	Vaseretic	ergotamine	Cafergot
maleate;		tartrate;	
hydrochlorothi-		caffeine	
azide		ergotamine	Ergostat
Enbrel	etanercept	tartrate	
encainide HCl	Enkaid	Ergotrate	ergonovine
Endep	amitriptyline HCl		maleate
Endocet	oxycodone HCl;	Ertaczo	sertaconazole
	acetaminophen	ertapenem	Invanz
Endrate	edetate disodium	sodium	
Enduron	methyclothiazide	Ery-Tab	erythromycin EC
enflurane	Ethrane	Erythrocin	erythromycin
enfuvirtide	Fuzeon	Stearate	stearate
Engerix-B	hepatitis B vaccine	erythromycin	E-Mycin
Enkaid	encainide HCl	erythromycin	PCE Dispertab
enoxaparin	Lovenox	base coated	
sodium		particles	
entacapone	Comtan	erythromycin;	Benzamycin
Entex LA	phenylpropanol-	benzoyl	
	amine HCl;	peroxide topical	
	guaifenesin SR	gel	

erythromycin EC	Ery-Tab
erythromycin estolate	Ilosone
erythromycin ethylsuccinate	E.E.S. 400
erythromycin ethylsuccinate; sulfisoxazole	Pediazole
erythromycin stearate	Erythrocin Stearate
escitalopram oxalate	Lexapro
Esclim	estradiol transdermal
Eserine Sulfate	physostigmine ophth ointment
Esidrix	hydrochlorothiazide
Esimil	guanethidine monosulfate; hydrochlorothiazide
Eskalith	lithium carbonate
esmolol HCl	Brevibloc
esomeprazole magnesium	Nexium
estazolam	ProSom
Estinyl	ethinyl estradiol
Estrace	estradiol
Estraderm	estradiol transdermal
estradiol	Estrace
estradiol hemihydrate vaginal tab	Vagifem
estradiol transdermal	Alora Climara Esclim Estraderm FemPatch Menostar Vivelle
estradiol vaginal ring	Estring
estradiol valerate	Delestrogen
estramustine phosphate sodium	Emcyt
Estratest	estrogens, esterified; methyltestosterone

Estratest H.S.	estrogens, esterified; methyltestosterone, half strength
Estring	estradiol vaginal ring
estrogens, conjugated	Premarin
estrogens conjugate, A synthetic	Cenestin
estrogens, conjugated; medroxyprogesterone acetate	Premphase Prempro
estrogens, esterified; methyltestosterone	Estratest
estrogens, esterified methyltestosterone, half strength	Estratest H.S.
estropipate	Ogen
Estrostep	norethindrone acetate; ethinyl estradiol
etanercept	Enbrel
ethacrynic acid	Edecrin
ethambutol HCl	Myambutol
ethchlorvynol	Placidyl
Ethezyme	papain; urea oint
ethinyl estradiol	Estinyl
ethinyl estradiol; levonorgestrel (91 day cycle)	Seasonale
ethionamide	Trecator-SC
Ethmozine	moricizine
ethopropazine HCl	Parsidol
ethosuximide	Zarontin
Ethrane	enflurane
ethyl chloride	ethyl chloride
ethynodiol diacetate; ethinyl estradiol	Demulen
Ethyol	amifostine
etidocaine HCl	Duranest
etidronate disodium	Didronel

E
R̸

etodolac	Lodine	Famvir	famciclovir
etodolac SR	Lodine XL	Fansidar	sulfadoxine; pyrimethamine
etomidate	Amidate		
etonogestrel; ethinyl estradiol vagina ring	NuvaRing	Fareston	toremifene citrate
		Faslodex	fulvestrant
		Fastin	phentermine HCl
etonogestrel implant	Implanon	fat emulsion	Intralipid Liposyn II and III
Etopophos	etoposide phosphate diethanolate		
		felbamate	Felbatol
		Felbatol	felbamate
etoposide	VePesid	Feldene	piroxicam
etoposide phosphate diethanolate	Etopophos	felodipine	Plendil
		Femara	letrozole
		Femhrt	norethindrone acetate; ethinyl estradiol
Etrafon	perphenazine; amitriptyline HCl		
		FemPatch	estradiol transdermal
Eulexin	flutamide		
Eurax	crotamiton	fenfluramine HCl (W)	Pondimin (W)
Euthroid (WA)	liotrix		
Eutonyl	pargyline HCl	fenofibrate	Tricor
Evista	raloxifene HCl	fenoldopam mesylate	Corlopam
Evoxac	cevimeline HCl		
Exelon	rivastigmine tartrate	fenoprofen calcium	Nalfon
exemestane	Aromasin	fentanyl citrate	Sublimaze
exisulind	Aposyn	fentanyl citrate; droperidol	Innovar
Ex-Lax	sennosides		
Extraneal	icodextrin 7.5% with electrolyte peritoneal dialysis soln	Fentanyl Oralet	fentanyl transmucosal
		fentanyl transdermal	Duragesic
ezetimibe	Zetia	fentanyl transmucosal	Actiq Fentanyl Oralet
ezetimibe; simvastatin	Vytorin		
		Feosol	ferrous sulfate
		Fer-In-Sol	ferrous sulfate
		Fergon	ferrous gluconate
		Feridex	ferumoxide HCl
	F	Ferrlecit	sodium ferric gluconate complex in sucrose inj
Fabrazyme	agalsidase beta		
Factive	gemifloxacin mesylate	ferrous gluconate	Fergon
		ferrous sulfate	Feosol Fer-In-Sol SlowFe
factor IX, concentrate	BeneFix		
Factrel	gonadorelin HCl	ferrous sulfate SR	SlowFe
famciclovir	Famvir		
famotidine	Pepcid	Fertinex	urofollitropin for inj
famotidine, oral disintegrating tablet	Pepcid RPD		
		ferumoxetil oral suspension	Gastromark

ferumoxide HCl	Feridex	flumazenil	Romazicon
fexofenadine HCl	Allegra	flunisolide	Aero Bid
		fluocinolone acetonide	Synalar
filgrastim	Neupogen		
finasteride	Propecia 1 mg tablet	fluocinonide	Lidex
		Fluor-I-Strip	fluorescein sodium strips
	Proscar 5 mg tablet	fluorescein sodium soln	Fluorescite
Finevin	azelaic cream		
Fioricet	butalbital; acetamino-phen; caffeine	fluorescein sodium strips	Fluor-I-Strip
		Fluorescite	fluorescein sodium soln
Fiorinal	butalbital; aspirin; caffeine	fluorometholone	FML
		Fluoroplex	fluorouracil cream; soln
Flagyl	metronidazole		
Flagyl ER	metronidazole SR	*fluorouracil inj*	*fluorouracil inj*
		fluorouracil cream; soln	Efudex
flavocoxid	Limbrel		Fluoroplex
flavoxate HCl	Urispas	Fluothane	halothane
Flaxedil	gallamine triethiodide	fluoxetine HCl	Prozac
			Sarafem
flecainide acetate	Tambocor	fluoxymesterone	Halotestin
Flexeril	cyclobenzaprine HCl	fluphenazine HCl	Permitil
			Prolixin
Flolan	epoprostenol sodium	flurazepam HCl	Dalmane
		flurbiprofen	Ansaid
Flomax	tamsulosin HCl	flutamide	Eulexin
Flonase	fluticasone propionate spray	fluticasone propionate spray	Flonase
			Flovent
Florinef	fludrocortisone acetate	fluticasone propionate cream & ointment	Cutivate
Florone	diflorasone diacetate		
Floropryl	isoflurophate	fluticasone propionate; salmeterol inhalation powder	Advair Diskus
Florotag	synopinine		
Flovent	fluticasone propionate spray		
Floxin	ofloxacin	fluvastatin sodium	Lescol
Floxin Otic	ofloxacin otic soln	fluvoxamine maleate	Luvox
floxuridine	FUDR		
fluconazole	Diflucan	FML	fluorometholone
flucytosine	Ancobon	Focalin	dexmethyl-phenidate HCl
Fludara	fludarabine phosphate		
		Folex PFS	methotrexate inj
fludarabine phosphate	Fludara	*folic acid*	Folvite
		Follistim	follitropin beta
fludrocortisone acetate	Florinef	follitropin alfa	Gonal-F
		follitropin beta	Follistim
Flumadine	rimantadine	Folvite	folic acid

fomepizole	Antizol	gallium nitrate	Ganite
fomivirsen sodium inj	Vitravene	Galzin	zinc acetate
fondaparinux sodium	Arixtra	Gamimune N	immune globulin intravenous
Foradil	formoterol fumarate	Gammagard S/D	immune globulin intravenous
Forane	isoflurane	ganciclovir	Cytovene
formoterol fumarate	Foradil	ganciclovir ophthalmic implant	Vitrasert
Fortaz	ceftazidime	ganirelix acetate	Antagon
Forteo	teriparatide	Ganite	gallium nitrate
Fortovase	saquinavir soft gel capsule	Gantanol (W)	sulfamethoxazole (W)
Fosamax	alendronate sodium	Garamycin	*gentamicin sulfate*
fosamprenavir calcium	Lexiva	Gastrocrom	cromolyn sodium
foscarnet	Foscavir	Gastromark	ferumoxetil oral suspension
Foscavir	foscarnet	gatifloxacin	Tequin
fosfomycin tromethamine	Monurol	gatifloxacin ophth soln	Zymar
fosinopril sodium	Monopril	gefitinib	Iressa
fosphenytoin sodium	Cerebyx	gemcitabine HCl	Gemzar
Fragmin	dalteparin sodium	gemfibrozil	Lopid
Frova	frovatriptan succinate	gemifloxacin mesylate	Factive
frovatriptan succinate	Frova	gemtuzumab ozogamicin	Mylotarg
FUDR	floxuridine	Gemzar	gemcitabine HCl
fulvestrant	Faslodex		
Fulvicin P/G	griseofulvin	GenEsa	arbutamine HCl
Fungizone	amphotericin B	Gengraf	cyclosporine capsules, (modified)
Furacin	nitrofurazone		
furosemide	Lasix	Genotropin	somatropin for inj
Fuzeon	enfuvirtide	*gentamicin sulfate*	Garamycin

G

		Geocillin	carbenicillin
		Geodon	ziprasidone HCl
gabapentin	Neurontin	Geref	sermorelin acetate
Gabitril	tiagabine HCl	glatiramer acetate	Copaxone
gadoteridol	ProHance		
gadoversetamide	OptiMark	Gleevec	imatinib mesylate
galantamine HBr	Reminyl	Gliadel	carmustine implantable wafer
gallamine triethiodide	Flaxedil	glimepiride	Amaryl
		glipizide	Glucotrol

glipizide SR	Glucotrol XL	guanabenz acetate	Wytensin
glipizide; metformin	Metaglip	guanadrel sulfate	Hylorel
GlucaGen	glucagon (rDNA origin)	guanethidine monosulfate	Ismelin
glucagon	glucagon	guanethidine monosulfate; hydrochlorothi-azide	Esimil
glucagon (rDNA origin)	GlucaGen		
Glucophage	metformin HCl	guanfacine HCl	Tenex
Glucophage XR	metformin HCl SR	Gynazole	butoconazole nitrate vaginal cream
Glucotrol	glipizide	Gyne-Lotrimin	clotrimazole
Glucotrol XL	glipizide SR		
Glucovance	glyburide; metformin HCl		
glyburide	DiaBeta Micronase		
glyburide; metformin HCl	Glucovance		

H

glyburide micronized	Glynase	Habitrol	nicotine transdermal system
glycerin ophth soln	Ophthalgan		
glycopyrrolate	Robinul	Haemophilus b conjugate vaccine reconstituted with diphtheria and tetanus toxoids and acellular pertussis vaccine adsorbed	ActHIB/Tripedia
Glynase	glyburide micronized		
Glyset	miglitol		
gold sodium thiomalate	Aurolate		
GoLYTELY	polyethylene glycol-electrolyte soln		
gonadorelin HCl	Factrel	Haemophilus b conjugate; Hepatitis B vaccine	Comvax
Gonal-F	follitropin alfa		
goserelin acetate implant	Zoladex		
graftskin	Apligraf	haemophilus b vaccine	Hib-Immune (W) HibTITER PedvaxHIB ProHIBiT
granisetron HCl	Kytril		
grepafloxacin HCl (W)	Raxar (W)		
Grifulvin V (W)	griseofulvin (W)	halcinonide	Halog
griseofulvin (W)	Fulvicin P/G (W) Grifulvin V	Halcion	triazolam
		Haldol	haloperidol
guaifenesin	Organidin NR Robitussin	Halfan	halofantrine HCl
		halofantrine HCl	Halfan
guaifenesin; codeine phosphate	Robitussin A-C Tussi-Organidin NR	Halog	halcinonide
		haloperidol	Haldol
		haloprogin	Halotex
guaifenesin; dextromethor-phan	Robitussin-DM	Halotestin	fluoxymesterone
		Halotex	haloprogin
		halothane	Fluothane

Havrix	hepatitis A vaccine, inactivated	Humalog	insulin, lispro (human)
Healon	sodium hyaluronate	Humalog Mix75/25	insulin lispro protamine susp 75%; insulin lispro inj 25% [rDNA origin]
Hectorol	doxercalciferol		
Helidac	bismuth subsalicylate; metronidazole; tetracycline HCl		
		Humatin	paromomycin sulfate
heparin sodium	*heparin sodium*	Humatrope	somatropin
hepatitis A inactivated; hepatitis B (recombinant) vaccine	Twinrix	Humira	adalimumab
		Humorsol	demecarium bromide
		Humulin 70/30	isophane insulin suspension 70%, insulin inj 30% (human)
hepatitis A vaccine, inactivated	Havrix Vaqta		
hepatitis B immune globulin (human)	NABI-HB	Humulin L	insulin zinc suspension (Lente) (human)
hepatitis B vaccine	Engerix-B Recombivax HB	Humulin N	isophane insulin suspension (NPH) (human)
Hepsera	adefovir dipivoxil		
Herceptin	trastuzumab	Humulin R	insulin inj (human)
Herplex (W)	idoxuridine (W)		
Hespan	hetastarch	Humulin U Ultralente	insulin zinc suspension, extended, (human)
hetastarch	Hespan		
hetastarch in lactated electrolyte inj	Hextend		
		Hurricane	benzocaine
Hetrazan	diethylcarbamazine citrate	Hyalgan	sodium hyaluronate
Hexadrol	dexamethasone		
Hexalen	altretamine	hyaluronidase	Wydase
Hextend	hetastarch in lactated electrolyte inj	Hycamtin	topotecan HCl
		Hydergine	ergoloid mesylates
Hib-Immune (WA)	haemophilus b vaccine	hydralazine HCl	Apresoline
Hibiclens	chlorhexidine gluconate	hydralazine HCl; hydrochlorothiazide	Apresazide
HibTITER	haemophilus b vaccine	hydralazine; hydrochlorothiazide; reserpine	Ser-Ap-Es
Hiprex	methenamine hippurate		
Hismanal (W)	astemizole (W)	Hydrea	hydroxyurea
Hivid	zalcitabine	*hydrochlorothiazide*	Esidrix
homatropine hydrobromide ophth	Isopto Homatropine		HydroDIURIL Microzide Oretic

hydrocodone bitartrate; acetaminophen	Anexsia 5/500
	Anexsia 7.5/650
	Lorcet 10/650
	Lorcet-HD (5/500)
	Lorcet plus (7.5/650)
	Lortab 2.5/500; 5/500; 7.5/500; 10/500
	Norco
	Vicodin
	Vicodin ES
	Zydone 5/400, 7.5/400, 10/400
hydrocodone bitartrate 7.5 mg; ibuprofen 200 mg	Vicoprofen
hydrocodone polistirex; chlorphenira-mine	Tussionex
hydrocortisone	Cortef
	Hydrocortone
hydrocortisone buteprate cream	Pandel
hydrocortisone sodium succinate	Solu-Cortef
Hydrocortone	hydrocortisone
HydroDIURIL	hydrochlorothia-zide
hydroflumethia-zide	Saluron
hydromorphone HCl	Dilaudid
hydromorphone HCl SR	Palladone XL
Hydromox (W)	quinethazone (W)
hydroquinone topical susp	Alustra
hydroquinone; tretinoin; fluocinolone cream	Tri-Luma
hydroxychloro-quine sulfate	Plaquenil
hydroxyurea	Droxia
	Hydrea
hydroxyzine HCl	Atarax
hydroxyzine pamoate	Vistaril
Hygroton	chlorthalidone
hylan G-F 20	Synvisc
Hylorel	guanadrel sulfate
hyoscyamine sulfate orally disintegrating tab	NuLev
hyoscyamine sulfate SR	Cystospaz-M
	Levbid
Hyperab (W)	rabies immune globulin, human
Hyperstat	diazoxide
Hyper-Tet (W)	tetanus immune globulin (human) (W)
Hytrin	terazosin HCl
Hyzaar	losartan potassium; hydrochlorothi-azide

I-J

ibandronate	Boniva
ibritumomab tiuxetan	Zevalin
ibuprofen	Advil
	Motrin
	Nuprin
ibutilide fumarate	Corvert
icodextrin 7.5% with electro-lyte peritoneal dialysis soln	Extraneal
Idamycin	idarubicin
idarubicin	Idamycin
idoxuridine (W)	Herplex (W)
IFEX	ifosfamide
ifosfamide	IFEX
Ilosone	erythromycin estolate
Imagent GI	perflubron
imatinib mesylate	Gleevec
imciromab pentetate	Myoscint

Imdur	isosorbide mono-nitrate SR
imiglucerase	Cerezyme
imipenem-cilastatin sodium	Primaxin
imipramine HCl	Tofranil
imiquimod cream	Aldara
Imitrex	sumatriptan
immune globulin intravenous	Gamimune N Gammagard S/D Sandoglobulin
Imodium	loperamide HCl
Imogam	rabies immune globulin, human
Implanon	etonogestrel implant
Imuran	azathioprine
inamrinone	Inocor
Inapsine	droperidol
indapamide	Lozol
Inderal	propranolol HCl
Inderide	propranolol HCl; hydrochlorothiazide
indinavir	Crixivan
indium In-111 pentetreotide	OctreoScan
Indocin	indomethacin
indomethacin	Indocin
Infasurf	calfactant intratracheal susp
INFeD	iron dextran inj
Infergen	interferon alfacon-1
infliximab	Remicade
Innohep	tinzaparin sodium
Innovar	fentanyl citrate; droperidol
Inocor	inamrinone
INOmax	nitric oxide for inhalation
Inspra	eplerenone
insulin aspart (rDNA origin)	NovoLog
insulin glargine (rDNA origin)	Lantus
insulin glulisine [rDNA origin]	Apidra
insulin inj (human)	Humulin R Novolin R Velosulin Human
insulin lispro (human)	Humalog
insulin lispro protamine susp 75%; insulin lispro inj 25% [rDNA origin]	Humalog Mix75/25
insulin zinc suspension (Lente) (human)	Humulin L Novolin L (WA)
insulin zinc suspension, extended (beef)	Ultralente U
insulin zinc suspension, extended, (human)	Humulin U Ultralente
Integrilin	eptifibatide
interferon alfa-2a	Roferon-A
interferon alfa-2b	Intron A
interferon alfa-n[1] lymphoblastoid	Wellferon
interferon alfa-n3 (human leukocyte derived)	Alferon
interferon alfacon-1	Infergen
interferon beta-la	Avonex Rebif
interferon beta-1b	Betaseron
interferon gamma 1-b	Actimmune
Intrachol	choline chloride inj
Intralipid	fat emulsion
Intron A	interferon alfa-2b
Intropin	dopamine HCl
Invanz	ertapenem sodium
Inversine	mecamylamine HCl
Invirase	saquinavir mesylate
iocetamic acid	Cholebrine
iodamide meglumine	Renovue 65
iodixanol	Visipaque

iohexol	Omnipaque
Ionamin	phentermine resin
iopamidol	Isovue
iopanoic acid	Telepaque
iopromide	Ultravist
iotrolan	Osmovist
ioversol	Optiray
ioxilan	Oxilan
Ipol	poliovirus vaccine inactivated
ipratropium bromide	Atrovent
ipratropium bromide; albuterol sulfate	Combivent
iprivask	Desirudin
irbesartan	Avapro
irbesartan; hydrochlorothi-azide	Avalide
Iressa	gefitinib
irinotecan HCl	Camptosar
iron dextran inj	INFeD Dexferrum
iron sucrose inj	Venofer
Ismelin	guanethidine monosulfate
ISMO	isosorbide mononitrate
isocarboxazid	Marplan
isoetharine HCl aerosol	Bronkometer
isoetharine HCl soln	Bronkosol
isoflurane	Forane
isoflurophate	Floropry l
isoniazid	Nydrazid
isoniazid; rifampin	Rifamate
isophane insulin suspension (NPH) (human)	Humulin N Novolin N
isophane insulin suspension (NPH) 70%, insulin inj 30% (human)	Humulin 70/30 Novolin 70/30
isoproterenol HCl	Isuprel
Isoptin	verapamil HCl
Isopto Carbachol	carbachol ophth

Isopto Carpine	pilocarpine HCl ophth
Isopto Homatropine	homatropine hydrobromide ophth
Isopto Hyoscine	scopolamine hydrobromide ophth
Isordil	isosorbide dinitrate
isosorbide dinitrate	Isordil
isosorbide mononitrate	ISMO
isosorbide mononitrate SR	Imdur
isotretinoin	Accutane
Isovue	iopamidol
isoxsuprine HCl	Vasodilan
isradipine	DynaCirc
Isuprel	isoproterenol HCl
itraconazole	Sporanox
ivermectin	Stromectol
IvyBlock	bentoquatam

K

Kadian	morphine sulfate SR
Kaletra	lopinavir; ritonavir
kanamycin sulfate	Kantrex
Kantrex	kanamycin sulfate
Kaon	potassium gluconate
Kaon-Cl	potassium chloride SR
Kayexalate	polystyrene sulfonate sodium
K-Dur	potassium chloride SR
Keflex	cephalexin
Keflin (W)	cephalothin sodium (W)
Keftab	cephalexin HCl
Kefurox	cefuroxime sodium

I

R̸

Kefzol (WA)	cefazolin sodium	Lac-Hydrin	lactic acid; ammonium lactate lotion
Kemadrin	procyclidine HCl		
Kenalog	triamcinolone acetonide	lactic acid; ammonium lactate lotion	Lac-Hydrin
Keppra	levetiracetam		
Kerlone	betaxolol	lactulose	Cephulac
Ketalar	ketamine HCl		Chronulac
ketamine HCL	Ketalar	Lamictal	lamotrigine
ketoconazole	Nizoral	Lamisil	terbinafine HCl
ketoprofen (W)	Orudis (W)	lamivudine	Epivir
ketoprofen SR	Oruvail		Epivir HBV
ketorolac tromethamine	Toradol		Epzicom
		lamivudine; abacavir sulfate	Epzicom
ketorolac tromethamine ophth	Acular		
		lamivudine; zidovudine	Combivir
ketotifen fumarate ophth soln	Zaditor	lamivudine; zidovudine; abacavir sulfate	Trizivir
Kineret	anakinra		
Klaron	sodium sulfacetamide lotion		
		lamotrigine	Lamictal
Klonopin	clonazepam	Lanoxicaps	digoxin capsules
Klor-Con 10	potassium chloride SR	Lanoxin	digoxin
		lansoprazole	Prevacid
K-Lyte	potassium bicarbonate; potassium citrate effervescent	lansoprazole; amoxicillin; clarithromycin	Prevpac
		Lantus	insulin glargine (rDNA origin)
K-Lyte/Cl	potassium chloride potassium bicarbonate effervescent	Lariam	mefloquine HCl
		Larodopa	levodopa
		laronidase	Aldurazyme
		Lasix	furosemide
Kogenate	antihemophilic factor (recombinant)	latanoprost	Xalatan
		leflunomide	Arava
		lepirudin	Refludan
Kolyum	potassium chloride; potassium gluconate	Lescol	fluvastatin sodium
		letrozole	Femara
		leucovorin calcium	Wellcovorin (WA)
Konsyl-D	psyllium	Leukeran	chlorambucil
Kwell (WA)	lindane	Leukine	sargramostim
Kytril	granisetron HCl	leuprolide acetate	Eligard
			Lupron
		leuprolide acetate implant	Viadur
L			
		Leustatin	cladribine
		levalbuterol HCl inhalation soln	Xopenex
labetalol HCl	Normodyne Trandate	levamisole HCl (W)	Ergamisol (W)

Levaquin	levofloxacin	Levoxyl	levothyroxine sodium
Levbid	hyoscyamine sulfate SR	Levulan Kerastick	aminolevulinic acid HCl topical soln
levetiracetam	Keppra		
Levitra	vardenafil HCl	Lexapro	escitalopram oxalate
Levlite	levonorgestrel; ethinyl estradiol	Lexiva	fosamprenavir calcium
levobupivacaine	Chirocaine	Lexxel	enalapril maleate; felodipine SR
levocabastine HCl ophth susp	Livostin	Librax	clidinium; chlordiaz-epoxide
Levo-Dromoran	levorphanol tartrate	Librium	chlordiazepoxide HCl
levobunolol HCl	Betagan	Lidex	fluocinonide
levocarnitine	Carnitor	lidocaine HCl	Xylocaine HCl
levodopa	Dopar	lidocaine patch	Lidoderm
	Larodopa	lidocaine; prilocaine cream	EMLA Cream
levodopa; carbidopa	Sinemet		
levodopa; carbidopa SR	Sinemet CR	Lidoderm	lidocaine patch
		Limbitrol	chlordiazepoxide HCl; amitrip-tyline HCl
levodopa, carbidopa, and entacapone	Stalevo		
levofloxacin	Levaquin	Limbrel	flavocoxid
levofloxacin ophth soln	Quixin	Lincocin	lincomycin HCl
		lincomycin HCl	Lincocin
levomethadyl acetate HCl	Orlaam	lindane	Kwell (WA) lindane
levonorgestrel	Plan B	linezolid	Zyvox
levonorgestrel; ethinyl estradiol	Alesse	Lioresal	baclofen
	Levlite	liothyronine sodium	Cytomel
	Nordette		
	Preven Emergency Contraceptive Kit	liothyronine sodium inj	Triostat
		liotrix	Thyrolar
	Tri-Levlen	Lipitor	atorvastatin calcium
	Triphasil		
levonorgestrel implant (W)	Norplant (W)	liposomal am-photericin B	AmBisome
levonorgestrel-releasing intrauterine system	Mirena	Liposyn II and III	fat emulsion
		lisinopril	Prinivil Zestril
Levophed	norepinephrine bitartrate	lisinopril; hydrochloro-thiazide	Zestoretic
levorphanol tartrate	Levo-Dromoran	lithium carbonate	Eskalith Lithobid
levothyroxine sodium	Levoxyl Synthroid	lithium citrate	Cibalith-S
		Lithobid	lithium carbonate

L

℞

425

Lithostat	acetohydroxamic acid	etabonate ophth susp	Lotemax
Livostin	levocabastine HCl ophth susp	Lotrel	amlodipine besylate; benazepril HCl
Lodine	etodolac	Lotrimin	clotrimazole
Lodine XL	etodolac SR	Lotrisone	betamethasone; clotrimazole cream
lodoxamide tromethamine ophth soln	Alomide	Lotronex (W)	alosetron (W)
Loestrin	norethindrone acetate; ethinyl estradiol	lovastatin	Mevacor
		lovastatin; niacin	Advicor
lomefloxacin	Maxaquin	Lovenox	enoxaparin sodium
Lomotil	diphenoxylate HCl; atropine sulfate		
lomustine	CeeNu	loxapine succinate	Loxitane
Loniten	minoxidil tablets	Loxitane	loxapine succinate
Lo/Ovral	norgestrel; ethinyl estradiol	Lozol	indapamide
		Ludiomil (W)	maprotiline HCl (W)
loperamide HCl	Imodium	Lufyllin	dyphylline
Lopid	gemfibrozil	LumenHance	manganese chloride
lopinavir; ritonavir	Kaletra		
Lopressor	metoprolol tartrate	Lunelle	medroxy-progesterone acetate; estradiol cypionate inj
Loprox	ciclopirox cream and lotion		
Lorabid	loracarbef	Lupron	leuprolide acetate
loracarbef	Lorabid	Luride	sodium fluoride
loratadine	Claritin	Luvox	fluvoxamine maleate
loratadine; pseudoephedrine sulfate	Claritin D	Luxiq	betamethasone valerate (foam)
lorazepam	Ativan	Lyme disease vaccine (W)	LYMErix (W)
Lorcet (various combinations)	hydrocodone bitartrate; acetaminophen	LYMErix (W)	Lyme disease vaccine (W)
Lortab (various combinations)	hydrocodone bitartrate; acetaminophen	lymphocyte immune globulin	Atgam
losartan potassium	Cozaar	lypressin (W)	Diapid (W)
losartan potassium; hydrochlorothi-azide	Hyzaar	Lysodren	mitotane

M

Maalox	aluminum hydroxide; magnesium hydroxide

Lotemax	loteprednol etabonate ophth susp
Lotensin	benazepril HCl
loteprednol	Alrex

Macrobid	nitrofurantoin macrocrystals and mono-hydrate
Macrodantin	nitrofurantoin macrocrystals
magaldrate	Riopan
manganese chloride	LumenHance
magnesium chloride SR	Slow-Mag
magnesium oxide	MAG-OX 400
magnesium sulfate	magnesium sulfate
MAG-OX 400	magnesium oxide
Malarone	atovaquone; proguanil HCl
Mandol	cefamandole nafate
mangofodipir trisodium	Teslascan
maprotiline HCl (W)	Ludiomil (W)
Marcaine HCl	bupivacaine HCl
Marinol	dronabinol
Marplan	isocarboxazid
Matulane	procarbazine HCl
Mavik	trandolapril
Maxalt	rizatriptan benzoate
Maxalt-MLT	rizatriptan oral disintegrating tablet
Maxaquin	lomefloxacin
Maxipime	cefepime HCl
Maxzide	triamterene 75 mg; hydro-chlorothiazide 50 mg
Maxzide-25MG	triamterene 37.5 mg; hydro-chlorothiazide 25 mg
mazindol	Sanorex
measles, mumps, rubella vaccines, combined	M-M-R II
Mebaral	mephobarbital
mebendazole	Vermox
mecamylamine HCl	Inversine

mechlorethamine HCl	Mustargen
Meclan	meclocycline sulfosalicylate
meclizine	Antivert
meclocycline sulfosalicylate	Meclan
meclofenamate sodium	Meclomen
Meclomen	meclofenamate sodium
Medrol	methylpredniso-lone
medroxyproges-terone acetate	Cycrin Provera Lunelle
medroxyproges-terone acetate; estradiol cypionate inj	
medroxyproges-terone acetate SR	Depo-Provera
mefenamic acid	Ponstel
mefloquine HCl	Lariam
Mefoxin	cefoxitin sodium
Megace	megestrol acetate
megestrol acetate	Megace
Mellaril	thioridazine HCl
meloxicam	Mobic
melphalan	Alkeran
memantine HCl	Namenda
menadiol sodium diphosphate	Synkayvite
Menostar	estradiol trans-dermal system
menotropins	Pergonal Repronex
Mentax	butenafine HCl
meperidine HCl	Demerol
mephentermine sulfate	Wyamine
mephenytoin	Mesantoin
mephobarbital	Mebaral
mepivacaine HCl	Carbocaine
meprobamate	Equanil (WA) Miltown
Mepron	atovaquone
mequinol; tretinoin	Solage
mercaptopurine	Purinethol
Meridia	sibutramine HCl monohydrate
meropenem	Merrem

M
℞

Merrem	meropenem
Meruvax II	rubella virus vaccine live attenuated
mesalamine	Asacol
	Rowasa
Mesantoin	mephenytoin
mesna	Mesnex
Mesnex	mesna
mesoridazine	Serentil
Mestinon	pyridostigmine bromide
Metadate ER	methylphenidate HCl SR
Metaglip	glipizide; metformin
Metamucil	psyllium
Metaprel	metaproterenol sulfate
metaproterenol sulfate	Alupent
	Metaprel
metaraminol bitartrate	Aramine
Metaret	suramin
Metastron	strontium-89 chloride inj
metformin HCl	Glucophage
metformin HCl SR	Glucophage XR
methadone HCl	Dolophine
methamphetamine HCl	Desoxyn
methazolamide	Neptazane
methenamine combination	Urised
methenamine hippurate	Hiprex
Methergine	methylergonovine maleate
methicillin sodium (W)	Staphcillin (W)
methimazole	Tapazole
methocarbamol	Robaxin
methohexital sodium	Brevital Sodium
methotrexate	Mexate
	Rheumatrex
	Trexall
methotrexate, preservative-free inj	Folex PFS
methoxamine HCl (W)	Vasoxyl (W)

methoxsalen	Oxsoralen
methoxsalen extracorporeal administration	Uvadex
methscopamine bromide	Pamine
methyclothiazide	Enduron
methyldopa	Aldomet
methyldopa; hydrochlorothiazide	Aldoril
methylergonovine maleate (W)	Methergine (W)
Methylin	methylphenidate HCl
Methylin ER	methylphenidate HCl SR
methylphenidate HCl	Methylin
	Ritalin
methylphenidate SR	Concerta
	Metadate ER
	Methylin ER
	Ritalin SR
methylprednisolone	Medrol
methylprednisolone acetate SR inj	Depo-Medrol
methylprednisolone sodium succinate inj	Solu-Medrol
methyltestosterone	*methyltestosterone*
methysergide maleate (W)	Sansert (W)
Meticorten	prednisone
metoclopramide HCl	Reglan
metolazone	Mykrox
	Zaroxolyn
Metopirone	metyrapone
metoprolol succinate SR	Toprol XL
metoprolol tartrate	Lopressor
MetroGel-Vaginal	metronidazole vaginal gel
metronidazole	Flagyl
metronidazole SR	Flagyl ER
metronidazole vaginal gel	MetroGel-Vaginal
metyrapone	Metopirone
metyrosine	Demser

Mevacor	lovastatin	Mirena	levonorgestrel-releasing intrauterine system
Mexate	methotrexate		
mexiletine HCl	Mexitil		
Mexitil	mexiletine HCl		
Mezlin (W)	mezlocillin (W)	mirtazapine	Remeron
mezlocillin (W)	Mezlin (W)	misoprostol	Cytotec
Miacalcin	calcitonin-salmon	Mithracin	plicamycin
mibefradil dihydrochloride (W)	Posicor (W)	mitomycin	Mutamycin
		mitotane	Lysodren
		mitoxantrone HCl	Novantrone
Micardis	telmisartan		
Micro K	potassium chloride SR	Mivacron	mivacurium chloride
miconazole nitrate	Monistat	mivacurium chloride	Mivacron
Micronase	glyburide	M-M-R II	measles, mumps, rubella vaccines, combined
Micronor	norethindrone		
Microzide	hydrochloro-thiazide		
Midamor	amiloride HCl	Moban	molindone HCl
midazolam HCl	Versed		
midodrine HCl	ProAmatine	Mobic	meloxicam
Mifeprex	mifepristone	modafinil	Provigil
mifepristone	Mifeprex	Moduretic	amiloride HCl; hydrochloro-thiazide
miglitol	Glyset		
miglustat	Zavesca		
Migranol	dihydroergota-mine mesylate nasal spray	moexipril HCl	Univasc
		moexipril HCl; hydrochloro-thiazide	Uniretic
milrinone lactate	Primacor		
Miltown	meprobamate	molindone HCl	Moban
Minipress	prazosin HCl	mometasone furoate topical	Elocon
Minocin	minocycline HCl		
minocycline HCl	Minocin	Mometasone furoate monohydrate nasal spray	Nasonex
minocycline HCl dental microspheres	Arestin		
		Monistat	miconazole nitrate
minoxidil tablets	Loniten		
minoxidil topical	Rogaine	Monocid (W)	cefonicid sodium (W)
Mintezol	thiabendazole		
Miochol E	acetylcholine ophth	Monopril	fosinopril sodium
MiraLax	polyethylene glycol 3350 powder	montelukast sodium	Singulair
		Monurol	fosfomycin tromethamine
Mirapex	pramipexole dihydrochloride	moricizine	Ethmozine
		morphine sulfate	Roxanol
Mircette	desogestrel; ethinyl estradiol and ethinyl estradiol	morphine sulfate extended-release liposome inj	DepoDur

M
R℞

morphine sulfate, immediate release concentrated oral soln — Roxanol-T

morphine sulfate inj — Duramorph

morphine sulfate SR — Avinza
Kadian
MS Contin
Oramorph SR
Roxanol SR

Motrin — ibuprofen

moxifloxacin HCl — Avelox

MS Contin — morphine sulfate SR

Mucomyst — acetylcysteine

multivitamins for infusion — Cernevit-12
Multi-12 (vial 1 and vial 2)

mupirocin nasal ointment — Bactroban

muromonab-CD3 — Orthoclone OKT3

Muse — alprostadil urethral suppository

Mustargen — mechlorethamine HCl

Mutamycin — mitomycin

M.V.I.-12 — vitamin, multiple inj

Myambutol — ethambutol HCl

Mycelex — clotrimazole

Mycifradin Sulfate — neomycin sulfate oral soln

Myciguent — neomycin sulfate ointment and cream

Mycolog Cream — nystatin; triamcinolone cream

mycophenolate mofetil — CellCept

mycophenolic acid — Myfortic

Mycostatin — nystatin

Mydriacyl — tropicamide

Myfortic — mycophenolic acid

Mykrox — metolazone

Myleran — busulfan

Mylicon — simethicone

Mylotarg — gemtuzumab ozogamicin

Myobloc — botulinum toxin type B

Myochrysine (WA) — gold sodium thiomalate

Myoscint — imciromab pentetate

Mysoline — primidone

N

NABI-HB — hepatitis B immune globulin (human)

nabumetone — Relafen

nadolol — Corgard

Nafcil (W) — nafcillin sodium

nafcillin sodium (W) — Nafcil (W)
Unipen (W)

nalbuphine HCl — Nubain

Nalfon — fenoprofen calcium

nalidixic acid — NegGram

nalmefene HCl — Revex

naloxone HCl — Narcan

naltrexone — ReVia

Namenda — memantine HCl

nandrolone phenpropionate (W) — Durabolin (W)

nandrolone decanoate — Deca-Durabolin

naphazoline ophth soln — Vasocon

Naprelan — naproxen sodium SR

Naprosyn — naproxen

naproxen — Naprosyn

naproxen sodium — Anaprox

naproxen sodium SR — Naprelan

naratriptan HCl — Amerge

Narcan — naloxone HCl

Nardil — phenelzine sulfate

Naropin — ropivacaine HCl

Nasacort — triamcinolone acetonide nasal inhaler

Nasalcrom	cromolyn sodium	Nesacaine	chloroprocaine HCl
Nascobal	cyanocobalamin nasal gel	nesiritide	Natrecor
Nasonex	Mometasone furoate monohydrate nasal spray	netilmicin sulfate	Netromycin
		Netromycin	netilmicin sulfate
nateglinide	Starlix	Neulasta	pegfilgrastim
Natrecor	nesiritide	Neumega	oprelvekin
Navane	thiothixene	Neupogen	filgrastim
Navelbine	vinorelbine tartrate	Neurolite	technetium Tc-99m bicisate kit
Nebcin	tobramycin sulfate	Neurontin	gabapentin
NebuPent	pentamidine isethionate aerosol	Neutrexin	trimetrexate glucuronate
		nevirapine	Viramune
nedocromil inhalation	Tilade	Nexium	esomeprazole magnesium
nedocromil ophth soln	Alocril	niacin SR	Niaspan
			Nicobid
nefazodone HCl (W)	Serzone (W)	Niaspan	niacin SR
NegGram	nalidixic acid	nicardipine HCl	Cardene
nelfinavir mesylate	Viracept	Niclocide	niclosamide
		niclosamide	Niclocide
Nembutal	pentobarbital sodium	Nicobid	niacin SR
		Nicorette	nicotine polacrilex
Neo-Synephrine	phenylephrine HCl		Nicotrol NS
neomycin sulfate ointment and cream	Myciguent	nicotine nasal spray	Nicorette
		nicotine polacrilex	
neomycin sulfate oral soln	Mycifradin Sulfate	nicotine transdermal	Habitrol Nicotrol Prostep
Neoral	cyclosporine capsules (modified) and oral soln	Nicotrol	nicotine transdermal
		Nicotrol NS	nicotine nasal spray
Neosar	cyclophosphamide	nifedipine	Adalat Procardia
Neosporin Cream	polymyxin; neomycin	nifedipine SR	Adalat CC Procardia XL
Neosporin Ointment	polymyxin; neomycin; bacitracin	Nilandron	nilutamide
		nilutamide	Nilandron
Neosporin ophth Ointment	polymyxin; neomycin; bacitracin	Nimbex	cisatracurium besylate
		nimodipine	Nimotop
Neosporin ophth soln	polymyxin; neomycin	Nimotop	nimodipine
		Nipent	pentostatin inj
neostigmine methylsulfate	Prostigmin	Nipride	nitroprusside sodium
		nisoldipine SR	Sular
Neptazane	methazolamide		

N
R

Novolin N	isophane insulin suspension (NPH) (human)	olanzapine	Zyprexa
		olanzapine; fluoxetine	Symbyaz
Novolin R	insulin inj (human)	olmesartan medoxomil	Benicar
NovoLog	insulin aspart (rDNA origin)	olmesartan medoxomil; hydrochloro-thiazide	Benicar HCT
NovoSeven	coagulation factor VII a (recombinant)		
Nubain	nalbuphine HCl	olopatadine HCl ophth soln	Patanol
NuLev	hyoscyamine sulfate orally disintegrating tab	olsalazine sodium	Dipentum
		Olux	clobetasol foam
Numorphan	oxymorphone HCl	omalizumab	Xolair
		omeprazole	Prilosec
Nupercainal	dibucaine	Omnicef	cefdinir
Nuromax	doxacurium chloride	Omnipaque	iohexol
		Oncaspar	pegaspargase
Nuprin	ibuprofen	OncoScint	satumomab pendetide
Nutropin	somatropin for inj		
		Oncovin	vincristine sulfate
Nutropin AQ	somatropin inj		
NuvaRing	etonogestrel; ethinyl estradiol vaginal ring	ondansetron	Zofran
		ondansetron orally disintegrating tab	Zofran ODT
Nydrazid	isoniazid		
nystatin	Mycostatin	Ontak	denileukin diftitox
nystatin topical powder	Nystop		
		Onxol	paclitaxel inj
nystatin; triamcinolone cream	Mycolog Cream	Ophthaine (WA)	proparacaine
		Ophthalgan	glycerin ophth soln
Nystop	nystatin topical powder		
		Ophthetic	proparacaine HCl
		opium; belladonna suppositories	B & O Supprettes
		oprelvekin	Neumega
		Opticrom	cromolyn sodium
O		OptiMark	gadoversetamide
		Optimine	azatadine maleate
OctreoScan	indium In-111 pentetreotide	Optiray	ioversol
		Optivar	azelastine HCl ophth soln
octreotide acetate	Sandostatin		
octreotide acetate susp for inj	Sandostatin LAR Depot	Orabase	benzocaine
		Orajel	benzocaine
		Oramorph SR	morphine sulfate SR
ofloxacin	Floxin		
ofloxacin otic soln	Floxin Otic	Orap	pimozide
		Oretic	hydrochlorothi-azide
Ogen	estropipate		

Orfadin	nitisinone	oxaprozin	Daypro
Organidin NR	guaifenesin	oxazepam	Serax
Orgaran	danaparoid sodium	oxcarbazepine	Trileptal
Orinase	tolbutamide	oxiconazole nitrate cream	Oxistat
Orlaam	levomethadyl acetate HCl	Oxilan	ioxilan
orlistat	Xenical	Oxistat	oxiconazole nitrate cream
Ornade Spansules	phenylpropanol-amine HCl; chlorphenir-amine maleate SR	Oxsoralen	methoxsalen
		oxtriphylline	Choledyl
		oxybate sodium	Xyrem
orphenadrine citrate	Norflex	oxybutynin chloride	Ditropan
orphenadrine citrate; aspirin; caffeine	Norgesic	oxychlorosene sodium	Clorpactin WCS-90
		oxycodone HCl	Percolone Roxicodone
Ortho-Cept	desogestrel; ethinyl estradiol	oxycodone HCl SR	OxyContin
		oxycodone HCl; acetaminophen	Percocet 5/325; 7.5/500; 10/650 Endocet Roxicet
Orthoclone OKT3	muromonab-CD3		
Ortho Evra	norelgestromin; ethinyl estradiol transdermal system	oxycodone HCl; aspirin	Percodan
		OxyContin	oxycodone HCl SR
		oxymetazoline HCl	Afrin nasal spray Dristan Long Lasting
Ortho-Novum (products)	norethindrone; ethinyl estradiol (or mestranol)		
		oxymetholone	Anadrol-50
		oxymorphone HCl	Numorphan
Ortho-Prefest	17β-estradiol; norgestimate	oxytocin	Pitocin
Ortho Tri-Cyclen	norgestimate; ethinyl estradiol (combinations)		

P

Orudis (W)	ketoprofen (W)		
Oruvail	ketoprofen SR		
Os-Cal 500	calcium carbonate	Pacis	BCG intravesical
oseltamivir phosphate	Tamiflu	paclitaxel	Onxol Taxol
Osmovist	iotrolan	palivizumab	Synagis
Otrivin	xylometazoline	Palladone XL	hydromorphone HCl SR
Ovidrel	choriogonado-tropin alfa	palonosetron HCl	Aloxi
Ovral	norgestrel; ethinyl estradiol	Pamelor	nortriptyline HCl
		pamidronate disodium	Aredia
oxaliplatin	Eloxatin	Pamine	methscopolamine bromide
Oxandrin	oxandrolone		
oxandrolone	Oxandrin		

Pancrease	pancrelipase EC	PedvaxHIB	haemophilus b vaccine
pancrelipase	Cotazym		
pancrelipase EC	Cotazym-S	pegaspargase	Oncaspar
	Pancrease	Pegasys	peginterferon alfa-2a
pancuronium bromide	Pavulon		
		pegfilgrastim	Neulasta
Pandel	hydrocortisone buteprate cream	peginterferon alfa-2a	Pegasys
Panretin	alitretinoin	peginterferon alfa-2b (recombinant)	PEG-Intron
pantoprazole	Protonix		
papain; urea oint	Accuzyme		
	Ethezyme	PEG-Intron	peginterferon alfa-2b (recombinant)
papaverine HCl SR	Pavabid		
paracetamol	acetaminophen	pegvisomant	Somavert
Paradione	paramethadione	pemetrexed disodium	Alimta
Paraflex	chlorzoxazone 250 mg		
		pemirolast potassium ophth soln	Alamast
Parafon Forte DSC	chlorzoxazone 500 mg		
paramethadione	Paradione	pemoline	Cylert
Paraplatin	carboplatin	penicillamine	Cuprimine
Parathar	teriparatide acetate	penciclovir cream	Denavir
paregoric	camphorated tincture of opium	penicillin G benzathine	Bicillin L-A (for IM use only) Permapen (for IM use only)
pargyline HCl	Eutonyl	penicillin G benzathine; penicillin G procaine	Bicillin C-R (for IM use only)
paricalcitol	Zemplar		
Parlodel	bromocriptine mesylate		
Parnate	tranylcypromine sulfate	penicillin G procaine	Wycillin (for IM use only)
paromomycin sulfate	Humatin	*penicillin V potassium*	Pen Vee K
paroxetine HCl	Paxil		
Parsidol	ethopropazine HCl	Penlac Nail Lacquer	ciclopirox soln
Paser	aminosalicylic acid		
		pentaerythritol tetranitrate	Peritrate
Patanol	olopatadine HCl ophth soln	pentagastrin	Peptavlon
		Pentam 300	pentamidine isethionate inj
Pavabid	papaverine HCl SR		
Pavulon	pancuronium bromide	pentamidine isethionate aerosol	NebuPent
Paxil	paroxetine HCl		
PBZ	tripelennamine HCl	pentamidine isethionate inj	Pentam 300
PCE Dispertab	erythromycin base coated particles	Pentaspan	pentastarch
		pentastarch	Pentaspan
Pediazole	erythromycin ethylsuccinate; sulfisoxazole	pentazocine HCl	Talwin
		pentazocine HCl; naloxone HCl	Talwin Nx

pentobarbital sodium	Nembutal	Phenaphen with Codeine (#2, 3, and 4) (WA)	acetaminophen 300 mg with Codeine Phosphate (15, 30, and 60 mg)
pentosan polysulfate sodium	Elmiron		
pentostatin inj	Nipent	phenazopyridine HCl	Pyridium
Pentothal	thiopental sodium		
pentoxifylline	Trental	phendimetrazine tartrate	Plegine
Pen Vee K	penicillin V potassium		
Pepcid	famotidine	phenelzine sulfate	Nardil
Pepcid RPD	famotidine, oral disintegrating tablet	Phenergan	promethazine HCl
Peptavlon	pentagastrin	phenobarbital	phenobarbital
Percocet 5/325; 7.5/500; 10/650	oxycodone HCl; acetaminophen	phenobarbital, ergotamine; belladonna	Bellergal-S
Percodan	oxycodone HCl; aspirin	phenoxybenza-mine HCl	Dibenzyline
Percolone	oxycodone HCl	phentermine HCl	Fastin
perflenapent emulsion	EchoGen		
perflubron	Imagent GI	phentermine resin	Ionamin
Pergonal	menotropins		
Periactin	cyproheptadine HCl	phentolamine mesylate (W)	Regitine (W)
Peri-Colace (W)	docusate sodium; casanthranol (W)	phenylbutyrate sodium	Buphenyl
Peridex	chlorhexidine gluconate mouth rinse	phenylephrine HCl	Neo-Synephrine
perindopril erbumine	Aceon	phenylpropanol-amine HCl; chlorphenir-amine maleate SR	Ornade
PerioChip	chlorhexidine gluconate		
Periostat	doxycycline hyclate 20 mg tab & cap	phenylpropanol-amine HCl; guaifenesin SR	Entex LA
Peritrate	pentaerythritol tetranitrate	Phenytek	phenytoin sodium extended
Permapen	penicillin G benzathine (for IM use only)	phenytoin	Dilantin
		phenytoin sodium extended	Phenytek
permethrin	Nix		
Permitil	fluphenazine HCl	Phospholine Iodide (W)	echothiophate iodide (W)
perphenazine	Trilafon	Photofrin	porfimer sodium
perphenazine; amitriptyline HCl	Etrafon Triavil	physostigmine ophth ointment	Eserine Sulfate
Persantine	dipyridamole		
petrolatum, white	Vaseline	physostigmine salicylate	Antilirium

phytonadione	AquaMEPHY-TON	pneumococcal vaccine	Pneumovax
pilocarpine HCl ophth	Isopto Carpine	pneumococcal 7-valent conjugate vaccine	Prevnar
pilocarpine HCl tablet	Salagen	Pneumovax	pneumococcal vaccine
pimecrolimus cream	Elidel	podofilox gel	Condylox
pimozide	Orap	Polaramine Repetabs	dexchlorphenir-amine maleate SR
pindolol	Visken		
pioglitazone HCl	Actos	poliovirus vaccine inactivated	Ipol
pipecuronium bromide	Arduan		
piperacillin sodium (W)	Pipracil (W)	polyethylene glycolelectro-lyte soln	CoLyte GoLYTELY
piperacillin sodium; tazobactam sodium	Zosyn	polyethylene glycol 3350 powder	MiraLax
Pipracil (W)	piperacillin sodium (W)	poly-l-lactic acid	Sculptra
piroxicam	Feldene	polymyxin B sulfate; trimethoprim ophth soln	Polytrim
Pitocin	oxytocin		
Pitressin	vasopressin		
Placidyl	ethchlorvynol		
Plan B	levonorgestrel	polymyxin; neomycin	Neosporin Cream Neosporin ophth soln
Plaquenil	hydroxy-chloroquine sulfate		
Plasbumin	albumin human	polymyxin; neomycin; bacitracin	Neosporin Ointment Neosporin ophth Ointment
plasma protein fraction	Plasma-Plex Plasmanate Plasmatein Protenate		
		polystyrene sulfonate sodium	Kayexalate
Plasma-Plex	plasma protein fraction	polythiazide (W)	Renese (W)
Plasmanate	plasma protein fraction	Polytrim	polymyxin B sulfate; trimethoprim ophth soln
Plasmatein	plasma protein fraction		
Platinol AQ	cisplatin	Pondimin (W)	fenfluramine HCl (W)
Plavix	clopidogrel bisulfate		
		Ponstel	mefenamic acid
Plegine	phendimetrazine tartrate	Pontocaine	tetracaine HCl
		poractant alpha intratracheal susp	Curosurf
Plenaxis	abarelix		
Plendil	felodipine		
Pletal	cilostazol	porfimer sodium	Photofrin
Plexion	sulfacetamide sodium and sulfur lotion		
		Posicor (W)	mibefradil dihydro-chloride (W)
plicamycin	Mithracin		

potassium bicarbonate; potassium citrate effervescent	K-Lyte	Preven Emergency Contraceptive Kit	levonorgestrel; ethinyl estradiol
potassium chloride; potassium bicarbonate effervescent	K-Lyte/Cl	Prevacid	lansoprazole
		Prevnar	pneumococcal 7-valent conjugate vaccine
potassium chloride SR	Kaon-Cl K-Dur Klor-Con 10 Slow-K Micro K	Preveon	adefovir dipivoxil
		Prevpac	lansoprazole; amoxicillin; clarithromycin
		Priftin	rifapentine
potassium chloride; potassium gluconate	Kolyum	Prilosec	omeprazole
		Primacor	milrinone lactate
		Primaxin	imipenemcila-statin sodium
potassium citrate tab	Urocit-K	primidone	Mysoline
		Primsol (W)	trimethoprim (W)
potassium gluconate	Kaon	Principen	ampicillin
		Prinivil	lisinopril
povidone iodine	Betadine	Priscoline	tolazoline
pralidoxime chloride	Protopam	ProAmatine	midodrine HCl
		Pro-Banthine	propantheline bromide
pramipexole dihydrochloride	Mirapex	probenecid	Benemid
		probenecid; colchicine	ColBENEMID (W)
pramoxine HCl	Tronothane HCl	procainamide	Pronestyl
		procainamide HCl SR	Procan SR Procanbid
Prandin	repaglinide	procaine HCl	Novocain HCl
prasterone	Aslera	Procan SR	procainamide HCl SR
Pravachol	pravastatin sodium		
pravastatin sodium	Pravachol	Procanbid	procainamide HCl SR
prazosin HCl	Minipress	procarbazine HCl	Matulane
Precedex	dexmedetomidine HCl inj	Procardia	nifedipine
		Procardia XL	nifedipine SR
Precose	acarbose	Prochieve	progesterone gel
prednisolone syrup	Prelone	prochlorperazine	Compazine
		Procrit	epoetin alfa
prednisone	Deltasone Meticorten	procyclidine HCl	Kemadrin
		progesterone gel	Crinone Prochieve
Prelone	prednisolone syrup	progesterone micronized	Prometrium
Premarin	estrogens, conjugated		
		Prograf	tacrolimus
Premphase	estrogens, conjugated	ProHance	gadoteridol
Prempro	estrogens, conjugated; medroxyproges-terone acetate	ProHIBiT	haemophilus b vaccine
Prepidil	dinoprostone gel		

Prokine (WA)	sargramostim	Prostin VR	alprostadil
Prolastin	alpha₁-proteinase inhibitor (human)	protamine sulfate	protamine sulfate
		Protenate	plasma protein fraction
Proleukin	aldesleukin	Protonix	pantoprazole
Prolixin	fluphenazine HCl	Protopam	pralidoxime chloride
Proloid (W)	thyroglobulin (W)		
promethazine HCl	Phenergan	Protopic	tacrolimus oint
		protriptyline HCl	Vivactil
Prometrium	progesterone micronized	Protropin	somatrem
		Protropin II	somatropin for inj
Pronestyl	procainamide	Proventil	albuterol
Propacet-100	propoxyphene napsylate; acetaminophen	Proventil HFA	albuterol sulfate inhalation aerosol
propafenone HCl	Rythmol	Proventil Repetabs	albuterol SR
propantheline bromide	Pro-Banthine		
		Provera	medroxyproges- terone acetate
proparacaine HCl	Ophthaine (WA)		
	Ophthetic	Provigil	modafinil
Propecia	finasteride tablets 1 mg	Prozac	fluoxetine HCl
		Prudoxin	doxepin HCl cream
Propine	dipivefrin		
propofol	Diprivan	Prussian blue	Radiogardase
propoxyphene HCl	Darvon	pseudoephedrine HCl	Sudafed
propoxyphene HCl; acetaminophen	Wygesic	pseudoephedrine HCl; bromphiramine maleate	Drixoral Syrup
propoxyphene HCl; aspirin; caffeine	Darvon Compound 65		
		psyllium	Konsyl-D Metamucil
propoxyphene napsylate; acetaminophen	Darvocet-N 100 Propacet-100	Pulmicort Turbuhaler	budesonide inhalation powder
propranolol HCl	Inderal	Pulmozyme	dornase alfa
propranolol HCl; hydrochlorothi- azide	Inderide	Purinethol	mercaptopurine
		Pyridium	phenazopyridine HCl
Propulsid (W)	cisapride (W)	pyridostigmine bromide	Mestinon
Proscar	finasteride tablets 5 mg		
ProSom	estazolam	pyrimethamine	Daraprim
ProstaScint	capromab pendetide	pyrimethamine; sulfadoxine	Fansidar
Prostep	nicotine transdermal system		
		Q	
Prostigmin	neostigmine methylsulfate		
Prostin E₂	dinoprostone vaginal suppositories	Quadramet	samarium SM 153 lexidronam

Quarzan (W)	clidinium bromide (W)	Raplon (W)	rapacuronium bromide (W)
Questran	cholestyramine	Raptiva	efalizumab
quetiapine fumerate	Seroquel	rasburicase	Elitek
		rattlesnake anti-venom	CroFab
Quinaglute	quinidine gluconate SR	Raxar (W)	grepafloxacin HCl (W)
quinapril HCl	Accupril	Rebetol	ribavirin
quinapril; hydrochloro-thiazide	Accuretic	Rebetron	ribavirin; inter-feron alfa-2b
quinethazone	Hydromox	Rebif	interferon beta-1a
Quinidex Extentabs	quinidine sulfate SR	reboxetine mesylate	Vestra
quinidine gluconate SR	Quinaglute	Recombivax HB	hepatitis B vaccine
quinidine sulfate	quinidine sulfate	Redux (W)	dexfenfluramine HCl (W)
quinidine sulfate SR	Quinidex Extentabs	Refacto	antihemophilic factor (recombinant)
quinupristin; dalfopristin	Synercid	Refludan	lepirudin
Quixin	levofloxacin ophth soln	Regitine (W)	phentolamine mesylate (W)
Qvar	beclomethasone diproprionate inhalation aerosol	Reglan	metoclopramide HCl
		Regranex	becaplermin gel
		Regroton	chlorthalidone; reserpine
		Relafen	nabumetone
R		Relenza	zanamivir for inhalation
		Relpax	eletriptan hydrobromide
RabAvert	rabies vaccine for human use	Remeron	mirtazapine
		Remicade	infliximab
rabeprazole sodium	Aciphex	remifentanil HCl	Ultiva
rabies immune globulin, human	Hyperab (W) Imogam	Reminyl	galanthamine HBr
		Remodulin	treprostinil sodium
rabies vaccine, adsorbed	rabies vaccine, adsorbed	Renagel	sevelamer HCl
rabies vaccine for human use	RabAvert	Renese (W)	polythiazide (W)
		Renova	tretinion topical
Radiogardase	Prussian blue	Renovue 65	iodamide meglumine
raloxifene HCl	Evista	ReoPro	abciximab
ramipril	Altace	repaglinide	Prandin
ranitidine bismuth citrate	Tritec	Repronex	menotropins
		Requip	ropinirole HCl
ranitidine HCl	Zantac	Rescriptor	delavirdine mesylate
rapacuronium bromide (W)	Raplon (W)	Rescula	unoprostone isopropyl ophth soln
Rapamune	sirolimus		

reserpine	Serpasil	rimexolone	Vexol
RespiGam	respiratory syncytial virus immune globulin intravenous (human)	Riopan	magaldrate
		risedronate sodium	Actonel
respiratory syncytial virus immune globulin intravenous (human)	RespiGam	Risperdal	risperidone
		risperidone	Risperdal
		Ritalin	methylphenidate HCl
		Ritalin SR	methylphenidate SR
Restasis	cyclosporine ophth emulsion	ritodrine HCl (W)	Yutopar (W)
		ritonavir	Norvir
Restoril	temazepam	Rituxan	rituximab
Retavase	reteplase	rituximab	Rituxan
reteplase	Retavase	rivastigmine tartrate	Exelon
Retin-A	tretinoin topical	rizatriptan benzoate	Maxalt
Retin-A Micro	tretinoin gel		
Retrovir	zidovudine	rizatriptan oral disintegrating tablet	Maxalt-MLT
Revex	nalmefene HCl		
ReVia	naltrexone	Robaxin	methocarbamol
Reyataz	atazanavir sulfate	Robinul	glycopyrrolate
Rezulin (W)	troglitazone (W)	Robitussin	guaifenesin
R-Gene	arginine HCl	Robitussin A-C	guaifenesin; codeine phosphate
Rheumatrex	methotrexate tablets		
Rhinocort	budesonide nasal inhaler	Robitussin-DM	guaifenesin; dextromethorphan
RH$_O$ (D) immune globulin	RhoGAM		
		Rocaltrol	calcitriol
RH$_O$ (D) immune globulin IV (human)	WinRho SD	Rocephin	ceftriaxone sodium
		rofecoxib (W)	Vioxx (W)
		Roferon-A	interferon alfa-2a
RhoGAM	RH$_O$ (D) immune globulin	Rogaine	minoxidil topical
		Romazicon	flumazenil
ribavirin	Rebetol Virazole	ropinirole HCl	Requip
		ropivacaine HCl	Naropin
ribavirin; interferon alfa-2b	Rebetron	Rosiglitazone maleate	Avandia
		rosiglitazone maleate; metformin HCl	Avandamet
Ridaura	auranofin		
Rifadin	rifampin		
Rifamate	isoniazid; rifampin	rosuvastatin calcium	Crestor
		Rotashield (W)	rotavirus (W) vaccine, live, oral, tetravalent
rifampin	Rifadin Rimactane		
rifapentine	Priftin	rotavirus vaccine, live, oral, (W) tetravalent	Rotashield (W)
rifaximin	Xifaxan		
Rilutek	riluzole		
riluzole	Rilutek		
Rimactane	rifampin	Rowasa	mesalamine
rimantadine	Flumadine		

Roxanol	morphine sulfate	saquinavir soft	Fortovase
Roxanol SR	morphine sulfate SR	gel capsule	
		Sarafem	fluoxetine
Roxanol-T	morphine sulfate, immediate release concentrated oral soln	sargramostim	Leukine Prokine (WA)
		satumomab pendetide	OncoScint
Roxicet	oxycodone HCl; acetaminophen	Sclerosol	talc, sterile aerosol
Roxicodone	oxycodone HCl	Scopace	scopolamine hydrobromide, soluble tab
rubella virus vaccine live attenuated	Meruvax II		
Rubex	doxorubicin HCl	scopolamine hydrobromide ophth	Isopto Hyoscine
Rythmol	propafenone HCl		
		scopolamine hydrobromide, soluble tab	Scopace

S

		scopolamine transdermal	Transderm Scop
sacrosidase	Sucraid	Sculptra	poly-l-lactic acid
Saizen	somatropin	Seasonale	ethinyl estradiol; levonorgestrel (91 day cycle)
Salagen	pilocarpine HCl tablet		
salbutamol sulfate	albuterol sulfate	Sectral	acebutolol HCl
		Seldane (W)	terfenadine (W)
salmeterol xinafoate	Serevent	Seldane D (W)	terfenadine; pseudoephedrine HCl (W)
salmeterol xinafoate inhalation powder	Serevent Diskus		
		selegiline HCl	Carbex Eldepryl
salsalate	Disalcid	selenium sulfide	Selsun Blue
Sal-Tropine	atropine sulfate tablets	Selsun Blue	selenium sulfide
		sennosides	Ex Lax
Saluron	hydroflumethiazide	sennosides	Senokot
		sennosides; docusate sodium	Senokot-S
samarium SM 153 lexidronam	Quadramet		
		Senokot	senna concentrates
Sanctura	trospium chloride		
Sandimmune	cyclosporine	Senokot-S	sennosides; docusate sodium
Sandoglobulin	immune globulin intravenous		
		Sensipar	cinacalcet HCl
Sandostatin	octreotide acetate	Septocaine	articaine; epinephrine
Sandostatin LAR Depot	octreotide acetate susp for inj		
		Septra	sulfamethoxazoletrimethoprim
Sanorex	mazindol		
Sansert (W)	methysergide maleate (W)		
		Ser-Ap-Es	hydralazine; hydrochlorothiazide; reserpine
Santyl	collagenase		
saquinavir mesylate	Invirase		

Serax	oxazepam	Slow-Mag	magnesium chloride SR
Serentil	mesoridazine		
Serevent	salmeterol xinafoate	sodium citrate; citric acid	Bicitra
Serevent Diskus	salmeterol xinafoate inhalation powder	sodium ferric gluconate complex in sucrose inj	Ferrlecit
Serlect	sertindole	sodium fluoride	Luride
sermorelin acetate	Geref	sodium hyaluronate	Amvisc Healon
Seromycin	cycloserine		Hyalgan
Seroquel	quetiapine fumarate	sodium oxybate	Xyrem
Serostim	somatropin (rDNA origin) for inj	sodium phenylbutyrate sodium phosphate tab	Buphenyl Visicol
Serpasil	*reserpine*	sodium sulfacetamide lotion	Klaron
sertaconazole	Ertaczo		
sertindole	Serlect		
sertraline HCl	Zoloft	sodium tetradecyl sulfate	Sotradecol
Serzone (W)	nefazodone HCl (W)		
sevelamer HCl	Renagel	Solage	mequinol; tretinoin
sevoflurane	Ultane		
short chain fatty acids enema	Colomed	Solaraze Solganal	diclofenac gel aurothioglucose
sibutramine HCl monohydrate	Meridia	Solu-Cortef	hydrocortisone sodium succinate
sildenafil citrate	Viagra		
Silvadene	silver sulfadiazine	Solu-Medrol	methylpredniso- lone sodium succinate
silver sulfadiazine	Silvadene	Soma	carisoprodol
simethicone	Mylicon	somatostatin	Zecnil
Simulect	basiliximab	somatrem	Protropin
simvastatin	Zocor	somatropin for inj	Genotropin
Sinemet	levodopa; carbidopa		Humatrope Norditropin
Sinemet CR	levodopa; carbidopa SR		Nutropin Protropin II Saizen
Sinequan	doxepin HCl		
Singulair	montelukast sodium	somatropin inj somatropin (rDNA origin) for inj	Nutropin AQ Serostim
sirolimus	Rapamune		
Skelid	tiludronate disodium	Somavert	pegvisomant
		Sonata	zaleplon
Slo-bid	theophylline SR	Soriatane	acitretin
Slo-Phyllin	theophylline	sotalol	Betapace
Slow Fe	ferrous sulfate SR	Sotradecol	sodium tetradecyl sulfate
Slow-K	potassium chloride SR		

S
Ŗ

sparfloxacin	Zagam	Sufenta	sufentanil citrate
stavudine	Zerit		
spectinomycin HCl	Trobicin	sufentanil citrate	Sufenta
Spectracef	cefditoren pivoxil	Sulamyd sodium	sulfacetamide sodium ophth
		Sular	Nisoldipine SR
Spiriva HandiHaler	tiotropium bromide inhalation powder	sulfacetamide sodium and sulfur lotion	Plexion
spironolactone	Aldactone	sulfacetamide sodium ophth	Sulamyd sodium
spironolactone; hydrochloroth-iazide	Aldactazide	sulfadoxine; pyrimethamine	Fansidar
Sporanox	itraconazole	sulfamethoxazole (W)	Gantanol (W)
Stadol	butorphanol tartrate inj	sulfamethoxazole-trimethoprim	Bactrim Cotrim co-trimoxazole Septra
Stadol NS	butorphanol tartrate nasal spray		
		sulfasalazine	Azulfidine
Stalevo	levodopa; carbidopa; entacapone	sulfinpyrazone	Anturane
		sulindac	Clinoril
		Sultrin	triple sulfa vaginal cream
stanozolol	Winstrol		
Staphcillin	methicillin sodium	sumatriptan	Imitrex
Starlix	nateglinide	Sumycin	tetracycline HCl
Stelazine	trifluoperazine HCl	Suprane	desflurane
Strattera	Atomoxetine HCl	Suprax (W)	cefixime (W)
Streptase	streptokinase	suramin	Metaret
streptokinase	Streptase	Surmontil	trimipramine maleate
streptomycin sulfate	streptomycin sulfate	Survanta	beractant
streptozocin	Zanosar	Sustiva	Efavirenz
Striant	testosterone buccal	Symbyax	olanzapine; fluoxetine
Stromectol	ivermectin	Symmetrel	amantadine HCl
strontium-89 chloride inj	Metastron	Synagis	palivizumab
Sublimaze	fentanyl citrate	Synalar	fluocinolone acetonide
Suboxone	buprenorphine HCl; naloxone HCl	Synercid	quinupristin; dalfopristin
Subutex	buprenorphine HCl	Synkayvite	menadiol sodium diphosphate
succinylcholine chloride	Anectine	synopinine	Florotag
		synthetic conjugated estrogens, A	Cenestin
Sucraid	sacrosidase		
sucralfate	Carafate	Synthroid	levothyroxine sodium
Sudafed	pseudoephedrine HCl	Synvisc	hylan G-F 20

S
R

444

T

tacrine HCl — Cognex
tacrolimus — Prograf
tacrolimus oint — Protopic
tadalafil — Cialis
Tagamet — cimetidine HCl
talc, sterile aerosol — Sclerosol
Talwin — pentazocine HCl
Talwin Nx — pentazocine HCl; naloxone HCl
Tambocor — flecainide acetate
Tamiflu — oseltamivir phosphate
tamoxifen citrate — Nolvadex
tamsulosin HCl — Flomax
Tapazole — methimazole
Targretin — bexarotene gel
Tarka — trandolapril; verapamil SR
tarzarotene gel — Tazorac
Tasmar — tolcapone
tasosartan — Verdia
Tavist — clemastine fumarate
Taxol — paclitaxel
Taxotere — docetaxel
Tazicef — ceftazidime
Tazidime — ceftazidime
Tazorac — tarzarotene gel
technetium Tc-99m bicisate kit — Neurolite
technetium Tc-99m red blood cell kit — Ultratag
technetium Tc-99m — Cardiotec
technetium Tc99m sestamibi teboroxime kit — Cardiolite
Teczem — enalapril maleate; diltiazem malate
tegaserod maleate — Zelnorm

Tegretol — carbamazepine
Teldrin — chlorpheniramine maleate SR
Telepaque — iopanoic acid
telmisartan — Micardis
temazepam — Restoril
Temodar — temozolomide
temozolomide — Temodar
tenecteplase — TNKase
Tenex — guanfacine HCl
teniposide — Vumon
tenofovir disoproxil fumarate — Viread
Tenoretic — atenolol; chlorthalidone
Tenormin — atenolol
Tensilon — edrophonium chloride
Tenuate — diethylpropion HCl
Tequin — gatifloxacin
Terazol — terconazole
terazosin HCl — Hytrin
terbinafine HCl — Lamisil
terbutaline sulfate aerosol — Brethaire
terbutaline sulfate tablets and inj — Brethine Bricanyl
terconazole — Terazol
terfenadine (W) — Seldane (W)
terfenadine; pseudoephedrine HCl (W) — Seldane D (W)
teriparatide — Forteo
teriparatide acetate — Parathar
Teslac — testolactone
Teslascan — mangofodipir trisodium
Testim — testosterone gel
Testoderm — testosterone transdermal
Testoderm TTS — testosterone transdermal
testolactone — Teslac
testosterone buccal — Striant
testosterone cypionate SR — DEPO-Testosterone
testosterone gel — AndroGel Testim

testosterone transdermal	Androderm Testoderm Testoderm TTS	tiagabine HCl Tiamate	Gabitril diltiazem maleate SR
tetracaine HCl	Pontocaine	Tiazac	diltiazem HCl SR
tetracycline HCl	Achromycin (WA) Sumycin	Ticar	ticarcillin disodium
tetrahydrozoline HCl ophth	Collyrium Visine Extra	ticarcillin disodium ticarcillin; clavulanic acid	Ticar Timentin
Teveten	eprosartan mesylate	TICE BCG	BCG intravesical
Teveten HCT	eprosartan mesy- late; hydro- chlorothiazide	Ticlid ticlopidine Tigan	ticlopidine Ticlid trimethobenz- amide HCl
thalidomide	Thalomid	Tikosyn	dofetilide
Thalomid	thalidomide	Tilade	nedocromil
Tham	tromethamine		inhalation
Theo-Dur	theophylline SR	tiludronate	Skelid
theophylline	Elixophyllin Slo-Phyllin	disodium Timentin	ticarcillin;
theophylline SR	Slo-bid Theo-Dur Uniphyl		clavulanic acid
TheraCys	BCG intravesical	timolol maleate ophth soln	Timoptic
Theragran-M	vitamins; minerals	timolol maleate ophth soln, gel forming	Timoptic-XE
thiabendazole	Mintezol		
thiethylperazine maleate	Torecan	timolol maleate	Blocadren
thioguanine	thioguanine	timolol maleate;	Cosopt
thiopental sodium	Pentothal	dorzolamide HCl	
Thioplex	thiotepa	Timoptic-XE	timolol maleate
thioridazine HCl	Mellaril		ophth soln, gel
thiotepa	Thioplex		forming
thiothixene	Navane	Timoptic	timolol maleate
Thorazine	chlorpromazine		ophth soln
Thrombate III	antithrombin III (human)	Tinactin Tindamax	tolnaftate tinidazole
thymalfasin	Zadaxin	Tine Test	tuberculin, old
Thymitaq	nolatrexed dihydrochloride	Tuberculin Old	
Thymoglobulin	anti-thymocyte globulin, (rabbit)	Tine Test PPD	tuberculin, purified protein
thyroglobulin (W)	Proloid (W)		derivative
thyroid	thyroid	tinidazole	Tindamax
Thyrogen	thyrotropin alpha	tinzaparin sodium	Innohep
Thyrolar	liotrix	TNKase	tenecteplase
thyrotropin (W)	Thytropar (W)	tioconazole	Vagistat-1
thyrotropin alpha	Thyrogen	tiotropium bromide inhalation powder	Spiriva HandiHaler
Thytropar (W)	thyrotropin (W)		

T
Rx

T
Rx

triamterene	Dyrenium	tripelennamine HCl	PBZ
triamterene 37.5 mg; hydro-chlorothiazide 25 mg	Maxzide -25MG Dyazide	Triphasil	levonorgestrel; ethinyl estradiol
triamterene 75 mg; hydro-chlorothiazide 50 mg	Maxzide	triple sulfa vaginal cream	Sultrin
		triprolidine HCl; pseudoephe-drine HCl	Actifed
Triavil	perphenazine; amitriptyline HCl	triptorelin pamoate	Trelstar Depot
triazolam	Halcion	triptorelin pamoate (3 month inj)	Trelstar LA
Tricor	fenofibrate		
Tri-Cyclen	norgestimate; ethinyl estradiol	Trisenox	arsenic trioxide
		Tritec	ranitidine bismuth citrate
Tridesilon	desonide		
Tridil	nitroglycerin inj	Tri-Vi-Flor	vitamins A, D, & C; fluoride
Tridione	trimethadione		
trifluoperazine HCl	Stelazine		
trifluridine	Viroptic	Trizivir	lamivudine; zidovudine; abacavir sulfate
trihexyphenidyl HCl (W)	Artane (W)		
Trileptal	oxcarbazepine	Trobicin	spectinomycin HCl
Trilafon	perphenazine		
Tri-Levlen	levonorgestrel; ethinyl estradiol	troglitazone (W)	Rezulin (W)
		tromethamine	Tham
		Tronothane HCl	pramoxine HCl
Trilisate	choline magnesium trisalicylate	TrophAmine	amino acid inj
		Tropicacyl	tropicamide
Tri-Luma	hydroquinone; tretinoin; fluocinolone cream	tropicamide	Mydriacyl Tropicacyl
		trospium chloride	Sanctura
trimethadione	Tridione	trovafloxacin	Trovan tablets
trimethaphan camsylate (W)	Arfonad (W)	Trovan tablet	trovafloxacin mesylate
trimethobenza-mide HCl	Tigan	Trovan inj	alatrofloxacin mesylate IV
trimethoprim (W)	Primsol (W)	Trusopt	dorzolamide HCl
trimetrexate glucuronate	Neutrexin	Truvada	emtricitabine; tenofovir disoproxil
trimipramine maleate	Surmontil	tuberculin, old	Tine Test, Tuberculin Old
Trimox	amoxicillin	tuberculin, purified protein derivative	Tine Test PPD
Tri-Nasal	triamcinolone acetonide nasal spray		
Triostat	liothyronine sodium inj	tuberculin skin test	Aplisol

T
Rx

tubocurarine	tubocurarine	Unipen (W)	nafcillin sodium (W)
Tucks	witch hazel pads	Uniphyl	theophylline SR
Tums	calcium carbonate	Uniretic	moexipril HCl; hydrochloro-thiazide
Tussi-Organidin NR	guaifenesin; codeine phosphate	Univasc	moexipril HCl
Tussionex	hydrocodone polistirex; chlorphenir-amine	Urecholine	bethanechol chloride
		Urised	methenamine combination
Twinrix	hepatitis A inactivated; hepatitis B (recombinant) vaccine	Urispas	flavoxate HCl
		urofollitropin	Bravelle
		urofollitropin for inj	Fertinex
		urokinase	Abbokinase
Tylenol	acetaminophen	unoprostone isopropyl ophth soln	Rescula
Tylenol with Codeine (#2, 3, and 4)	acetaminophen 300 mg with Codeine Phosphate (15, 30, and 60 mg)		
		UroXatral	alfuzosin
		Uprima	apomorphine HCl
		Urocit-K	potassium citrate tab
Typhim Vi	typhoid Vi polysaccharide vaccine	URSO	ursodiol
		ursodiol	Actigall URSO
typhoid Vi polysaccharide vaccine	Typhim Vi	Uvadex	methoxsalen extracorporeal administration
tyropanoate sodium	Bilopaque		

T
Rx

U

V

		Vagifem	estradiol hemihydrate vaginal tab
UbiQGel	coenzyme Q10		
Ultane	sevoflurane		
Ultiva	remifentanil HCl	Vagistat-1	tioconazole
Ultracet	tramadol HCl; acetaminophen	valacyclovir	Valtrex
		Valcyte	valganciclovir
Ultralente U	insulin zinc suspension, extended (beef)	valdecoxib	Bextra
		valganciclovir	Valcyte
		Valium	diazepam
Ultram	tramadol HCl	valproate sodium inj	Depacon
Ultratag	technetium Tc-99m red blood cell kit		
		valproic acid	Depakene
		valrubicin, (for intravesical use)	Valstar
Ultravist	iopromide		
Unasyn	ampicillin sodium; sulbactam sodium	valsartan	Diovan
		valsartan; hydro-chlorothiazide	Diovan HCT

449

Valstar	valrubicin, (for intravesical use)	verapamil HCl SR bedtime formulation	Covera HS Verelan PM
Valtrex	valacyclovir	Verdia	tasosartan
Vancenase	beclomethasone dipropionate	Verelan	verapamil HCl SR
Vancenase AQ Nasal	beclomethasone dipropionate	Verelan PM	verapamil HCl SR bedtime formulation
Vanceril	beclomethasone dipropionate	Verluna	nofetumomab
Vancocin	vancomycin HCl	Vermox	mebendazole
vancomycin HCl	Vancocin	Versed	midazolam HCl
Vaniqa	eflornithine HCl cream	verteporfin inj	Visudyne
Vantin	cefpodoxime proxetil	Vesanoid	tretinoin capsules
Vaponefrin	epinephrine racemic	Vestra	reboxetine mesylate
		Vexol	rimexolone
Vaqta	hepatitis A vaccine, inactivated	Vfend	voriconazole
		Viactiv	calcium carbonate; vitamin D and K chewable
vardenafil HCl	Levitra		
varicella virus vaccine	Varivax	Viadur	leuprolide acetate implant
Varivax	varicella virus vaccine	Viagra	sildenafil citrate
Vascor (W)	bepridil (W)	Vibramycin	doxycycline hyclate
Vaseline	petrolatum, white		
Vaseretic	enalapril maleate; hydrochloro-thiazide	Vicodin	hydrocodone bitartrate; acetaminophen
Vasocon	naphazoline ophth soln	Vicoprofen	hydrocodone bitartrate 7.5 mg; ibuprofen 200 mg
Vasodilan	isoxsuprine HCl		
vasopressin	Pitressin	vidarabine monohydrate	Vira-A
Vasotec	enalapril maleate		
Vasoxyl (W)	methoxamine HCl (W)	Vidaza	azacitidine
		Videx	didanosine
vecuronium bromide	Norcuron	Videx EC	didanosine SR
		vinblastine sulfate	Velban
Velban	vinblastine sulfate		
Velcade	bortezomib	vincristine sulfate	Oncovin
Velosef	cephradine		
Velosulin Human	insulin inj (human)	vindesine sulfate	Eldisine
		vinorelbine tartrate	Navelbine
venlafaxine HCl	Effexor		
venlafaxine HCl SR	Effexor XR	Vioform	clioquinol
		Vioxx (W)	rofecoxib (W)
Venofer	iron sucrose inj	Vira-A	vidarabine monohydrate
Ventolin	albuterol		
VePesid	etoposide	Viracept	nelfinavir mesylate
verapamil HCl	Isoptin		
verapamil HCl SR	Calan SR Verelan	Viramune	nevirapine

Virazole	ribavirin
Viread	tenofovir disoproxil fumarate
Viroptic	trifluridine
Visicol	sodium phosphate tab
Visine Extra	tetrahydrozoline HCl ophth
Visipaque	iodixanol
Visken	pindolol
Vistaril	hydroxyzine pamoate
Vistide	cidofovir
Visudyne	verteporfin inj
Vitravene	fomivirsen sodium inj
Vivelle	estradiol trans-dermal system
Volmax	albuterol SR
Voltaren	diclofenac sodium
Voltaren-XR	diclofenac sodium SR
voriconazole	Vfend
Vumon	teniposide
Vytorin	ezetimibe; simvastatin

W

warfarin sodium	Coumadin
Welchol	colesevelam HCl
Wellbutrin	bupropion HCl
Wellbutrin SR	bupropion HCl SR
Wellcovorin (WA)	*leucovorin calcium*
Wellferon	interferon ALFA-n[1] lymphoblastoid
WinRho SD	RH$_O$ (D) immune globulin IV (human)
Winstrol	stanozolol
witch hazel pads	Tucks
Wyamine	mephentermine sulfate
Wycillin (for IM use only)	penicillin G procaine (for IM use only)
Wydase	hyaluronidase

Wygesic	propoxyphene HCl; acetaminophen
Wymox	amoxicillin
Wytensin	guanabenz acetate

XYZ

Xalatan	latanoprost
Xanax	alprazolam
Xeloda	capecitabine
Xenical	orlistat
Xifaxan	rifaximin
Xigris	drotrecogin alfa
Xolair	omalizumab
Xopenex	levalbuterol HCl inhalation soln
Xylocaine HCl	lidocaine HCl
xylometazoline	Otrivin
Xyrem	oxybate sodium
Yasmin	drospirenone; ethinyl estradiol
Yutopar (W)	ritodrine HCl (W)
Zadaxin	thymalfasin
Zaditor	ketotifen fumarate ophth soln
zafirlukast	Accolate
Zagam	sparfloxacin
zalcitabine	Hivid
zaleplon	Sonata
Zanaflex	tizanidine HCl
zanamivir for inhalation	Relenza
Zanosar	streptozocin
Zantac	ranitidine HCl
Zarontin	ethosuximide
Zaroxolyn	metolazone
Zavesca	miglustat
Zecnil	somatostatin
Zelnorm	tegaserod maleate
Zemplar	paricalcitol
Zenapax	daclizumab
Zerit	stavudine
Zestoretic	lisinopril; hydrochloro-thiazide
Zestril	lisinopril
Zetar	coal tar product
Zetia	ezetimibe

V
R̸

Zevalin	ibritumomab tiuxetan	Zoloft	sertraline HCl
Ziac	bisoprolol fumarate; hydrochloro- thiazide	zolpidem tartrate	Ambien
		Zometa	zoledronic acid for inj
		Zomig	zolmitriptan
Ziagen	abacavir sulfate	Zomig-ZMT	zolmitriptan orally disintegrating tablet
zidovudine	Retrovir		
zidovudine; lamivudine	Combivir		
zileuton	Zyflo	Zonegram	zonisamide
Zinacef	cefuroxime sodium	zonisamide	Zonegram
zinc acetate	Galzin	Zosyn	piperacillin so- dium; tazobac tam sodium
Zinecard	dexrazoxane		
ziprasidone HCl	Geodon		
Zithromax	azithromycin	Zovirax	acyclovir
Zocor	simvastatin	Zyban	bupropion HCl SR
Zofran	ondansetron		
Zofran ODT	ondansetron orally disintegrating tab	Zydone 5/400, 7.5/400, 10/400	hydrocodone bitartrate; acetaminophen
		Zyflo	zileuton
Zoladex	goserelin acetate implant	Zyloprim	allopurinol
		Zymar	gatifloxacin opth soln
zoledronic acid for inj	Zometa	Zyprexa	olanzapine
zolmitriptan	Zomig	Zyrtec	cetirizine HCl
zolmitriptan orally disintegrating tablet	Zomig-ZMT	Zyrtec-D	cetirizine HCl; pseudo- ephedrine HCl SR
		Zyvox	linezolid

References

1. Facts and Comparisons. St. Louis: Facts and Comparisons, Inc. (published monthly and online)
2. Billup NF, Billup SM. American drug index. St. Louis: Facts and Comparisons, Inc.yw (published yearly)
3. Sweetman SC. Ed. Martindale: 33rd edition. The Pharmaceutical Press. London, 2002.

Chapter 9

Normal Laboratory Values*

In the following tables, normal reference values for commonly requested laboratory tests are listed in traditional units and in SI units. The tables are a guideline only. Values are method dependent and "normal values" may vary between laboratories.

	Blood, Plasma or Serum	
	Reference Value	
Determination	Conventional Units	SI Units
Ammonia (NH_3) — diffusion	20–120 mcg/dl	12–70 mcmol/L
Ammonia Nitrogen	15–45 mcg/dl	11–32 μmol/L
Amylase	35–118 IU/L	0.58–1.97 mckat/L
Anion Gap ($Na^+ - [Cl^- + HCO_3^-]$) (P)	7–16 mEq/L	7–16 mmol/L
Antinuclear antibodies	negative at 1:10 dilution of serum	negative at 1:10 dilution of serum
Antithrombin III (AT III)	80–120 units/dl	800–1200 units/L
Bicarbonate: Arterial Venous	21–28 mEq/L 22–29 mEq/L	21–28 mmol/L 22–29 mmol/L
Bilirubin: Conjugated (direct) Total	≤0.2 mg/dl 0.1–1 mg/dl	≤4 mcmol/L 2–18 mcmol/L
Calcitonin	<100 pg/mL	<100 ng/L
Calcium: Total Ionized	8.6–10.3 mg/dl 4.4–5.1 mg/dl	2.2–2.74 mmol/L 1–1.3 mmol/L
Carbon dioxide content (plasma)	21–32 mmol/L	21–32 mmol/L
Carcinoembryonic antigen	<3 ng/mL	<3 mcg/L
Chloride	95–110 mEq/L	95–110 mmol/L
Coagulation screen: Bleeding time Prothrombin time Partial thromboplastin time (activated) Protein C Protein S	3–9.5 min 10–13 sec 22–37 sec 0.7–1.4 μ/mL 0.7–1.4 μ/mL	180–570 sec 10–13 sec 22–37 sec 700–1400 units/mL 700–1400 units/mL
Copper, total	70–160 mcg/dl	11–25 mcmol/L
Corticotropin (ACTH adrenocorticotropic hormone) — 0800 hr	<60 pg/mL	<13.2 pmol/L
Cortisol: 0800 hr 1800 hr 2000 hr	5–30 mcg/dl 2–15 mcg/dl ≤50% of 0800 hr	138–810 nmol/L 50–410 nmol/L ≤50% of 0800 hr
Creatine kinase: Female Male	20–170 IU/L 30–220 IU/L	0.33–2.83 mckat/L 0.5–3.67 mckat/L
Creatine kinase isoenzymes, MB fraction	0–12 IU/L	0–0.2 mckat/L
Creatinine	0.5–1.7 mg/dl	44–150 mcmol/L
Fibrinogen (coagulation factor I)	150–360 mg/dl	1.5–3.6 g/L

Normal Laboratory Values (Cont.) Blood

	Blood, Plasma or Serum (Cont.)	
	Reference Value	
Determination	**Conventional Units**	**SI Units**
Follicle-stimulating hormone (FSH):		
Female	2–13 mIU/mL	2–13 IU/L
Midcycle	5–22 mIU/mL	5–22 IU/L
Male	1–8 mIU/mL	1–8 IU/L
Glucose, fasting	65–115 mg/dl	3.6–6.3 mmol/L
Glucose Tolerance Test (Oral)	mg/dL	mmol/L
	Normal	Normal
Fasting	70–105	3.9–5.8
60 min	120–170	6.7–9.4
90 min	100–140	5.6–7.8
120 min	70–120	3.9–6.7
	Diabetic	Diabetic
Fasting	>140	>7.8
60 min	≥200	≥11.1
90 min	≥200	≥11.1
120 min	≥140	≥7.8
(γ) − Glutamyltransferase (GGT):		
Male	9–50 units/L	9–50 units/L
Female	8–40 units/L	8–40 units/L
Haptoglobin	44–303 mg/dl	0.44–3.03 g/L
Hematologic tests:		
Fibrinogen	200–400 mg/dl	2–4 g/L
Hematocrit (Hct), female	36%–44.6%	0.36–0.446 fraction of 1
male	40.7%–50.3%	0.4–0.503 fraction of 1
Hemoglobin A_{1C}	5.3%–7.5% of total Hgb	0.053–0.075
Hemoglobin (Hb), female	12.1–15.3 g/dl	121–153 g/L
male	13.8–17.5 g/dl	138–175 g/L
Leukocyte count (WBC)	3800–9800/mcl	$3.8–9.8 \times 10^9$/L
Erythrocyte count (RBC), female	$3.5–5 \times 10^6$/mcl	$3.5–5 \times 10^{12}$/L
male	$4.3–5.9 \times 10^6$/mcl	$4.3–5.9 \times 10^{12}$/L
Mean corpuscular volume (MCV)	80–97.6 mcm^3	80–97.6 fl
Mean corpuscular hemoglobin (MCH)	27–33 pg/cell	1.66–2.09 fmol/cell
Mean corpuscular hemoglobin concentrate (MCHC)	33–36 g/dl	20.3–22 mmol/L
Erythrocyte sedimentation rate (sedrate, ESR)	≤30 mm/hr	≤30 mm/hr
Erythrocyte enzymes:	250–5000 units/10^6 cells	250–5000 mcunits/cell
Glucose-6-phosphate dehydrogenase (G-6-PD)		
Ferritin	10–383 ng/mL	23–862 pmol/L
Folic acid: normal	>3.1–12.4 ng/mL	7–28.1 nmol/L
Platelet count	$150–450 \times 10^3$/mcl	$150–450 \times 10^9$/L
Reticulocytes	0.5%–1.5% of erythrocytes	0.005–0.015
Vitamin B_{12}	223–1132 pg/mL	165–835 pmol/L
Iron: Female	30–160 mcg/dl	5.4–31.3 mcmol/L
Male	45–160 mcg/dl	8.1–31.3 mcmol/L
Iron binding capacity	220–420 mcg/dl	39.4–75.2 mcmol/L
Isocitrate Dehydrogenase	1.2–7 units/L	1.2–7 units/L
Isoenzymes		
Fraction 1	14%–26% of total	0.14–0.26 fraction of total
Fraction 2	29%–39% of total	0.29–0.39 fraction of total
Fraction 3	20%–26% of total	0.20–0.26 fraction of total
Fraction 4	8%–16% of total	0.08–0.16 fraction of total
Fraction 5	6%–16% of total	0.06–0.16 fraction of total
Lactate dehydrogenase	100–250 IU/L	1.67–4.17 mckat/L

Normal Laboratory Values (Cont.) Blood

Blood, Plasma or Serum (Cont.)		
	Reference Value	
Determination	**Conventional Units**	**SI Units**
Lactic acid (lactate)	6–19 mg/dl	0.7–2.1 mmol/L
Lead	≤50 mcg/dl	≤2.41 mcmol/L
Lipase	10–150 units/L	10–150 units/L
Lipids:		
Total Cholesterol		
Desirable	<200 mg/dl	<5.2 mmol/L
Borderline-high	200–239 mg/dl	<5.2–6.2 mmol/L
High	>239 mg/dl	>6.2 mmol/L
LDL		
Desirable	<130 mg/dl	<3.36 mmol/L
Borderline-high	130–159 mg/dl	3.36–4.11 mmol/L
High	>159 mg/dl	>4.11 mmol/L
HDL (low)	<35 mg/dl	<0.91 mmol/L
Triglycerides		
Desirable	<200 mg/dl	<2.26 mmol/L
Borderline-high	200–400 mg/dl	2.26–4.52 mmol/L
High	400–1000 mg/dl	4.52–11.3 mmol/L
Very high	>1000 mg/dl	>11.3 mmol/L
Magnesium	1.3–2.2 mEq/L	0.65–1.1 mmol/L
Osmolality	280–300 mOsm/kg	280–300 mmol/kg
Oxygen saturation (arterial)	94%–100%	0.94–1 fraction of 1
PCO_2, arterial	35–45 mm Hg	4.7–6 kPa
pH, arterial	7.35–7.45	7.35–7.45
PO_2, arterial: Breathing room air[1]	80–105 mm Hg	10.6–14 kPa
On 100% O_2	<500 mm Hg	
Phosphatase (acid), total at 37°C	0.13–0.63 IU/L	2.2–10.5 IU/L or 2.2–10.5 mckat/L
Phosphatase alkaline[2]	20–130 IU/L	20–130 IU/L or 0.33–2.17 mckat/L
Phosphorus, inorganic,[3] (phosphate)	2.5–5 mg/dl	0.8–1.6 mmol/L
Potassium	3.5–5 mEq/L	3.5–5 mmol/L
Progesterone		
Female	0.1–1.5 ng/mL	0.32–4.8 nmol/L
Follicular phase	0.1–1.5 ng/mL	0.32–4.8 nmol/L
Luteal phase	2.5–28 ng/mL	8–89 nmol/L
Male	<0.5 ng/mL	<1.6 nmol/L
Prolactin	1.4–24.2 ng/mL	1.4–24.2 mcg/L
Prostate specific antigen	0–4 ng/mL	0–4 ng/mL
Protein: Total	6–8 g/dl	60–80 g/L
Albumin	3.6–5 g/dl	36–50 g/L
Globulin	2.3–3.5 g/dl	23–35 g/L
Rheumatoid factor	<60 IU/mL	<60 kIU/L
Sodium	135–147 mEq/L	135–147 mmol/L
Testosterone: Female	6–86 ng/dl	0.21–3 mmol/L
Male	270–1070 ng/dl	9.3–37 nmol/L

[1]Age dependent
[2]Infants and adolescents up to 104 IU/L
[3]Infants in the first year up to 6 mg/dl

Normal Laboratory Values (Cont.) Blood

	Blood, Plasma or Serum (Cont.)	
	Reference Value	
Determination	**Conventional Units**	**SI Units**
Thyroid Hormone Function Tests:		
Thyroid-stimulating hormone (TSH)	0.35–6.2 mcU/mL	0.35–6.2 mU/L
Thyroxine-binding globulin capacity	10–26 mcg/dl	100–260 mcg/L
Total triiodothyronine (T_3)	75–220 ng/dl	1.2–3.4 nmol/L
Total thyroxine by RIA (T_4)	4–11 mcg/dl	51–142 nmol/L
T_3 resin uptake	25%–38%	0.25–0.38 fraction of 1
Transaminase, AST (aspartate aminotransferase, SGOT)	11–47 IU/L	0.18–0.78 mckat/L
Transaminase, ALT (alanine aminotransferase, SGPT)	7–53 IU/L	0.12–0.88 mckat/L
Transferrin	220–400 mg/dL	2.20–4.00 g/L
Urea nitrogen (BUN)	8–25 mg/dl	2.9–8.9 mmol/L
Uric acid	3–8 mg/dl	179–476 mcmol/L
Vitamin A (retinol)	15–60 mcg/dl	0.52–2.09 mcmol/L
Zinc	50–150 mcg/dl	7.7–23 mcmol/L

Normal Laboratory Values—Urine

	Urine	
	Reference Value	
Determination	**Conventional Units**	**SI Units**
Calcium[1]	50–250 mcg/day	1.25–6.25 mmol/day
Catecholamines: Epinephrine	<20 mcg/day	<109 nmol/day
Norepinephrine	<100 mcg/day	<590 nmol/day
Catecholamines, 24-hr	<110 mcg	<650 nmol
Copper[1]	15–60 mcg/day	0.24–0.95 mcmol/day
Creatinine: Child	8–22 mg/kg	71–195 μmol/kg
Adolescent	8–30 mg/kg	71–265 μmol/kg
Female	0.6–1.5 g/day	5.3–13.3 mmol/day
Male	0.8–1.8 g/day	7.1–15.9 mmol/day
pH	4.5–8	4.5–8
Phosphate[1]	0.9–1.3 g/day	29–42 mmol/day
Potassium[1]	25–100 mEq/day	25–100 mmol/day
Protein		
Total	1–14 mg/dL	10–140 mg/L
At rest	50–80 mg/day	50–80 mg/day
Protein, quantitative	<150 mg/day	<0.15 g/day
Sodium[1]	100–250 mEq/day	100–250 mmol/day
Specific Gravity, random	1.002–1.030	1.002–1.030
Uric Acid, 24-hr	250–750 mg	1.48–4.43 mmol

[1]Diet dependent

Normal Laboratory Values—Drug Levels

	Drug Levels†		
		Reference Value	
	Drug Determination	**Conventional Units**	**SI Units**
Aminoglycosides	Amikacin		
	(trough)	1–8 mcg/mL	1.7–13.7 mcmol/L
	(peak)	20–30 mcg/mL	34–51 mcmol/L
	Gentamicin		
	(trough)	0.5–2 mcg/mL	1–4.2 mcmol/L
	(peak)	6–10 mcg/mL	12.5–20.9 mcmol/L
	Kanamycin		
	(trough)	5–10 mcg/mL	nd
	(peak)	20–25 mcg/mL	nd
	Netilmicin		
	(trough)	0.5–2 mcg/mL	nd
	(peak)	6–10 mcg/mL	nd
	Streptomycin		
	(trough)	<5 mcg/mL	nd
	(peak)	5–20 mcg/mL	nd
	Tobramycin		
	(trough)	0.5–2 mcg/mL	1.1–4.3 mcmol/L
	(peak)	5–20 mcg/mL	12.8–21.8 mcmol/L
Antiarrhythmics	Amiodarone	0.5–2.5 mcg/mL	1.5–4 mcmol/L
	Bretylium	0.5–1.5 mcg/mL	nd
	Digitoxin	9–25 mcg/L	11.8–32.8 nmol/L
	Digoxin	0.8–2 ng/mL	0.9–2.5 nmol/L
	Disopyramide	2–8 mcg/mL	6–18 mcmol/L
	Flecainide	0.2–1 mcg/mL	nd
	Lidocaine	1.5–6 mcg/mL	4.5–21.5 mcmol/L
	Mexiletine	0.5–2 mcg/mL	nd
	Procainamide	4–8 mcg/mL	17–34 mcmol/mL
	Propranolol	50–200 ng/mL	190–770 nmol/L
	Quinidine	2–6 mcg/mL	4.6–9.2 mcmol/L
	Tocainide	4–10 mcg/mL	nd
	Verapamil	0.08–0.3 mcg/mL	nd
Anti-convulsants	Carbamazepine	4–12 mcg/mL	17–51 mcmol/L
	Phenobarbital	10–40 mcg/mL	43–172 mcmol/L
	Phenytoin	10–20 mcg/mL	40–80 mcmol/L
	Primidone	4–12 mcg/mL	18–55 mcmol/L
	Valproic acid	40–100 mcg/mL	280–700 mcmol/L
Antidepressants	Amitriptyline	110–250 ng/mL[3]	500–900 nmol/L
	Amoxapine	200–500 ng/mL	nd
	Bupropion	25–100 ng/mL	nd
	Clomipramine	80–100 ng/mL	nd
	Desipramine	115–300 ng/mL	nd
	Doxepin	110–250 ng/mL[3]	nd
	Imipramine	225–350 ng/mL[3]	nd
	Maprotiline	200–300 ng/mL	nd
	Nortriptyline	50–150 ng/mL	nd
	Protriptyline	70–250 ng/mL	nd
	Trazodone	800–1600 ng/mL	nd
Antipsychotics	Chlorpromazine	50–300 ng/mL	150–950 nmol/L
	Fluphenazine	0.13–2.8 ng/mL	nd
	Haloperidol	5–20 ng/mL	nd
	Perphenazine	0.8–1.2 ng/mL	nd
	Thiothixene	2–57 ng/mL	nd

†The values given are generally accepted as desirable for treatment without toxicity for most patients. However, exceptions are not uncommon.
[3]Parent drug plus N-desmethy7l metabolite
nd — No data available

Drug Levels†		
	Reference Value	
Drug Determination	**Conventional Units**	**SI Units**
Amantadine	300 ng/mL	nd
Amrinone	3.7 mcg/mL	nd
Chloramphenicol	10–20 mcg/mL	31–62 mcmol/L
Cyclosporine[1]	250–800 ng/mL (whole blood, RIA)	nd
	50–300 ng/mL (plasma, RIA)	nd
Ethanol[2]	0 mg/dl	0 mmol/L
Hydralazine	100 ng/mL	nd
Lithium	0.6–1.2 mEq/L	0.6–1.2 mmol/L
Salicylate	100–300 mg/L	724–2172 mcmol/L
Sulfonamide	5–15 mg/dl	nd
Terbutaline	0.5–4.1 ng/mL	nd
Theophylline	10–20 mcg/mL	55–110 mcmol/L
Vancomycin		
(trough)	5–15 ng/mL	nd
(peak)	20–40 mcg/mL	nd

Miscellaneous

†The values given are generally accepted as desirable for treatment without toxicity for most patients. However, exceptions are not uncommon.
[1]24 hour trough values
[2]Toxic: 50–100 mg/dl (10.9–21.7 mmol/L)

Reorder and Prices for the 12th Edition

Medical Abbreviations: 26,000 Conveniences at the
Expense of Communication and Safety
by Neil M Davis
(ISBN 0-931431-12-3)

1–19 copies	$24.95 each plus S&H
20 or more copies	$17.50 each plus S&H

Plus U.S. Shipping and Handling Charges

Number of Books Ordered	U.S. S&H charges to be added to each **order**
1	$5.00 + price shown above
2	$7.00 + price shown above
3–6	$9.00 + price shown above
7–11	$12.00 + price shown above
12–20	$16.00 + price shown above
21–40	$28.00 + price shown above
41 or more	$42.00 + price shown above

Orders shipped to Pennsylvania must add 6% sales tax.
No sales tax for other states (subject to change).
Purchase orders are accepted.

Payable by–

Visa   MasterCard   Discover
American Exp.   Check   Money Order

Order from and make check payable to–

Neil M. Davis Associates
2049 Stout Drive, B-3
Warminster PA 18974-3861

Orders may be mailed to above address or

Phone 215 442 7430 or 888 333 1862
Fax 215 442 7432 or 888 333 4915
Secure Web site www.medabbrev.com
E-mail med@neilmdavis.com

Where applicable, please have ready credit card number and
expiration date, phone number, and mailing address. A PO
box address is <u>not</u> acceptable for orders as they are shipped
via UPS.

Reorder and Price Information—continued

Outside of the United States

- Pay by credit card (VISA, MasterCard, Discover, American Express), or in U.S. dollars through a corresponding U.S. bank, or an International Money Order in U.S. currency.
- Prices as shown on the previous page plus shipping costs.
- To obtain shipping cost, fax query to 1 215 442 7432 or E-mail to ev@neilmdavis.com

Information Needed on Order Form

PLEASE PRINT OR TYPE

Name _____

Address (PO Box addresses not acceptable) _____

_____

City _____ State _____ Zip Code _____

Phone (___) _____

Attention (If Applicable) _____

Number of copies ordered _____ PO # (If Applicable) _____

Method of payment:

_____ Check or money order enclosed

_____ Visa _____ MasterCard

_____ Discover _____ American Express

Card Number _____

Exp. Date _____

Cardholder's Name _____

Signature _____

Internet Access

Each book purchased includes, at no extra cost, a single-user access license for the website version of this 12th edition, which is updated monthly (see preface). This license is valid for 24 months from the date of the initial log-in. Multi-User Site Licenses are available. To obtain a copy of the Multi-User Site License, call 1 888 333 1862, FAX 1 888 333 4915 or E-mail to ev@neilmdavis.com

To Order the PDA Versions

Palm OS or Pocket PC PDA versions of "Medical Abbreviations: 26,000 Conveniences at the Expense of Communication and Safety," the 12th edition, 2005, by Neil M Davis, are available from Lexi-Comp Inc., at either:

Their website	www.lexi.com
Phone	1 800 837 5394
Fax	330 656 4308

The PDA versions are updated with 80 new entries per month. The Palm version is approximately 1.7MB. The Pocket PC version is approximately 2.2MB.

Pricing: If you list on the Lexi-Comp website order form or mention on the telephone or FAX order, the Promotion Code **"KT8BK"** you will be given a 10% discount, lowering the price to $31.50 for one year. The normal price is $35.00.

Additions

Please forward additional meanings for these abbreviations, additional abbreviations and their meanings, or corrections to the author so that the web-version, PDA versions, and book can be updated. Thank you. Dr. Neil M Davis, 2049 Stout Drive, B-3, Warminster, PA 18974. FAX 215 442 7432 or 888 333 4915. E-mail med@neilmdavis.com

Additions

(See the preface for instructions on how to access to the web-version of this book which is updated each month with about 80 new entries. Your suggestions are appreciated.)

_____

_____

_____

_____

_____

_____

_____

_____

_____

_____

_____

_____

_____

_____

_____

_____

_____

_____

_____

_____

_____

_____

_____

_____

Additions (See the preface for instructions on how to access to the web-version of this book which is updated each month with about 80 new entries. Your suggestions are appreciated.)

_____

_____

_____

_____

_____

_____

_____

_____

_____

_____

_____

_____

_____

_____

_____

_____

_____

_____

_____

_____

_____

_____

_____

_____

Additions

(See the preface for instructions on how to access to the web-version of this book which is updated each month with about 80 new entries. Your suggestions are appreciated.)

_____

_____

_____

_____

_____

_____

_____

_____

_____

_____

_____

_____

_____

_____

_____

_____

_____

_____

_____

_____

_____

Additions

(See the preface for instructions on how to access to the web-version of this book which is updated each month with about 80 new entries. Your suggestions are appreciated.)

_____

_____

_____

_____

_____

_____

_____

_____

_____

_____

_____

_____

_____

_____

_____

_____

_____

_____

_____

_____

_____

_____

_____

Additions

(See the preface for instructions on how to access to the web-version of this book which is updated each month with about 80 new entries. Your suggestions are appreciated.)

_____

_____

_____

_____

_____

_____

_____

_____

_____

_____

_____

_____

_____

_____

_____

_____

_____

_____

_____

_____

_____

_____

_____

Additions (See the preface for instructions on how to access to the web-version of this book which is updated each month with about 80 new entries. Your suggestions are appreciated.)

_____

_____

_____

_____

_____

_____

_____

_____

_____

_____

_____

_____

_____

_____

_____

_____

_____

_____

_____

_____

_____

_____

_____

Additions

(See the preface for instructions on how to access to the web-version of this book which is updated each month with about 80 new entries. Your suggestions are appreciated.)

_____

_____

_____

_____

_____

_____

_____

_____

_____

_____

_____

_____

_____

_____

_____

_____

_____

_____

_____

_____

_____

_____

_____

Additions

(See the preface for instructions on how to access to the web-version of this book which is updated each month with about 80 new entries. Your suggestions are appreciated.)

_____

_____

_____

_____

_____

_____

_____

_____

_____

_____

_____

_____

_____

_____

_____

_____

_____

_____

_____

_____

_____

_____

_____

_____

Additions

(See the preface for instructions on how to access to the web-version of this book which is updated each month with about 80 new entries. Your suggestions are appreciated.)

_____

_____

_____

_____

_____

_____

_____

_____

_____

_____

_____

_____

_____

_____

_____

_____

_____

_____

_____

_____

_____

_____

_____

_____

_____

Additions

(See the preface for instructions on how to access to the web-version of this book which is updated each month with about 80 new entries. Your suggestions are appreciated.)

_____
_____
_____
_____
_____
_____
_____
_____
_____
_____
_____
_____
_____
_____
_____
_____
_____
_____
_____
_____
_____
_____
_____
_____

Additions, Corrections, and Suggestions are Welcomed

Please send them via any means shown below:

Neil M Davis
2049 Stout Drive, B-3
Warminster PA 18974-3861

FAX 1 888 333 4915 or 1 215 442 7432
Email med@neilmdavis.com
Web site www.medabbrev.com

Thank you for your help in the past.

Have You Used the Web-Version of This Book?

- It is instantaneously searchable for the meanings of abbreviations
- It is reverse searchable (search for all the abbreviations containing a particular word)
- Each month, about 80 new entries are added

See the preface (page vii) for access instructions. A two-year, single-user access is included in the purchase price of the book.

PDA Versions are Available

See pricing and ordering information in the pricing section on page 461.

Multi-User Site Licenses are Available

Medical facilities can substitute their own "Do Not Use" list of dangerous abbreviations for the one present. This list would be controlled by the facility. Demonstrations and pricing information are available by calling 1 888 333 1862 or 1 215 442 7430 or via an e-mail request to ev@neilmdavis.com